FRONTIERS IN ANTIOXIDANTS RESEARCH

FRONTIERS IN ANTIOXIDANTS RESEARCH

HAROLD V. PANGLOSSI
EDITOR

Nova Science Publishers, Inc.
New York

For permission to use material from this book please contact us:
Telephone 631-231-7269; Fax 631-231-8175
Web Site: http://www.novapublishers.com

Library of Congress Cataloging-in-Publication Data

Frontiers in antioxidants research / Harold V. Panglossi (editor).
p. ; cm.
Includes index.
ISBN 1-60021-273-5
1. Antioxidants--Research. I. Panglossi, Harold V.
[DNLM: 1. Antioxidants. QV 325 F935 2006]
RB170.F76 2006
613.2'86--dc22 2006017579

Published by Nova Science Publishers, Inc. ✢New York

CONTENTS

PREFACE

In biological systems, the normal processes of oxidation (plus a minor contribution from ionizing radiation) produce highly reactive free radicals. These can readily react with and damage other molecules. In some cases the body uses free radicals to destroy foreign or unwanted objects, such as in an infection. However, in the wrong place, the body's own cells may become damaged. Should the damage occur to DNA, the result could be cancer. Antioxidants decrease the damage done to cells by reducing oxidants before they can damage the cell. Virtually all studies of mammals have concluded that a restricted calorie diet extends the lifespan of mammals by as much as 100%. This remarkable finding suggests that food is actually more damaging than smoking. As food produces free radicals (oxidants) when metabolized, antioxidant-rich diets are thought to stave off the effects of aging significantly better than diets lacking in antioxidants. The reduced levels of free radicals, resulting from a reduction in their production by metabolism, is thought to be a major cause of the success of caloric restriction in increasing life span. Antioxidants consist of a group of vitamins including vitamin C, vitamin E, selenium and carotenoids, (such as beta-carotene, lycopene, and lutein). This new book brings together the latest research in this dynamic field.

There is extensive evidence for the protective role by antioxidants (AOs) against oxidative insults in humans, as discussed in chapter 1. Among the numerous endogenous and exogenous AOs are the principal ones, vitamin C, vitamin E, and glutathione, whose action mechanism is addressed. Literature on miscellaneous AOs is included. Oxidative stress (0S) often arises from electron transfer (ET) reactions which give rise to reactive oxygen species, which can form from carcinogens, abused drugs, industrial chemicals, pesticides, herbicides, metal compounds, and medicinals. Classes of ET functionalities include quinones (or precursors), metal complexes, aromatic nitro compounds (or reduced derivatives), and imine or iminium species. The main portion of this review is devoted to the countering influence of AOs to OS generated in various body constituents: the cardiovascular system, central nervous system, reproductive system, liver, kidney, and mitochondria. A similar approach is presented concerning a number of illnesses, such as, cancer, diabetes, lupus, Down's syndrome, Bloom's syndrome, and Fanconi's anemia. Rationale is provided for the pro-oxidant effects of principal AOs which are observed under certain conditions.

Chapter 2 reviews that the results of large-scale trials on antioxidant vitamin supplementation in cardiovascular disease (CVD) have been disappointing and failed to prove any protective effect of these vitamins (especially vitamin E and beta-carotene). However, the oxidative theory of atherosclerosis has aroused much hope for more than fifteen years in these antioxidant treatments. Indeed, according to this theory, oxidative modification of lipoproteins, especially low density lipoproteins (LDL), increases their atherogenicity. Several *in vitro* and *in vivo* studies suggest that LDL oxidation promotes endothelial cell damage, foam cell accumulation and thrombosis, and interferes with normal vasomotor regulation. Antioxidant vitamins represent one of the many nonenzymatic antioxidant defense systems. Vitamin E (of which α-tocopherol is the major component) is an abundant antioxidant that is widely studied, but several other dietary antioxidants have shown a preventive role *in vitro* in limiting or inhibiting LDL oxidation, especially by scavenging free radicals; however, no prevention of experimental atherogenesis has been demonstrated in animal. In fact, basic research only provides insight into the potential mechanisms of antioxidants in limiting the development of atherosclerosis, but descriptive, analytical and intervention studies are needed to try to establish the relationship between the activity of these antioxidants and the prevention of atherogenesis. Randomized trials generally provide the best data on the benefit and risk from an intervention, and thus are required for developing preventive strategies.

In contrast with supplementation studies, many cross-sectional, case-control, and cohort studies have found an association between antioxidant consumption (especially vitamin E) and a reduced risk of coronary heart disease; moreover, people who consume a diet rich in fruits and vegetables have lower risks of CVD. This addresses the question whether the use of antioxidant supplements to reduce cardiovascular risk is advisable. The relative inefficiency of the antioxidant vitamin supplementation probably results partly from the fact that atherosclerosis is a progressive arterial disease which develops during several years, so that an antioxidant treatment would hardly be effective on already oxidized cell targets. Besides, recent findings support the fact that oxidants may be beneficial under some conditions, for example play a role in regulating very low density lipoprotein (VLDL) secretion and also as signalling molecules. Other factors, such as the dose, the duration of treatment, the kind of vitamin E used, the association with other antioxidants, but also the initial antioxidant status of the patients included in the studies, likely play a key role in the results obtained.

As far as now, there is no sufficient data from randomized trials to justify establishment of recommendations regarding the use of vitamin E for CVD prevention. The best is to recommend a balanced diet (as proposed by the American Heart Association –AHA–) with antioxidant-rich fruits and vegetables. Anyway, even if future clinical trials could demonstrate a beneficial role of antioxidant supplementation in the reduction of CVD, the use of these supplements should be always considered as adjunct therapies, with a strict respect of the classical cardioprotective behaviors (physical activity, control of blood pressure and dyslipidemia, avoidance of obesity and smoking abstention).

Erythrocytes export electrons across the cell membrane to external oxidants (such as ferryicyanide) through a redox system that remains still unknown, as discussed by the authors of chapter 3. The rate of ferricyanide reduction varies as a function of cytoplasmic electron donor concentration. Indeed, the pathway is linked to a set of intracellular redox couples including $NADH/NAD^+$, GSSG/SGSH, and ascorbate/vitamin C.

Since the activity of membrane electron transport systems appears to be closely related to the redox homeostasis and the metabolic state of the cell, our aim was to characterise the membrane reducing system in healthy and in type 1 diabetes (T1DM) families and its relationship with nutritional indicators and oxidative biomarkers. Particularly, present research work aimed at evaluating in healthy and T1DM families: (a) the rate of erythrocyte electron transport in relation with body mass and metabolic efficiency, (b) modulating effects of diet and lifestyle on erythrocyte electron transfer system.

The authors measured the erythrocyte electron transport to extracellular ferricyanide (RBC vfcy) in 100 healthy controls and 99 non-diabetic relatives of type 1 diabetics. Erythrocyte Na/H exchange (RBC NHE), RBC glutathione (GSH), plasma thiols, plasma and RBC malondialdheyde were also determined, in addition to plasma glucose, insulin, lipids, HbA1c, creatinine clearance, and urinary albumin. Moreover, we assessed dietary habits and lifestyle of 76 relatives and 95 healthy subjects by using the European Prospective Investigation of Cancer and Nutrition questionnaires.

A. Among healthy controls, individuals with BMI$\leq$25 kg/m^2 had lower rates of electron transport in comparison with age-gender-matched subjects who were overweight or obese. Indeed, RBC vfcy correlated positively with two indices of fat body mass (BMI and circulating triglycerides), and negatively with an index of lean body mass (24-hour urinary creatinine excretion). Moreover, RBC vfcy showed a negative association with RBC NHE and plasma MDA. On the contrary, among relatives, RBC vfcy did not change significantly with BMI. It showed a positive association with RBC MDA, negative with RBC GSH.
B. Both Spearman's rank correlation and stepwise multiple regression analyses including lifestyle information found different independent variables to be positively associated with RBC vfcy: daily dietary intake of vitamin C among healthy controls, whereas time spent in regular exercise among relatives.

In conclusion, (a) electron transfer catalysed by the transmembrane ferricyanide reductase activity may reflect the functional state of membrane proton pumps that modulate cellular metabolism by regulating the intracellular redox levels. In the case we should have a useful tool to indirectly evaluate some aspects of energy balance in human metabolic diseases by using easily accessible cells and simple laboratory procedure. Moreover, the transport system, that seems functionally normal, contributes to oxidation in T1DM families, whereas in healthy people it protects from oxidation. Furthermore, (b) dietary intake of vitamin C and sporting activities modulate erythrocyte electron transfer efficiency. In the cytosol, ascorbic acid or vitamin C can donate electrons to trans-plasma membrane electron transfer activity in erythrocytes. Thus, intracellular electron donors available from dietary sources can be very important in maintaining the redox environment of a cell, i.e. the summation of the products of the reduction potential and reducing capacity of the linked redox couples present. Our data also support indirect evidence suggesting that regular exercise may improve electron transport efficiency. However, the reason why independent lifestyle variables associated with RBC vfcy markedly differed among population subgroups remains unknown.

Chapter 4 reviews that high sympathetic and low vagal activity have a determinant role in the genesis of sudden cardiac death (SCD). Particularly in chronic heart failure (CHF), low baroreflex sensitivity and heart rate variability are risk factors for SCD. Recent investigations show that in normal subjects nitric oxide (NO) modulates cardiovascular autonomic control. Conversely, in various conditions including aging, CHF, hypertension, metabolic syndrome, and diabetes, NO synthesis is altered. Three different isoforms of NO synthase (NOS) produce NO: endothelial NOS (eNOS), neuronal NOS (nNOS), and cytokine-inducible NOS (iNOS). Many studies showed that eNOS and nNOS are both expressed in cardiomyocytes, while nNOS is widely distributed in central and peripheral sites of the autonomic nervous system. In vitro studies show that eNOS and nNOS attenuate sympathetic and increase parasympathetic sinus responses. Human studies confirmed this behavior, but failed to clarify the underlying mechanism and the cell types stimulated. In healthy subjects, during NOS inhibition, high-frequency power, a sinus spectral marker of vagal modulation, decreases, and in patients with CHF, during infusion of the NO substrate L-arginine, the same spectral component increases. Ample evidence indicates that ascorbic acid improves endothelial function by increasing NO. The numerous mechanisms involved in preserving NO are largely hypothetical. For example, an open question is whether ascorbic acid acts as an antioxidant, diminishing oxidative stress, or whether it acts directly on NOS. Recent data indicate that in patients with CHF, who typically have low baroreflex sensitivity and decreased heart rate variability, acute administration of L-arginine and ascorbic acid improves sympathovagal control. Furthermore, in elderly subjects, infusion of ascorbic acid at high doses increases baroreflex sensitivity. Although all these results suggest that ascorbic acid might improve the age-related and disease-related imbalance of autonomic control, studies using chronic oral administration have so far yielded disappointing results. Our aim in this review is to consider possible interactions between NO and ascorbic acid and to examine their influence on autonomic control and the possible benefits of administering ascorbic acid.

The authors of chapter 5 discusses that cardiovascular diseases develop on the background of the marked oxidative stress, erythrocytes being an important "target" for reactive oxygen species. The effect of reactive oxygen species on erythrocytes causes a pathological increase in their aggregation and a decrease in deformability. The disturbance of the rheological properties of erythrocytes induced by reactive oxygen species contributes to the formation of the high blood viscosity syndrome developing in cardiovascular diseases.

During in vitro experiments under blood hyperviscosity model conditions there has been established a hemorheological effect of dihydroquercetin (a bioflavonoid isolated from larch wood) and ascorbic acid. This effect has manifested itself by reduction in hyperaggregation of erythrocytes and improvement in their deformability. A synergistic effect of a combination of dehydroquercetin and ascorbic acid has been demonstrated, it being more pronounced than individual effects of the antioxidants studied. Under the same conditions optimal ratio of antioxidant concentrations in the compound have been selected.

In experiments on spontaneously hypertensive rats with high blood viscosity syndrome, the use of the antioxidant complex (AOC) comprising dihydroquercetin and ascorbic acid (20 mg/kg and 50 mg/kg, respectively) during 14 days improved the reduced erythrocytes deformability and decreased their hyperaggregation. It was shown that the mechanism due to which the AOC had a beneficial effect on rheological properties of erythrocytes was mediated by its action on the morphofunctional state of these cells. The AOC decreased a high level of lysophospholipids in erythrocyte membranes in the spontaneously hypertensive rats, promoted preservation of the normal phospholipid spectrum and phospholipid balance in the external and internal layers of erythrocyte membranes. The capacity of the AOC to preserve the lipid composition of erythrocyte membranes provided an increase in the number of discocytes and a decrease in pathological shapes of erythrocytes in their population.

A clinical study of the AOC involved patients suffering essential hypertension grades I–II with manifestation of high blood viscosity syndrome. During 21 days the patients received Ascovertin (20 mg dihydroquercetin and 50 mg ascorbic acid in a tablet) 3 times a day in addition to a standard antihypertensive therapy. A group of clinically healthy people (10 volunteers) was used as normotensive control. By day 21 of treatment Ascovertin application resulted in decreased contents of lipid peroxidation products in erythrocyte membranes and in blood plasma. In this period the patients with arterial hypertension experienced abatement of high blood viscosity syndrome manifestations mainly because of a beneficial effect of the preparation on the cellular rheological indices, i.e. improvement in deformability of erythrocytes and a decrease in their aggregation. A correlation between a decrease in the amount of conjugated dienes in erythrocyte membranes and improvement of erythrocyte deformability was established. An integral effect of the hemorheological therapy with Ascovertin was a reduction in blood viscosity resulting in a moderate decrease of systolic and diastolic arterial blood pressure and of peripheral resistance. In addition, the patients demonstrated a decrease in manifestation of discirculatory encephalopathy clinical signs and improvement in cognitive and neurodynamic functions.

Formation of reactive oxygen species (ROS) is a natural process during oxidative metabolism. ROS play an important role not only in pathological processes of human organism as usually presented but less attention is paid to their proper important role in cell signaling, biosynthesis or non-specific antiinfectious defence, as reviewed in chapter 6. Overproduction of ROS during numerous pathological situations in presence of insufficient antioxidant protection leads to substantial oxidative changes of lipids, proteins, sugars, and also DNA. Protection against ROS is assured by different extracellular or intracellular antioxidant mechanisms as studied during last decades. Antioxidant enzymes rectifying the oxidative damage are studied with regard to their different activities and usefulness in body protection. Their genetic polymorphisms are certainly involved in different response to oxidative stress.

Special attention should be devoted to the topic of oxidative nuclear and mitochondrial DNA damage and its restoring via DNA repair process, especially base excision repair (BER). A large scale of antioxidant enzymes is involved in correction of DNA oxidative damage. Natural trend of worsened DNA repair is usually associated with aging. Other pathologies related with deficient DNA repair are susceptibility to carcinogenesis (lack of apoptosis control) or degenerative diseases.

Oxidative stress is involved in the pathophysiology of diabetes mellitus (DM – oxidative stress of mainly metabolic origin) and inflammatory bowel diseases (IBD – oxidative stress of mainly inflammatory origin). In spite of confirmed OS in DM or IBD, the substantial information about the intensity of DNA repair and its possible relationship to the disease course and development of chronic complications is missing.

Our pilot studies completed both in adult and pediatric patients with DM or IBD confirmed an increased oxidative stress as well as oxidative DNA damage examined with comet assay. The surprising findings were ascertained in intensity of DNA repair (analysed with modified comet assay). DNA repair process was stimulated in Type 1 diabetes adults without diabetic microvascular complications and still more in diabetic children with short disease duration. On the other hand adults with Type 2 diabetes had substantially increased oxidative DNA damage and extremely low DNA repair. This finding could be the link to increased susceptibility of Type 2 DM patients to cancerogenesis. Patients with IBD (Crohn´s disease - both children and adults) had similar tendencies in OS intensity and oxidative DNA damage and repair but less intensive.

Large population studies in DM or IBD studying intensity of OS and expression of DNA repair enzymes are needed in order to get the correlation between individual repair enzymes expression and the long-term course and occurence of complications in DM or IBD.

In: Frontiers in Antioxidants Research
Editor: Harold V. Panglossi, pp. 1-38

ISBN 1-60021-273-5

Chapter 1

BENEFICIAL EFFECTS OF ANTIOXIDANTS IN RELATION TO CARCINOGENS, TOXINS, AND VARIOUS ILLNESSES

Peter Kovacic[1]* and Ratnasamy Somanathan[2]
[1]San Diego State University, San Diego, CA
[2]Centro de Graduados e Investigación del Instituto Tecnológico de Tijuana, Mesa Otay, Baja California, México.

ABSTRACT

There is extensive evidence for the protective role by antioxidants (AOs) against oxidative insults in humans. Among the numerous endogenous and exogenous AOs are the principal ones, vitamin C, vitamin E, and glutathione, whose action mechanism is addressed. Literature on miscellaneous AOs is included. Oxidative stress (0S) often arises from electron transfer (ET) reactions which give rise to reactive oxygen species, which can form from carcinogens, abused drugs, industrial chemicals, pesticides, herbicides, metal compounds, and medicinals. Classes of ET functionalities include quinones (or precursors), metal complexes, aromatic nitro compounds (or reduced derivatives), and imine or iminium species. The main portion of this review is devoted to the countering influence of AOs to OS generated in various body constituents: the cardiovascular system, central nervous system, reproductive system, liver, kidney, and mitochondria. A similar approach is presented concerning a number of illnesses, such as, cancer, diabetes, lupus, Down's syndrome, Bloom's syndrome, and Fanconi's anemia. Rationale is provided for the pro-oxidant effects of principal AOs which are observed under certain conditions.

* Corresponding author, Tel.: +1 619 594 5595; fax: +1 619 594 4634. E-mail address: pkovacic@sundown.sdsu.edu

INTRODOUCTION

The seeds of antioxidant (AO) knowledge and use were planted years ago [1]. The crucial roles of vitamins C and E in nutrition have long been recognized. More than fifty years ago, lack of vitamin C was associated with various problems of aging. At that time, a number of investigators suggested higher intakes of the vitamin. The use of AOs (mainly vitamin C, E and beta carotene) for prevention of illnesses of aging, e.g., cancer, stroke and heart attacks, has attracted an abundance of recent attention in research and news media. These findings are based on the hypothesis that OS is an important contributor to the distresses commonly associated with the aging process.

The supporting evidence for AO effectiveness has been characterized as overwhelming. However, there is disagreement concerning proper supplementation for the general public. Some advise waiting until more information is available, whereas others feel that supplementation should immediately be a part of the daily diet. Also, debate continues with regard to the preferred form of the protective agents, namely, tablets or fruits and vegetables. The marked increase in laboratory work has been augmented in recent years by epidemiological studies. Generally, the population statistics indicate a beneficial influence on a variety of aging illnesses. For a smaller number of cases, adverse effects have been reported, e.g., in the highly publicized Finnish study. The investigators observed a higher incidence of lung cancer among men who received beta carotene than among those who did not. Serious flaws in the study have been pointed out. Since AOs can also function as pro-oxidants in certain situations, the proposal appears reasonable that beta carotene may be generating ROS species in the lungs of smokers (see pro-oxidant section)

Advances in the AO field have often gone hand–in–hand with research on the toxic effects of free radicals which generate OS. The fundamental framework of the OS theory was laid down by four groups in the 1950's in connection with the mechanism of carcinogenesis [1]. It is remarkable that the essential features still provide a cogent base even though the experimental, supporting evidence at the time was quite limited. Several corollaries were advanced, including protection by AOs. Hence, these reports appear to provide the first mechanistic links between OS and attenuation by AOs. Although little attention was paid to the theory in the ensuing 10-15 years, a surge of activity began in the 1970's, with dramatic, continuing escalation starting in the 1980's. Electron transfer (ET) and reactive oxygen species (ROS) have been increasingly implicated in a variety of conditions brought on by endogenous and exogenous agents, such as, anti-infective drugs [2], anticancer drugs [3,4] , carcinogens [1], reproductive toxins [5], nephrotoxins[6], hepatotoxins [7], cardiovascular toxins [8], nerve toxins [9], mitochondrial toxins [10], abused drugs [11], and various others [12]. The most common ROS are superoxide (SO), hydrogen peroxide, hydroxyl radical, and peroxyl radicals, which are often formed by ET, and the most frequently encountered reactive nitrogen species (RNS) are nitric oxide (NO) and peroxynitrite (PN). ET functionalities include quinones (or precursors), metal complexes (or chelators), aromatic nitro compounds (or reduction products) and imines (or iminiums), which may undergo redox cycling with oxygen to form ROS. Many bioactive substances or usually their metabolites contain ET groups. OS can produce beneficial results, as with therapeutics, or unwanted side effects in the case of toxins.

This review is concerned with the beneficial effects of AOs. Initially, structure and mechanism are discussed for the principal AOs, namely, vitamins C and E, glutathione (GSH), superoxide dismutase (SOD), and catalase. The main portion of this chapter is devoted to countering influences of AOs to oxidative insults on body constituents, including the kidney, cardiovascular system, reproductive system, central nervous sytem (CNS), liver, mitochondria, and miscellaneous others. Also included are beneficial effects in relation to abused drugs and various illnesses (cancer, diabetes, lupus, Down's syndrome, Bloom's syndrome, and Fanconi's anemia). In recent years, there has been increasing evidence for pro-oxidant reactions elicited by AOs. Rationale is provided for these unusual phenomena.

Since the amount of literature in the area is overwhelming, this summary can only deal with a portion of the research. Of the many reports forthcoming during the last three decades, focus is on material from more recent years. Often original articles can be found in review citations. Although our approach deals mainly with AOs in relation to ET-ROS-OS, it should be rcognized that in vivo reactions are often complex, with a number of factors involved in a multifaceted fashion.

Antioxidant Structure and Mechanism

During the past 30 years, large numbers of articles, reviews, and books have appeared dealing with the subject of AOs, including natural and synthetic types. Although the category encompasses many members, this review will concentrate on principal ones namely, vitamin C (an enol) **1**, vitamin E (a phenol) **2**, thiols (mainly glutathione, GSH) **3**, superoxide dismutase (SOD), and catalase. In relation to mechanism, the AOs can be fitted into two classes. The first three terminate harmful redox cycling chains by reducing peroxyl radicals through hydrogen donation. Specificity pertains since the resultant AO radical must not function as a redox chain initiator. In the case of the vitamins, radical delocalization diminishes activity for propagation. Another contributing feature is transformation of the radical into a stable, non-radical product, e.g., donation of two hydrogens from vitamin C with production of dehydroascorbic acid, and dimerization of thiyl radicals to give disulfides. An important aspect that applies to vitamin E is reduction of the aroyloxy radical by vitamin C resulting in regeneration of the parent AO. With regard to formation of the AO radicals, two pathways compete, one entailing hydrogen atom abstraction, and the other comprising electron donation and proton loss. Apparently, the second route can proceed either stepwise or in a concerted manner. In many cases, there is not definitive evidence to permit a decision for mechanistic choice. In a recent review, there are numerous examples presented in addition to discussion of action mode [13].

In consideration of SOD and catalase, these beneficial endogenous AOs guard against insult by converting dangerous ROS into less harmful species [12]. Catalase efficiently decomposes hydrogen peroxide with formation of oxygen and water. For SOD, superoxide is transformed into oxygen and hydrogen peroxide. In both cases, the reaction entails dismutation (disproportionation). Also, additional factors should be taken into account, such as, solubility, concentration, and metal ions (see pro-oxidant section).

Antioxidant Prevention of Organ Toxicity

Cardiovascular (CV) System (Toxins and AOs)

The ET-OS-ROS framework serves nicely as a unifying mechanistic theme for the preponderance of CV toxins, including medicinal drugs, abused drugs, industrial chemicals, metal compounds, carcinogens, endogenous substances, and miscellaneous types. Extensive evidence points to depletion of AO pools, and beneficial effects of added AOs.

Antioxidant Protection

Endogenous and synthetic antioxidants, such as iron-chelating agents, N-acetyl-L-cysteine, apocynin, probucol, and edaravone, are useful in preventing CV injury and diseases [8]. Endogenous antioxidants in the myocardium include vitamins C and E, cysteine and the enzymes, SOD, catalase and glutathione peroxidase. In cases where events such as ischemia and hypoxia have compromised the cardiac cell's natural defense mechanisms, synthetic antioxidants such as N-acetyl-L-cysteine, a thiol-containing compound, have proved successful in protection against OS on reperfusion. Secondary plant metabolites containing flavonoids and coumaric acid derivatives from spinach are effective against OS in the rat heart [14]. Targets for AO therapy include NADPH oxidase, a source of superoxide and peroxides. Apocynin, a NADPH oxidase inhibitor, decreased levels of malondialdehyde and NADPH-oxidase activity in rat heart [15]. Another target for AOs is LDP in atherosclerosis. Probucol, a strong, hydrophobic AO of the phenolic class, has proven clinically to lower serum cholesterol. Aspirin has been used for more than 100 years and provides protection from OS, partly as a cyclo-oxygenase inhibitor. Initiating aspirin therapy within 24 h after acute myocardial infarction reduces the risk of nonfatal reinfarction, nonfatal stroke and CV death [16]. Edaravone, a free radical scavenger, inhibits vascular endothelial cell injury and ameliorates neuronal damage in ischemia , and provides modest cardiac protection in diabetes mellitus [17]. This unusual AO may operate by hydrogen donation yielding a benzylic radical that is highly resonance stabilized by the three adjacent substituents. AOs acted as defense system against ROS induced tissue damage during development of atherosclerosis [18]. A 2005 review on stroke addressed the aspect of oxidative damage, AO defense systems, and the possibilities of combined therapy including AOs [19]. Clinical trials testing the efficiency of AOs in patients suffering stroke have been reviewed [20]. The results are promising for use of AOs for the treatment of ischemic stroke.

Evidence demonstrates that the optimal use of AO therapy in cardiac disease and injury is preventative and ameliorating. Avoiding smoking and maintaining a sufficient intake of fruits and vegetables, rich sources of AOs, evidently is important for CV health [12]. When needed, supplementation should be implemented. In addition to the AOs listed, many others both exogenous and endogenous are available for cardioprotection.

1. Flavonoids

A study of the elderly found a decreased risk of mortality from heart disease in subjects with elevated flavonoid intake, including correction for β-carotene and vitamins C and E [12]. There are many flavonoid sources, including red wine and tea. Flavonoids found in cocoa and chocolate have a variety of beneficial actions, including AO protection and moderation of vascular homeostasis [21]. This apparent cardioprotective effect may be due to inhibition of lipid peroxidation. Several modes of action are available for the AO property. One involves the common effect of hydrogen atom donation by the phenol to the ROS. Another entails chelation of OS-producing iron [12].

2. Vitamin E

In an epidemiological study of nurses, those in the top 20% of dietary vitamin E intake showed 23 to 50% less heart disease [12]. A similar result was noted for United States male health professionals. However, other investigations gave inconsistent results [8]. The AO properties of this fat-soluble vitamin are widely documented for many situations of OS.

3. Vitamin C

Although several investigations revealed no association between vitamin C intake and lower risk of coronary disease, high doses of this supplement are reported to improve vascular function in some cases. Data indicating little effect of vitamin C on CV disease may possibly be a reflection of the already good vitamin C status of the US population [12].

4. Probucol

This phenolic drug, which exhibits AO properties, slows the progression of atherosclerosis in animals and in some human studies [12]. Protection is reported against adriamycin cardiotoxicity. Mechanistically, by hydrogen atom donation, the AO may operate by breaking harmful redox cycling chains that produce OS. Apparently, the generated AO radical can be recycled back to the parent phenol by vitamin C, as has been demonstrated for the related vitamin E.

5. Ubiquinol

This hydroquinone derivative, the reduced form of coenzyme Q (CoQ) may act as an AO in vivo [12]. Long-term supplementation of humans raised CoQH2 levels appreciably in plasma and LDL with resultant enhancement in resistance to peroxidation of LDL.

6. Selenium

There are reports that low blood selenium might predispose to CV disease and other illnesses [12]. Selenium can exert a desirable effect as an AO at the appropriate concentration.

Additional reports on desirable influence of AOs can be found in the following sections on individual toxins.

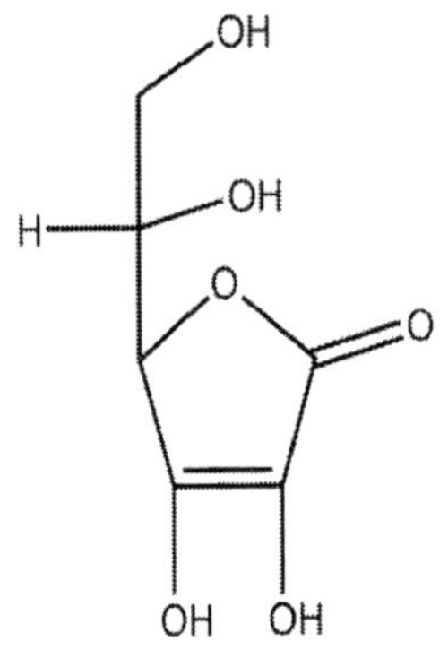
OH
H
OH
O
O
OH OH

1

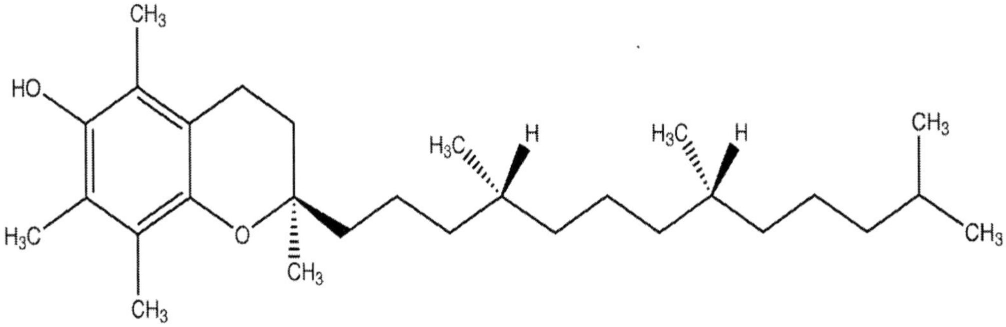
CH3
HO
H3C
CH3
O
CH3
H3C
H
H3C
H
CH3
CH3

2

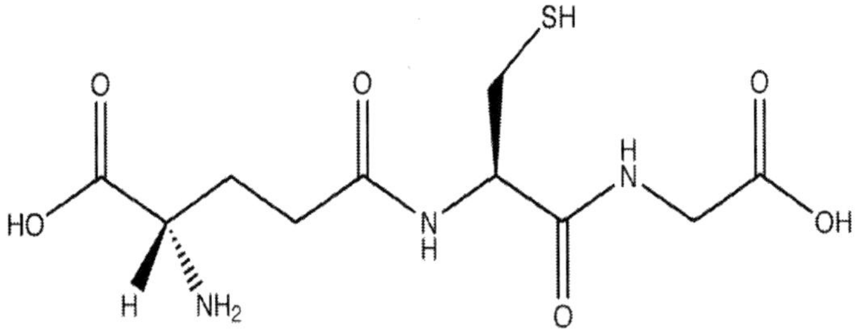
SH
O
O
O
HO
H
NH2
N
H
H
N
O
OH

3

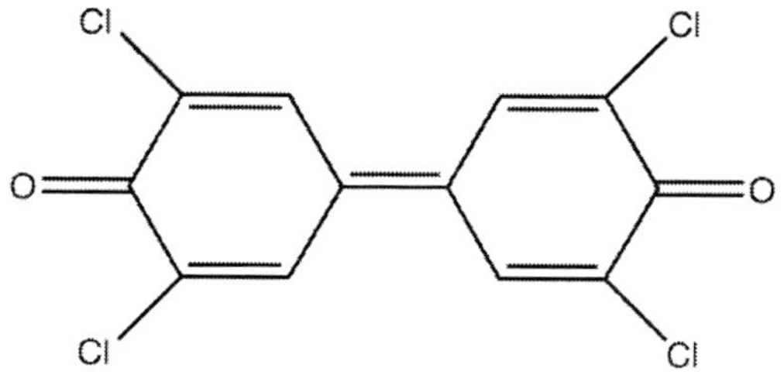

4

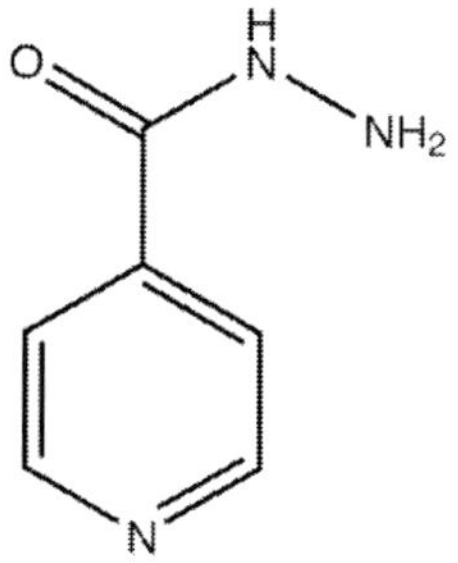

5

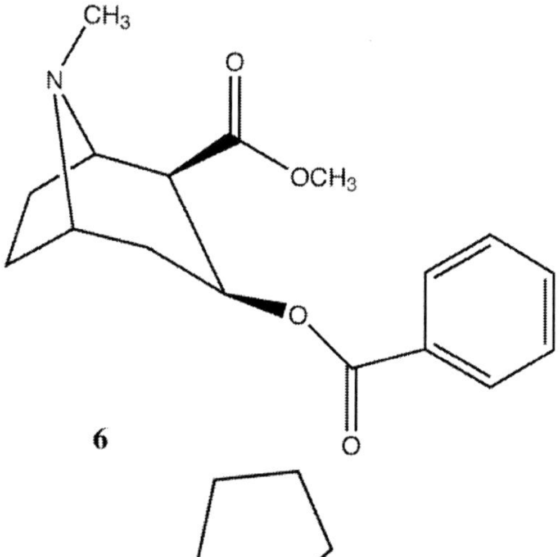

6

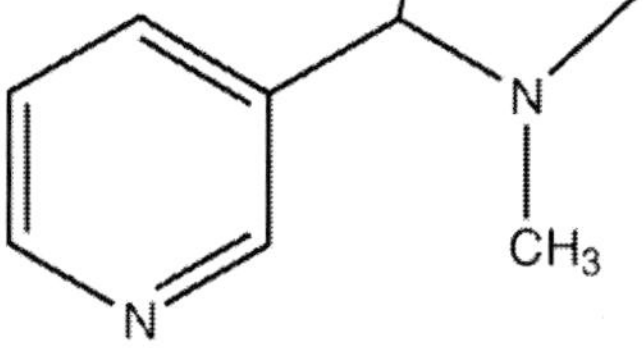

7

Medicines (Anthracyclines)

Cardiotoxicity, the main limiting factor in their use, includes congestive heart failure and arrhythmia. OS is widely believed to be a factor in the cardiac insult [12]. Analogs with less toxicity evidently undergo less redox cycling in vitro. ROS might be formed from redox cycling of the derived semiquinone. Enhanced lipid peroxidation has been reported in the hearts of rats treated with doxorubicin [2,4]. Alternatively, OS could arise from redox cycling by the corresponding iron derivatives; anthracyclines are avid chelators. The suggestion that iron plays an important part in anthracycline cardiotoxicity is examined in a recent review [22]. The approach is strengthened by the observation that the chelator, dexrazoxane, elicits a potent cardioprotective effect. The OS thesis enjoys additional support from AO studies [2].

Metal Compounds

A significant number of metal substances, including those of Cd, Co, Pb, Mn, Ni, V, As, Cr, Cu, and Hg, adversely affect the cardiovascular system giving rise to various toxicities which are summarized [23]. Most members of this class have been addressed in prior reviews on toxins [5,6], and carcinogens [1]. The heavy metal compound functionality, a familiar one capable of ET, usually displays a reduction potential favorable for in vivo ET. The toxicities are characterized by generation of various ROS, lipid peroxidation, DNA cleavage, and decrease in AO concentration. The effects are alleviated by AOs of various types. Intravenous infusion of deferoxamine, an Fe chelator, produced improved cardiovascular function in patients with coronary artery disease.

Paraquat

Although evidence exists for vascular damage in lungs and brain [8], other work reveals nontoxicity to the heart [8]. This much-studied herbicide readily undergoes redox cycling with generation of various ROS [5]. In addition to induction of MDA and DNA strand breaks, AO protection is reported. The dipyridinium compound fits into the iminium-like ET category.

Industrial Chemicals

1. Acrolein

The unsaturated aldehyde is formed in various ways in vivo, including metabolism of allylamine, and commonly from degradation during lipid peroxidation [8]. Heart perfusion resulted in irregular beats and denaturation of creatine kinase [8]. ROS were formed, which are likely responsible for induction of lipid peroxidation. GSH depletion by Michael addition to acrolein could also elevate OS. The glutathionyl propionaldehyde adduct also enhances oxy radical levels, even more so than for acrolein itself. Goodly numbers of studies with various organs reveal the protective effects of AOs [8,24,25].

2. Allylamine

This simple amine brings about vascular lesions in aorta and arteries [8]. Evidently, the compound itself can generate OS since metabolic deamination is accompanied by formation of hydrogen peroxide. However, toxicity has generally been attributed to the acrolein metabolite (see acrolein). After allylamine treatment, hydroxyl radical levels were enhanced in aorta. Preferential damage occurs to aortic mitchondria, accompanied by marked depletion of thiol content and striking increase in TBRS.

Polychlorinated Biphenyls (PCBs)

Investigations with cardiac myocytes showed a negative inotropic effect [26]. Enhancement of lipid peroxidation occurs in erythrocytes [8]. Lipid peroxidation was observed in various animals. The more recent reports in the cardiac area buttress the earlier findings in relation to OS and AO effects [8,27]. Oxidative metabolism leads to a diphenoquinone **4** with a reduction potential amenable to in vivo ET [1,5,6].

Dioxins

They display a variety of toxic effects with similarity to syndromes produced by PCBs [1,5,6]. A number of reports deal with effects of 2,3,7,8-tetrachlorodibenzo-p-dioxin (TCDD), the most toxic member, on the heart. . Various ROS were reported that can give rise to lipid peroxidation. Concomitantly, decreased levels of sulfhydryls resulted. Additional relevant observations include DNA insult and interference with respiration. The damaging effects of OS can be alleviated by AOs [8,28].

Silicates

Silicates, e.g. talc, induce pulmonary arteriolar thrombosis and emboli [8]. Quartz dust has also been cited as a carcinogen [1]. Since high doses of vitamin E are claimed to be beneficial in thrombotic vascular disease [12], this might comprise additional support for an OS role. However, the claim is disputed due to inconsistent results.

Natural Toxins

In the case of snake venom, a cardiotoxin which causes systolic arrest and disruption of membrane and myofibrils [8], various reports point to the participation of OS. Studies performed with the AO 2-hydroxy-4-methoxybenzoic acid showed that it effectively neutralized inflammation induced by viper venom and efficiently protected against insult by ROS [8]. With another AO, both the elevated malondialdehyde and the reduction in viper venom clotting time were blocked when erythrocytes were treated with the phenolic compound, N-allylsecoboldine. The findings suggest that hypercoagulability is associated with peroxidative lipid damage.

Other CV Toxins

A 2000 review addresses the relationship of lipoperoxidation and antioxidants to cardiovascular disease [29]. Elsewhere in the chapter is relevant material on other cardiotoxins, e.g. abused drugs, ROS, other medicinals, and other industrial chemicals, accompanied by AO effects.

In conclusion, there is overwhelming evidence in support of a role for ET-ROS-OS in the action of cardiovascular toxins, both endogenous and xenobiotic. All major classes of diverse types are involved, including many miscellaneous ones, as well as various illneses. Major insults comprise lipid peroxidation, DNA attack, as well as injury to other body components. The benefits and limitations of AO use for prevention and amelioration are addressed.

Central Nervous System (CNS) (Toxins and AOs)

There is much prior literature dealing with ET-ROS-OS participation involving nerve toxins, of which there are many [9]. This portion of the chapter deals with accompanying AO effects.

Antioxidant Protection

Substantial evidence for a beneficial role for AOs may be found in the following sections. The OS-ROS-ET theme is further buttressed by additional observations on neuroprotection by appreciable numbers of AOs, both natural and synthetic, including tocopherol analogs [9]. Mechanistically, the phenolic types apparently terminate harmful redox cycle chains by electron or hydrogen atom donation with accompanying formation of radical species unable to function in chain propagation [12]. A problem with AO effectiveness is penetration of the blood-brain barrier [9].

Ebselen, a seleno-organic substance, prevents neuronal damage in ischemia and reperfusion [9]. Its beneficial effects include inhibiting both NO synthase and lipid peroxidation, deactivating hydrogen peroxide and lipid peroxide, and scavenging endoperoxides. With the much investigated selegiline, inhibition of monoamine oxidase β is accompanied by decreased formation of SO, hydrogen peroxide, and hydroxyl radicals [9]. The compound displays AO properties independent of enzyme deactivation.

In the case of melatonin, synthesis in the pineal gland is followed by migration to the brain [9]. Protection from CNS damage, including that of DNA, evidently arises from scavenging of hydroxyl and peroxyl radicals. Other beneficial attributes comprise induction of GSH peroxidase and inhibition of NO synthase. A net result appears to be reduction in loss of brain neurons. Another AO is α-lipoic acid (and reduced thiol form) which quenches SO, hydroxyl radicals, peroxyl radicals, and singlet oxygen [9]. Hence, lipid peroxidation and DNA insult are avoided. Other roles include maintenance of the favorable redox status of other AOs, such as vitamins C and E, and GSH, in addition to metal chelation. In the clinical area, application is found in treatment of diabetic polyneuropathy.

Other AOs that exert protective effects are spin trapping agents and exifone [9]. In additional work, antioxidants are very effective in the treatment of animal paradigms, and they selectively protect neurochemical functioning in rats overproducing ROS [9]. In a 2002 summary, the status of AO therapy in acute CNS injury was addressed, including results from a large number of the more common protectors [30]. Also in a similar study it was shown that high dietary intake of vitamin C and E may lower the risk of Alzheimer's disease [31]. The beneficial effects of melatonin, together with low toxicity and ability to increase levels of AO enzymes, suggest its supplemental use in the treatment of neurological disorders in which OS is involved [32]. Although a few of the AOs demonstrated some efficacy in animals or in small clinical trials, the data were not verified by comprehensive, controlled trials in humans. Possible reasons for the discrepancy were presented. Much research remains to be done in order to determine more definitively the effectiveness of AO regimens [9].

Additional examples of toxic xenobiotics are provided, together with effects of AOs.

Medicinals

1. Cytosine Arabinoside

The nucleoside analog produces significant neurotoxicity in cancer patients undergoing chemotherapy [33]. Apoptosis of cerebral cortical neurons is mediated by OS. Cell death is reduced by various free radical scavengers, and is increased following depletion of GSH stores.

2. Cyclosporin A

Patients treated with this agent may experience adverse events entailing sensory or motor functions [9]. Appreciable data provide evidence for formation of ROS, lipid peroxidation, depletion of GSH, and beneficial effects of AOs [6]. The metal complexor desferrioxamine produced marked improvement in nephrotoxicity.

Cyanide

This well-known poison displays neurotoxicity which is accompanied by increases in SO and lipid peroxidation [9]. The adverse effects are attenuated by aspirin. Part of the pro-oxidant effect may reflect inhibition of AO enzymes, such as SOD and catalase [12].

Pesticides

1. Pyrethroid

Pyrethrins are insecticidal constituents of pyrethrum flowers; a large variety of synthetic pyrethroid analogues have been reported. In mammals these chemicals inhibit a variety of CNS enzymes, and disrupt the voltage sensitive channels [34]. Oxidative damage in brain and liver of developing young and adult exposed rats has been studied. Decreased levels of ACHE and GSH were seen along with high amounts of malondialdehyde from lipid oxidation. Vitamin E supplementation showed a beneficial AO effect [9].

2. Organophosphates

Methidathion, one of the most widely used insecticides, promotes lipid peroxidation which is alleviated by the AO vitamins C and E [35]

3-Nitropropionic acid (NPA) and Nitropropanol [9]

3-Nitropropionic acid and nitropropanol, widely distributed in the genera Astragalus (Leguminasae), also called "Locoweeds", are nerve toxins, affecting cattle and sheep. NPA not only inhibits succinate dehydrogenase, but also brings about reduction in the intracellular level of GSH, which probably contributes to the oxidative damage in both neurons and astrocytes. NPA, a mycotoxin, induces mitochondrial dysfunction and neurodegeneration, evidently with involvement of ROS, including PN and hydroxyl radicals. OS was attenuated by AOs, such as thiols and vitamin E.

Cannabinoids

Cannabinoids were shown to better protect against oxidative damage to neurons than other AOs, as well as against glutamate neurotoxicity [9].

3,3′ – Iminodipropionitrile (IDPN)

IDPN, HN(CH2CH2CN)2, an industrial intermediate, is used as an experimental nerve toxin [9]. Administration of the toxin produced a significant increase in MDA and decrease in vitamin E and GSH, suggesting a role for ROS in toxicity. Concurrent use of Se significantly inhibited IDPN-induced neurobehavioral changes in rats, and reduced TBARS production, evidently through attenuation of toxicity by decreased lipid peroxidation. Co-treatment with cysteamine protected rats against dyskinesia by IDPN. Depletion of vitamin E and GSH through toxic action was alleviated by the thiolamine as AO. Similarly, adjuvant use of salicylate decreased abnormal neurobehavior and reversed GSH depletion, presumably by AO action of the phenol [36].

Metal Compounds

1. Tin

Metal compounds in this category produce adverse effects involving the CNS [9]. Stannous chloride can elicit either stimulation or depression. ROS are a possible cause of lesions. Inhibition or disappearance of toxic symptoms resulted from use of ROS scavengers or metal chelators.

2. Cadmium

There are recent reports on OS from the nerve toxin Cd, with inhibition by thiol [37] and by AOs on brain lipid oxidation [9].

3.Copper

Copper is an essential metal exhibiting both toxic effects, antiinfective properties, and AO activity. At low doses, Cu blocks quinolinic acid neurotoxicity, which evidently involves ROS [38].

Reproductive System (Toxins and AOs)

There are large numbers of toxins which inflict insults upon the reproductive system, A 2001 summary documents widespread participation of ET-ROS-OS [5]. In many cases, beneficial effects of AOs are observed, some of which are discussed herein.

Metals

There is general discussion of this class in the cardiovascular section.

1. Lead [5]

There is a great deal of evidence that indicates involvement of OS in lead metabolism. In two studies, lead(II) created ROS, conceivably by redox cycling with oxygen, which was alleviated by AOs. Lead induced lipid peroxidation. Inhibition of SOD, GSH depletion and formation of SO have also been observed.

2. Cadmium

Emerging evidence indicates that OS plays a role in the toxicity. Chronic cadmium administration adversely affects GSH levels and causes lipid peroxidation, which was decreased by vitamin E [5].

3. Nickel

Oxidative paths are implicated in the in vivo toxicity. Various ROS have been observed, apparently via redox cycling and Fenton type reactions [39]. DNA damage via hydroxyl radical formation is suspected, as well as lipid peroxidation and protein carbonyl formation [12], which can be alleviated by vitamin C [5].

4. Manganese [5]

Reports of OS involving manganese exposure are few. However, some sources indicate an indirect role. Certain ROS- inducing neurotransmitters, like dopamine, are increased upon absorption of the metal. Quinones and semiquinones , the suspected metabolites, are reportedly involved. Free radical pathways were also noted which were mitigated by SOD, CAT, and vitamin E.

Organic solvents

1. Carbon tetrachloride

Metabolic studies demonstrate formation of ROS. In relation to the effects of exogenous and endogenous antioxidants, vitamin E decreased the level of liver injury [12], and the fruit antioxidant, schisandrin B, also protected, presumably by maintaining the GSH/GSSG ratio [5]. Depletion of SOD has also been noted [5].

2. Trichloroethylene (TCE) and Perchloroethylene [5,40]

TCE is a prevalent indoor air pollutant, widely used in building materials and consumer products. Metabolic studies point to the epoxide as the initial product formed by the mixed-function oxidase enzyme system. The highly reactive ether may attack nucleic acids. In the case of perchloroethylene which behaves in a similar fashion biochemically, vitamin E exerted a protective effect, presumably as an AO.

3. Benzene

It is readily metabolized to more reactive species, e.g., various phenols, hydroquinones, semiquinones and quinones [1]. The presence of ROS, Fe, or Cu increases the DNA damage, whereas ascorbate and GSH inhibited binding and damage.

Insecticides

1. Organochlorines [5]

Many literature sources indicate an OS role in organochlorine function. The antioxidants BHA (butylated hydroxyanisole), vitamin E, vitamin C, ellagic acid, and cysteine attenuate the oxidative effects of chlordane and endrin .

2. Organophosphates [5]

Employed as chemical warfare nerve agents, these types are also widely used as insecticides to protect crops. Several studies indicate a role of OS in the toxicity. The mutagenic effects of Rogor can be mitigated by vitamin C, suggesting an oxidative component.

Anticancer Drugs

1. Methotrexate

Possible modes of action, including a role for ET-OS, have been discussed [4,5,41]. Other relevant observations concerning methotrexate action include chromosomal damage, induction of lipoperoxidation, and alleviation of toxicity by the reducing agent ascorbate.

2. Daunorubicin

Teratogenic properties are associated with this antitumor-antibiotic agent. Although the mode of action is controversial for this anthraquinone category, some believe that induction of OS is responsible for most, if not all, biological activity [4,5]. Various lines of evidence buttress the contention, such as production of ROS, lipid peroxidation, and protection by AOs. The drugs readily chelate metals, e.g., iron and copper, resulting in DNA damage probably resulting from ET-ROS by the metal complex.

3. 3'-Azido-3'-deoxythymidine (AZT)

AZT is commonly used as a nucleoside analog in the viral treatment of patients with HIV. As to the mode of action, mitochondria and DNA appear to be targets. OS is part of the picture, including generation of ROS and increase in 8-oxo dG. Vitamins C and E protect the host from OS by AZT [2,12].

4. Isoniazid

Many modes of action have been proposed [2,42] for the antitubercular drug **5**, most of which entail interference with NAD+ and the ET system. Extensive metabolism, leading to free radical intermediates, gives rise to lipid peroxidation and DNA damage. The drug exhibits a high affinity for metals, particularly copper, which may result in ET reactions. Toxic manifestations in patients are alleviated by AOs.

5. Acetaminophen

The agent, used to alleviate pain, has found increasing use as an aspirin substitute. In cases of overdose, usually rescue can be accomplished by administering N-acetylcysteine as antidote. Metabolism and molecular sources of toxicity have been summarized [5,12].

Vitamin A Congeners

The retinoids are designated as potent teratogens. A recent report indicates that pro-oxidant ability may be responsible for toxicity in an investigation of carcinogenicity [1]. Retinol and retinal caused cellular DNA damage, evidently with involvement of H_2O_2, SO, and carbon radicals. Cu(II) could be involved as a mediator, and CAT acted as an inhibitor

[43]. Pro-oxidant activity was also observed in an investigation involving high oxygen tension, which resulted in protein oxidation [44]. AOs exerted a beneficial influence.

Liver

An earlier book [7] summarizes the role of ROS in hepatotoxicity along with the beneficial effects of AOs. Three principal agents which provide endogenous AO defenses are GSH and vitamins C and E. Various mimics of naturally occurring AOs have been examined, including those of SOD, GSH, organoselenium compounds, vitamin C, and vitamin E. Included are variations of classic AOs, such as, BHA and BHT. There is discussion of the interrelation between vitamins C and E, as well as between vitamin E and glutathione peroxidase. Radical species generated from vitamin C in rat hepatocytes were investigated. In a report on vitamin C, lipid peroxidation in rat hepatocytes was completely blocked. Pretreatment of animals with this vitamin was effective in preventing alcohol-mediated damage to hepatocytes (see abused drugs). The treatise includes extensive treatment of the natural AO GSH. In the category of other AOs are SOD and the thiol reductant, dithiothreitol.

Additional reports can be cited which deal with the beneficial effects of AOs in relation to hepatotoxicity. Experimental and chemical studies suggest that xenobiotic hepatotoxicity with variable depletion of AOs can be avoided or ameliorated by administration of a high dosage of zinc or by a combination of AOs above daily requirements [45]. Hepatic injury by carbon tetrachloride, entailing lipid peroxidation, is accompanied by formation of isoprostane and prostaglandin metabolites which can be regulated by AO nutrients [46]. Grape seed proanthocyanidin AOs shielded against drug induced cytotoxicity in human liver cells [47]. Glycine, an AO nutrient, diminished liver injury caused by hepatotoxic drugs [48]. S-Adenosylmethionine, which replenshed GSH, reduced mortality in patients with cirrhosis [49]. The rosemary plant (hepatoprotective) contains constituents, some that are phenolic, which have AO effects [50]. Eugenol, the active principle of clove, protected against hepatotoxicity induced by carbon tetrachloride, perhaps by anti-peroxidative activity [51]. The flavonoid silymarin guards liver cell membrane against hepatotoxic agents and prevents or inhibits membrane peroxidation [52].

Kidney [6]

As with other major organs, the kidney is subjected to attack by a variety of toxins, many of which are discussed in the sections on other organs, in addition to those below. In vivo administration of H_2O_2 produced proximal tubular injury associated with decreased renal function. H_2O_2 can also react with certain drugs to yield radical intermediates, as in the case of ibuprofen. Various phenolic AOs, such as vitamin E, prevented lipid peroxidation. Since desferrioxamine decreased lipid peroxidation, iron-dependency was implicated

Radiocontrast Agents [6]

Renal agents, which are used to visualize various organs for diagnostic purposes, have been connected to nephrotoxicity. 2,4,6-Triiodobenzoic acid derivatives are the primary radiocontrast agents used for medicinal puposes. The production of ROS may be involved in some of the toxic manifestations. Studies also indicate that the use of various AOs may attenuate the decline in renal function induced by these agents. Mannitol, used as a preventive measure, maintains the glomerular filtration rate in rats and prevents ischemic renal failure in dogs. When nifedipine was used, human patients had an increase in glomerular filtration rate and renal plasma flow.

Cyclosporin A (CsA) [6]

Cyclosporin A, a widely used immunosuppressant in organ transplantation, is also effective in treatment of autoimmune diseases. However, clinical use is limited by unwanted side effects, the most severe of which is nephrotoxicity. Considerable data point to a role for OS. Following ischemic insult which is identified with enhanced OS, there is increase in CsA nephrotoxicity. Invovement of ROS has been suggested, e.g., in increased lipid peroxidation. Appreciable numbers of publications, provide evidence for formation of ROS, lipoperoxidation, depletion of GSH, and attenuation by AOs. The metal complexor desferrioxamine produced marked improvement in toxicity pointing to an adverse role by metal ions.

Alloxan [6]

This toxin, widely used experimentally as a diabetogenic drug, also gives rise to lipid peroxidation in the kidney, which is a likely source of subsequent insult. Further, these adverse effects can be alleviated by addition of AOs, e.g., SOD, catalase, and scavengers of hydroxyl radicals.

Mitochondria

Mitochondria, vital constituents of the body, employ ET for energy production [10]. A side reaction generates harmful ROS via ET to oxygen with production of SO. This section summarizes the aspect of endogenous and exogenous AO agents in their beneficial roles.

Antioxidants

It is not surprising that the situation for mitochondria involving endogenous and exogenous AOs is similar to that for many other body components subject to OS. This is especially true since ROS are being generated continually in close proximity to the ETC. AO enzymes normally present include GSH peroxidase, but not catalase (except heart mitochondria). Mixed disulfides, GSSR, in equilibrium with GSH, accumulate during mitochondrial oxidative stress. α-Tocopherol depletion may also occur [12]. A number of investigations have been performed with added AOs. Endogenous ROS formation, including that from mitochondria, was inhibited by ROS scavengers and deferoxamine [53]. Ascorbate reduces superoxide production and improves mitochondrial respiratory chain function in human fibroblasts with electron transport chain deficiencies [54]. The cytoprotective effect of CoQ in mitochondrial diseases, e.g., neurodegenerative disorders, requires reduction to the AO dihydro form [55]. The relatively high levels of ubiquinol in most membranes are believed to protect against pro-oxidant damage.

In diet supplementation, antioxidants, such as coenzyme Q10, α-lipoic acid, thioproline, and N-acetylcysteine, may protect the mitochondria against respiration-linked OS, resulting in preservation of genomic and structural integrity with concomitant increase in functional life span [56]. Various lines of evidence indicated that conjugated linoleic acid is more effective than vitamin A in protecting rat liver mitochondria from nonenzymatic peroxidative damage [57]. In U937 cells and mice exposed to ionizing radiation, α-phenyl-N-tert- butylnitrone (spin trap) reduced mitochondrial damage as reflected by the altered permeability transition, ROS production, ATP generation, and morphological changes [58]. AO use may be a practical means of preventing illness arising from mitochondrial insult by ROS. In the following, several additional AOs are described.

1. Quercetin

Quercetin, a polyphenolic flavonol, decreased the impairment of cardiac function following ischemia- reperfusion, which is apparently associated with improved mitochondrial function [59].

2. Ebselen

Ebselen, an organoselenium compound and a mimic of GSH peroxidase, prevents drastic structural and functional changes induced by OS in mitochondria [60].

3. Ginkgo

Ginkgo biloba protected mitochondria from attacks by H_2O_2, and decreased ROS levels and apoptosis due to OS [61]. The neuroprotective properties are probably due to the AO effects on mitochondria.

4. 1,4-Dihydropyridines

The antioxidant and ROS scavenging protective effects of anti-inflammatory 1,4-dihydropyridine derivatives was assessed for mitochondria [62]. Cerebrocrast and diethone could provide protection against oxidative damage in mitochondria. The role of this class of electron donors has been discussed [63].

Mitochondrial Medicine [10]

Therapeutic intervention to prevent mitochondrial oxidative stress toxicity is also available and includes various antioxidants, such as tocopherol analogues, CoQ, as well as bioenergetic factors, e.g. acetyl-L-carnitine, which supplies acetyl CoA for the citric acid cycle and carnitine to shuttle fatty acids into the mitochondria for β–oxidation. The earlier dihydropyridine section is relevant. The favorable effects of AOs discussed in prior sections could well serve in disease prevention.

Aging [10]

With regard to the free radical theory of aging, an expansion was proposed in a recent review designated the mitochondrial theory of aging. Senescence may be linked to OS injury to the genome and membranes of mitochondria. Further details are provided in the AO section.

Diseases [10]

The mitochondrial ETC is considered to be the major source of ROS that have been implicated in a number of diseases and disorders. Mitochondrial dysfunction may predispose a person to a witch's brew of medical problems. The defects include obesity, propensity to diabetes, high blood pressure, heart attack, and stroke. A number of books deal with the disease link.

Other Organs

Due to space limitations, similar OS reports for organs, including others, will be given from ref. [10]: liver, kidney, testes, ovary, pancrease, and esophagus.

Classes of Toxins

Carcinogens [1]

Considerable research over the past decades supports the thesis of ET-ROS-OS involvement in carcinogenesis. Concomitant data, presented herein, indicate an important role for AOs in prevention.

The following sections provide more detail on individual AOs.

Radiation [1]

UV radiation, a mostly non-ionizing type, can homolytically cleave hydrogen peroxide to form hydroxyl radicals, and can also generate singlet oxygen and, indirectly, 8-OHdG. CAT, GSH, vitamin C, ubiquinol, and vitamin E may play a role in radiation protection. Dietary beta carotene and caffeine are also beneficial.

Peroxides [1]

Various peroxides have long been associated with carcinogenesis [66]. Enzymatic and non-enzymatic cleavage of peroxides generates three predominant types of radicals: alkoxyl, peroxyl, and hydroxyl. Evidence indicates that peroxide cleavage comes about most aggressively in the presence of certain metals. Cu, Fe, and Ni enhanced DNA oxidative damage via Fenton reactions with hydrogen peroxide, whereas EDTA, a metal chelator, was significantly protective. Additional protective effects of various AOs have been observed, e.g., melatonin, an endogenous type, inhibited H_2O_2-induced DNA damage; beta-carotene decreased strand breaks by tertiary-butyl-hydroperoxide, and vitamin E ameliorated oxidation of DNA pyrimidines and purines by H_2O_2.

Carbon Tetrachloride [1]

CCl_4 and other haloalkanes (HAs) are widely used industrial solvents. The carcinogenicity and toxicity associated with CCl_4 exposure is well established. Metabolic steps leading to ROS are well known. In relation to the effects on exogenous and endogenous antioxidants, vitamin E decreased the level of liver injury, and the fruit antioxidant, schisandrin B, also protected, presumably by maintaining the GSH/GSSG ratio. Depletion of SOD has also been noted.

Quinones [1]

Quinones are widely distributed in plants and animals, and are also incorporated into various medicinals . Adriamycin and daunomycin are reported carcinogens. In many cases, the quinone is generated metabolically from a precursor. Redox cycling generates ROS. Metal chelators and oxygen radical scavengers ameliorated the harmful effects.

Phenols [1]

Pentachlorophenol (PCP), an herbicide, wood preservative, and insecticide, is a probable carcinogen. Evidence indicates that 8-OHdG is formed via ROS created from the hydroquinone metabolite, which in the presence of oxygen, can give rise to SO via redox reactions, resulting in hydrogen peroxide and hydroxyl radicals. GSH depletion and induction of p53 oncogenic proteins were also noted. Catechin, a green tea AO, mitigated against PCP damage. o-Phenylphenol (OPP), a disinfectant and fungicide, is a carcinogen that can alkylate DNA and generate ROS. The quinone metabolites, working in concert with SO, and mediated by CYP450, are suspected moieties for generating ROS and 8-OHdG. CAT, GSH, and ascorbic acid were protective by inhibiting oxidation. Dietary administration of 2(3)-tert-butyl-4-hydroxyanisole (BHA) resulted in a protective effect in chemical carcinogenesis.

Flavonoids are polyphenolic molecules present in fruits and vegetables. Flavonoids inhibit the promotion stage of carcinogenesis by inhibiting ROS-forming enzymes [64]. Quercetin acts as a carcinogen, via ROS and oxidative DNA damage in the presence of Cu(II). However, Fenton catalysis is not probable since hydroxyl radical scavengers were ineffective. CAT, however, was protective, indicating the involvement of hydrogen peroxide.

Since natural and synthetic estrogens exhibit much of the reaction behavior already described, their metabolites are suspected to play a role in breast and endometrial cancer, Estradiol, hexestrol, and diethylstilbesterol undergo oxidation to catechols or hydroquinones, semiquinones, and quinones. Redox cycling and the generation of ROS then ensue, followed by lipid peroxidation. Cu chelators, CAT, and singlet oxygen scavengers were preventive.

Aromatic Nitro Compounds [1]

Certain monocyclic and polycyclic aromatic nitro compounds are implicated in carcinogenesis. Nitrobenzene is readily reduced by NADH to reactive entities, namely, C_6H_5NHOH, $C_6H_5NHO\bullet$, and C_6H_5NO which are implicated in oxidative DNA damage. CAT prevented DNA cleavage suggesting that H_2O_2 plays a crucial role. In vivo experimentation with polycycles, including the diesel exhaust constituents 1-nitropyrene and 2-nitrofluorene, resulted in nitroso species, as well as DNA adducts. Nitropyrenes (NPs) possess favorable reduction potentials, making for possible involvement in ET and redox cycling. The nitroso form exhibited superior ability in electron uptake. The antioxidants beta-carotene, as well as other carotenoids, and catechin were protective against the deleterious effects of NPs, as were bean derived flavonoids. In the heteroaromatic category, 4-nitroquinoline N-oxide (4-NQO), which also incorporates an iminium type entity, is a carcinogen. Reduction to the hydroxylamine, acylation, and then electrophilic attack on DNA is a possible mechanistic route. DNA strand breaks have been observed, possibly from free radical intermediates detected by ESR. Moreover, SO activity was noted, which was inhibited by SOD. Electron reduction of 4-NQO and ensuing redox cycling with oxygen have been reported.

Aromatic Amines

1. Hydrocarbon Types [1]

A recent review incorporates a large body of knowledge concerning aromatic amines and their link to cancer. Among the more familiar ones are benzidine, naphthylamines, and aminofluorenes. Relevant metabolic routes are oxidation to hydroxylamines and aminophenols, leading to OS. Some studies suggest a role for ROS in carcinogenicity. Catechin, an antioxidant, proved to be beneficial.

2. Heterocyclic Types [1]

Pyrolysis of food can create several types of heterocyclic amines, many of which are suspected in carcinogenesis. Carcinogenic mechanisms involve ring epoxidation to form a phenol, or a multi-step process beginning with N-hydroxylation to create the RNHOH moiety which is esterified to RNHOCOR. Recently, other pathways have been offered for the metabolism and carcinogenicity, several of which include a role by ROS. The RNHOH functionality, has been implicated in the formation of ROS. Endogenous and exogenous AOs can be helpful, e.g., GSH, caffeine, vitamin E, and certain dietary phenols.

Hydrazines [1]

Humans are exposed to hydrazines, many of which are carcinogenic and teratogenic, via mushrooms, herbicides, medicinals, rocket fuel, tobacco, and other sources. Studies have noted DNA alkylation, as well as other DNA lesions, perhaps via the carbocation and carbon radical-O2 interactions to form ROS. ET, involving CYP450, seems to be a major player leading to DNA strand scission by radicals. Free radical scavengers alleviated the deleterious effects.

N-Nitroso compounds [1]

At least 300 carcinogens containing this functionality are known. Human exposure comes about primarily through foods and tobacco, but also from various agricultural and industrial chemicals, cosmetics, and medicinals. Several studies indicate participation of OS, e.g., N-nitrosamines promote inflammation and, indirectly, are responsible for phagocytic oxidative damage which was countered by vitamin E and, to a lesser extent, beta-carotene. Vitamin E also prevents DNA alkylation and oncogene induction by an N- nitrosonicotine.

Tobacco [1]

Cancer caused by tobacco is one of the most familiar. In addition to the usual in vivo problems, the diversity of carcinogens within tobacco gives rise to difficulties in pinpointing mechanisms and principal causative agents. Indications that OS is occurring are: decreases in GSH, increases in malondialdehyde and 8-OHdG, and quenching in the presence of SOD and CAT. Many types of AOs have proven protective against the effects of smoking. Vitamins A, C, and E, red ginseng, and AO combinations significantly reduced tobacco-mediated damage.

Hydrogen peroxide and SO are components of cigarette smoke. Cr(VI) and cigarette smoke exhibited a synergistic effect in DNA strand breaks, presumably via •OH formation in Fenton-like reactions with H2O2. Mannitol, DMSO, and hydroxyl radical scavengers were preventive.

Metals [1]

Large numbers of metals induce cancer, including Ni, Cr, Pb, Cd, and Be. In 1986, a unifying hypothesis of participation by ROS was advanced [65]. There has been mounting evidence to buttress this theme. In two studies, lead(II) created ROS, conceivably by redox cycling with oxygen, which was alleviated by AOs.

Asbestos [1]

There have been numerous case studies correlating cancer, especially that of the lung, with exposure to mineral fibers, particularly asbestos. Another study addressed the effect of ornithine decarboxylase (ODC) which is responsible for polyamination in DNA repair and replication. Upon exposure to asbestos, ODC is activated, which suggests DNA damage. CAT acted as an inhibitor.

Inorganic Agents

Inorganic ROS, such as peroxides, are treated in another section. One can regard active oxygen as a universal carcinogen.

1. Ozone

This powerful oxidant and major pollutant occurs both naturally and by acts of man. It behaves both as a direct carcinogen and a cocarcinogen, and exhibits synergistic action with ionizing radiation [1]. Studies reveal a number of metabolic products in the ROS category, including: macromolecular peroxides, hydrogen peroxide, ozonides (via addition across double bonds), •OH, singlet oxygen, as well as formation of 8-OHdG [12]. Ascorbate, GSH, SOD, and CAT are inhibitors of ozone insult.

2. Potassium Bromate

KBrO3, an inorganic oxidant used as a food additive, displays cancer-inducing properties [1]. There is oxidative DNA damage and increase in lipoperoxidation. AOs which act as radical scavengers exert a protective effect.

Other Aspects

1. Other Antioxidants

A 2005 study supports an inverse association of colorectal cancer with fish intake [66]. Fish oils contain unsaturated omega--fatty acids that may act as free radical scavengers that protect against OS [67].

Olive oil, which contains beta-sitosterol, exerts remarkable preventive effects on the development of cancer and cardiovascular disorders [68]. The paradoxical effects of isothiocyanates appear to occur in tandem: first acute increase in stress, followed by a lasting increase in protection against oxidants and carcinogens [69].

The general effectiveness of AOs as cancer inhibitors buttresses the OS theory for carcinogenesis.

2. Oncogenes [1]

Recent experimentation reveals a major role of OS in the activation of oncogenes. Antioxidants protect against the effect which also suggests the involvement of ROS.

3. Viruses [1]

The toxicity of ROS and reactive nitrogen species may be the mechanism of tissue injury observed in many viral infections, including hepatitis and influenza. The possible mitigating effects of AOs taken during infection are currently being investigated.

4. Other

One must use caution in distinguishing between anticancer agents used for prevention and those used to combat tumors already established. For example, some time ago, vitamin C was claimed to produce measurable benefits in the treatment of cancer [1]. However, evidence indicates that it must never be regarded as an alternative to proven, conventional methods of cancer treatment since its efficacy is still unproven. On the other hand, sufficient evidence has now accumulated to conclude that this AO, as inhibitor, is linked to a reduced risk of virtually all cancers.

Abused Drugs

Cocaine [70]

1. Introduction

Cocaine **6** is one of the major drugs of abuse [1]. Evidence was provided in support of the contention that oxidative metabolites of cocaine play a role in toxicity and addiction involving OS, ROS, and ET. The metabolites include norcocaine and norcocaine derivatives: nitroxide, N-hydroxy, and nitrosonium, plus cocaine iminium and formaldehyde. Cocaine is mainly metabolized by two distinct pathways in humans. The minor route is an oxidative one involving the amine moiety, which has attracted most attention relative to some toxic responses.

2. Electrochemistry [10]

Electrochemical studies with nitroxide yielded a reduction potential indicating a conceivable role in redox cycling in vivo with production of OS via ROS. Only a small quantity of minor metabolite is required to generate large quantities of ROS since the operation is catalytic.

3. Metabolites and Oxidative Stress [10]

Brain microsomal reduction of norcocaine nitroxide generates SO (21). Incubation of liver microsomes with either the nitroxide or the N-hydroxy derivative leads to lipid peroxidation, the degree of which is greater for the metabolites than for cocaine itself, indicating the crucial role of the metabolites in toxicity. Redox cycling involving the metabolites is believed to take place, accompanied by formation of SO and lipid peroxyl radicals. Immunotoxicity in rats is promoted by N-oxidative metabolism, evidently via OS, accompanied by depletion in GSH. Formaldehyde, an oxidative metabolite of (19), is reported to produce ROS.

4. Body Components: OS and AO Protection

a. Liver [70]

Various studies of hepatotoxicity revealed the generation of ROS, including lipid peroxides [71, 72]. Much evidence was garnered pointing to depletion of the common AOs, and prevention by thiol and deferoxamine [70].

b. Central nervous system

Increased OS induced by cocaine can lead to neurodegeneration (71,72). In studies of the brain, multiple low doses of cocaine generated ROS, such as the hydroxyl radical; the AO salicylate may offer protection (73).

c. Cardiovascular system

Intraperitoneal injection of the drug increased cardiac OS, partly by compromising AO defense systems (74). Hydroxyl radical formation was noted after multiple low doses, with protection by the AO salicylate (75).

d. Reproductive system

Fetal membrane damage by cocaine is apparently due to peroxidation [76]. The effect, countered by vitamin E, resulted in depletion of AO defenses, including GSH in rat testis [70].

e. Mitochondria

Evidence was presented that cocaine cytotoxicity involves mitochondrial damage in which ROS participate [78]. Deferoxamine and N-acetylcysteine acted as protective agents.

5. Apoptosis

In cocaine use, OS has been linked to apoptosis [70,73]. In another study, protective effects of thiol and deferoxamine confirmed involvement of ROS [78].

•

Nicotine

Cigarette smoke is responsible for large numbers of deaths in the US annually. Included among the many harmful components is nicotine **7** which is both addictive and toxic to most organs, particularly the lung and cardiovascular system.

1. Metabolism

A recent review [79] provides evidence of a role for iminium metabolites.

2. Electrochemistry

In 1990 reduction potentials were reported for various nicotine metabolites belonging to the ET conjugated iminium category, which fall in the range ameable to in vivo ET [79].

3. Generation of Reactive Oxygen Species

Extensive documentation exists for formation of ROS from interaction of nicotine or its metabolites with various organs [79]

4. Organ Toxicity, OS and AO Protection

a. Insult Prevention by Antioxidant [79]

The dietary consumption of fruits and vegetables rich in AOs is inversely correlated with the incidence of various illnesses, such as lung cancer and cardiovascular disease. Vitamin E and S-allyl cysteine sulfoxide (from garlic) were examined for their ability to combat peroxidative damage induced by nicotine in liver, lungs and heart of rats. Administration of the AOs resulted in decreased concentrations of TBARS, hydroperoxides and conjugated dienes.

b. Lung [79]

Chronic inflammation may promote the toxic effect through generation of ROS. The toxic nitrosamine matabolites caused a significant increase in DNA strand breakage. Pretreatment with vitamin E or beta-carotene provided significant protection against DNA scission. Oxygen radical scavengers (SOD, CAT, mannitol) appreciably reduced the DNA damage, indicating that hydroxyl radicals could be playing an important role. Also, human lung cells were pretreated with nicotine and with stimulated human phagocytes. In this situation, epigallocatechin galleate, a main AO constituent of green tea, afforded marked protection against genetic damage.

c. Cardiovascular System [79]

Leukocyte adhesion was significantly attenuated by pretreatment with SOD suggesting a key role for SO. There was impairment of arteriolar function by way of a mechanism entailing ROS; SOD exerted a beneficial effect.

d. Central Nervous System

Various reports document OS, ROS, TBARS, lipid peroxidation, and alleviation by AO [79].

Alcohol [80]

Alcohol is one of the most dangerous and economically damaging of the abused drugs.

1. Metabolism

The pathways have been fairly well elucidated. The majority of the drug is metabolized in the liver by dehydrogenase enzymes to acetaldeyde which is rapidly converted for the most part by a dehydrogenase to acetic acid. ROS are generated, and the common symptoms of OS have been noted, such as lipid peroxidation, accumulation of conjugated dienes, decreased SOD activity, and reduction in GSH.

Much of the toxicity is believed to arise from acetaldehyde. Scant attention has been paid to the products of the aldehyde side reactions, which mainly fall in the C4 category, namely, diacetyl, acetoin, and 2,3-butanediol.

2. Electrochemistry

Values for diacetyl and its imine derivatives (iminium form) fall within the range amenable to ET in vivo. Imines could readily be formed non-enzymatically in vivo by condensation of diacetyl with pri-amino groups of protein.

3. α-Dicarbonyl stress

Recent reports address cellular damage by α-dicarbonyls, including diacetyl, in a process designated the Maillard reaction which yields advanced glycation end products (AGEs). These species can exert their adverse effects by increasing OS, thereby generating a vicious cycle involving ROS and α-dicarbonyls.

4. Organ Toxicity, OS and AOs

In relation to alcohol exposure, there is discussion of the following major organs: CNS, liver, reproductive system, cardiovascular system, and liver. Adverse effects include carcinogenesis, mutagenesis, and enzyme inhibition. There are the usual reports of OS, ROS, lipid peroxidation, AO depletion, and toxicity prevention by AOs. Some of the insults have been attributed to participation of diacetyl. An increasing body of evidence points to OS as a major player in the multi-faceted toxicity, which entails several possible mechanisms, most of which involve ROS. Lipid peroxidation and protein oxidation have been observed. Vitamin E, beta carotene, and ascorbic acid have proven effective in combating ethanol toxicity. A recent study centered on association of alcohol, particularly large amounts, with brain insult. The toxicity was rationalized by linkage with ROS and lipid peroxidation which apparently are responsible for brain injury. Pretreatment with vitamin E prevented vascular damage and brain pathology.

Phencyclidine (PCP) [11]

Several studies on apoptosis indicate involvement of ROS. SO is believed to play a role; treatment with a SOD mimetic prevented apoptosis. Expression of haem oxygenase –1, a heat shock protein, is induced by OS after exposure to PCP. Pretreatment with 1,3-dimethylthiourea, an AO, significantly reduced protein induction.

Methylenedioxymethamphetamine (MDMA) [11]

ROS appear to be involved since hydroxyl radicals were detected and SOD provided protection, as did nitrone AOs. The neurotoxicity is minimized in transgenic mice that express human CuZnSOD. The conclusion was drawn that free radical formation is responsible for neurotoxicity which was prevented by the AO α-lipoic acid.

Morphine and Heroin [11]

Various studies of OS-ROS from morphine and heroin have been reported. In the case of morphine, macrophage apoptosis was associated with generation of SO and NO, with protection provided by AOs, such as N-acetyl cysteine (81). A similar result occurred in an investigation of renal injury (82).

Delta-9-tetrahydocannabinol (THC) [11]

THC induces neurotoxicity which has been attributed to generation of free radicals. Neuronal cell death was inhibited by aspirin, vitamin E, and other AOs, another indication of OS.

Others

Other sections contain treatment of additional categories of toxins, such as, industrial chemicals, metals, pesticides, herbicides, and medicinals.

ILLNESSES

All of the following maladies possess the common characteristic of OS arising from generation of excess ROS [12]. Therefore, it is logical to expect benefits from AO application. As a result, appreciable numbers of investigations have been carried out.

Diabetes

AOs (N-acetyl cysteine, vitamins C and E) can exert positive effects in diabetes, e.g., suppression of in vivo beta-cell function. The finding suggests a potential usefulness of AOs in treating diabetes [83]. Exposure of diabetic rats to AOs (vitamin C and thioactic acid) attenuated the manifestations of OS. Thus, AOs may serve as useful tools in alleviating pathological effects [84]. AO application with vitamin E, probucol, lipoic acid, or taurine normalized diabetes-induced renal and glomerular dysfunctions [85]. On the other hand, large-scale clinical trials with classic AOs failed to show any benefit for diabetes patients [86]. Others proposed that additional long-term AO studies are needed in order to assess with greater cetainity the possible beneficial effects [87].

Systemic Lupus Erythematosus (SLE) and Other Autoimmune Diseases [88]

This illness mainly affects younger women who display a variety of symptoms. A review tabulates more than 60 xenobiotics in the SLE category [89]. A recent report documents involvement of ROS and AOs [12].

1. Prevention and Amelioration by AOs [88]

Various reports demonstrate positive effects of AOs versus SLE in humans and other animals. SOD and copper chelates that can destroy SO have proven helpful. A study, entailing vitamins C and E, and β-carotene revealed beneficial effects. A significant increase in serum 8-OHdG was detected in SLE patients, which may be lessened by vitamin C. Other AOs in the form of thiols, such as cysteamine and N-acetylcysteine, suppressed immune damage. High levels of ROS and low AO status have been implicated in the pathogenesis. Inclusion of AOs into the multi-modality therapy has been suggested. Other references incorporate relevant information. It is important that large-scale investigations of AOs be initiated so that the general population, as well as those afflicted, might benefit.

2. Cadmium [88]

Upon exposure to this toxin, depletion of GSH ensues due to induction of a pro-oxidant state. Chronic administration resulted in lipid peroxidation which was attenuated by incorporation of ascorbate.

3. Paraquat [88]

It is generally accepted that redox cycling leading to OS is responsible for toxic manifestations. The favorable reduction potential gives rise to ROS, such as SO and H_2O_2, as well as HO• which is believed to be responsible for DNA damage. Alleviation by AOs, e.g., Se and SOD, is in line with involvement of OS. The compound, a member of the iminium ET family and an herbicide, has been extensively investigated as a redox-cycling agent.

4. Cisplatin [88]

Cisplatin, $Cl_2Pt(NH_3)_2$, finds use in chemotherapy, but, as usual, toxicity enforces limits. The various modes of action have been critically analyzed. There is widespread consensus that activity results from intra- and inter-strand cross-links that bend and unwind DNA, resulting in attractions of certain proteins with resultant interference with excision repair and other vital DNA processes. However, it appears that binding alone is not sufficient and that some mechanism which occurs after the Pt species attaches itself to DNA must account for the anticancer activity. Since considerable evidence indicates that many other metals operate by ET-OS, it is reasonable to propose a similar mode of action in this case. Appreciable support has appeared for this thesis which has attracted little attention. Involvement of radicals and lipoperoxidation have been observed in various systems accompanied by decrease in antioxidant levels. SO arises from interaction with DNA. Also, resistance to the drug is associated with increase in levels of GSH. Plausibility for this rationale is provided by recent reports that ROS are involved in the cytotoxicity which is enhanced by GSH depletion. In addition, cisplatin is known to activate macrophages. Electrochemical data lend additional credence to this chemical viewpoint. The drug induces apoptosis, which may arise from radicals generated in the vicinity of DNA. Cisplatin displays radiation sensitizer properties, which usually entail ET reactions. Free radical damage has been proposed for the nephrotoxicity which is ameliorated by AOs.

A number of examples are provided involving various drugs and other exogenous substances that produce the condition, along with favorable effects by AOs.

5. Aminoglycosides [88]

Familiar members of this anti-infective class are streptomycin, associated with SLE, and gentamycin. Radical species likely play a role in the toxic effects. There has been controversy about whether a free-radical mechanism is involved because aminoglycosides are considered to be redox-inactive. However conversion into a redox-active form may occur, which can undergo ET with molecular targets. Aminoglycosides act as chelating agents by binding to metal ions, such as iron, with subsequent induction of ROS and lipid peroxidation. Hydroxyl radicals from hydrogen peroxide may affect mitochondrial function since catalase has been found to inhibit alterations in mitochondrial respiration in vitro. There is a decrease in gentamicin-induced lipid peroxidation in the kidney upon administration of vitamin E, supporting the proposal of radical involvement.

6. Nitrofurans [88]

This class, best known for anti-infective properties, induces kidney tumors. The metabolic transformations are well documented and enjoy broad consensus as being involved in bioactivity. Various lines of evidence point to generation of the radical anion which may be an important player. A correlation is observed between electron affinity and radio-sensitization, hypoxic cell toxicity, and chronic aerobic toxicity, suggesting that redox processes play an important role. In an aerobic environment the intermediate nitro radical anion readily conveys an electron to oxygen. For example, nitrofurantoin, an SLE inducer, stimulated the uptake of oxygen in hepatic incubations, which was partially reversed by SOD and catalase; this suggested the presence of superoxide and H_2O_2. Activated oxygen may be responsible for toxic effects. In other cases, including anaerobic conditions, the radical anion exerts its effect by another route, presumably interference with normal ET. Both the favorable effect and the liabilities might be intimately related to the ease of ET.

7. Chlordane [88]

Oxidative addition to the pesticide double bond yields an epoxide metabolite that conceivably produces OS by DNA alkylation. There is implication of various ROS and in DNA cleavage. The adverse oxidative effects are attenuated by AOs.

Down's Syndrome

This syndrome has a high incidence of chromosomal disorders and is a predisposing factor for leukemia. GVS-111, which apparently operates by an AO mechanism, exhibited significantly higher neuroprotection compared to Piracetum or to the more common AOs, such as, vitamin E, propyl gallate, and nitrone spin trap [90]. Hence GVS-111 may prove useful in combating mental retardation and chronic neurodegenerative disorders present in this pathology.

Bloom's Syndrome

Patients with this condition exhibit a high incidence of cancer and possess cells with a high frequency of chromosome damage and sister chromatid exchange (SCE) [91]. Treatment with AOs decreased the level of SCE.

Fanconi's Anemia

In this illness, there is breakdown of the hereditary apparatus and derangement of membrane structure. AO investigations were carried out with SOD and catalase. From the results, the authors concluded that AOs might be applied in the therapy for patients with Fanconi's anemia [92].

Others

Additional illnesses, e.g. cancer, are discussed in prior sections.

Other Antioxidant Effects

In this section AOs are cited without discussion for beneficial influence on various body constituents: cells exposed to radiation, BHT and trolox [93], Mn porphyrin complex [94], beta-carotene [95]; lung, peroxiredoxin [96]; mitochondria [10,97]; diabetic cells, probucol [98]; lipids, EDTA [99]; plasma, Zn [100]; ear, 7 AOs and Fe chelators [101]; lipids, S-adenosylmethionine [102]; LDL, cocoa and chocolate [103], prenylchalcones and prenylflavanones [104].

This section contains investigations on protection by natural AOs against OS on body constituents: membranes, yacon leaves (phenols) [105]; mayloid β-protein, cocoa (phenols) [106]; brain liposomes, plantago (flavonoids) [107]; neuronal cells, strawberry (phenols) [108]; LDL citrus limonoids and flavonoids [109]; atherosclerosis, wine phenolics [110]; protein, anthocyanins [111]; LDL, wheat (phenols) [112]; liposome, fruits and vegetables (flavonoids) [113]; dietary red meat, dietary polyphenols [114]; neurons, quercetin (flavonoid) [115]; cardiac hypertrophy, red wine polyphenols [116]; mammary cells (carcinogenesis), grapes (phenols) [117]; anti-inflammatory and immunomodulatory, mango stem bark extract [118].

Pro-Oxidant Effects

This supposed dichotomy is another example of balance in nature. Apparently, conditions are important in determining whether the substance behaves mainly as an AO or as pro-oxidant.

Vitamin E [12]

1. Since the phenol can reduce higher valence states of Fe and Cu, it can exert pro-oxidant effects in certain in vitro systems (see vitamin C).
2. The phenoxyl radical acts as a weak promoter of lipid oxidation under certain conditions.
3. The quinone metabolite possesses the potential for redox cycling usually associated with the quinone class.

Vitamin C [12]

1. Reduction of Fe (III) or Cu (II) produces metal ions capable of Fenton catalysis leading to the hydroxyl radical.
2. The oxidized form of vitamin C is an α-dicarbonyl. Electrochemical studies with analogs reveal reduction potentials favorable for in vivo ET which could lead to ROS [119].

GSH

The pro-oxidant effect that occurs in the presence of transition metal ions (see above) also applies to GSH [12]. In addition, thiols can produce such an effect via generation of ROS by interaction of various metabolic sulfur radicals with oxygen [120].

Selenium

The AO-pro-oxidant behavior has been reported [10].

Flavonoids

This class, similar to vitamin E, is mainly known for its AO properties. However, the ability to generate OS through ROS has attracted increasing attention [121]. Mechanistically, the pro-oxidant effects can reasonably be associated with metabolites, namely, aryloxy radicals and quinones.

CONCLUSION

Antioxidants play an important role in preventing or ameliorating oxidative damage to body organs by various toxins. Oxidative stress is commonly generated by reactive oxygen species formed via redox reactions involving electron transfer functionalities. These toxic entities participate in a variety of illnesses. Mechanistic insight should aid in the design of synthetic antioxidants. Further studies are required in order to determine effectiveness in humans by the antioxidants and optimum dosage. The recent area of pro-oxidant activity requires additional elucidation.

REFERENCES

[1] Kovacic, P; Jacintho, JD. Mechanisms of carcinogenesis: focus on oxidative stress and electron transfer *Curr. Med.Chem.,* 2001, 8, 773-796.

[2] Kovacic, P; Becvar, LE. Mode of action of anti-infective agents: emphasis on oxidative stress and electron transfer. *Curr. Pharmaceut. Des.,* 2000, 6, 143-167.

[3] Kovacic, P; Wakelin, LPG. DNA Molecular electrostatic potential: Novel perspective for the mechanism of action of anti-cancer drugs invoving electron transfer and oxidative stress. Anticanc. *Drug Des.,* 2001,16,175-184.

[4] Kovacic, P; Osuna,JA, Mechanisms of anticancer agents: emphasis on oxidative stress and electron transfer. *Curr. Pharmaceut. Des.,* 2000, 6, 277-309.

[5] Kovacic, P; Jacintho, JD. Reproductive toxins: Pervasive theme of oxidative stress and electron transfer. *Curr. Med. Chem.,* 2001, 8, 863-892.

[6] Kovacic, P; Sacman, A; Wu-Weis, M. Nephrotoxins: Widespread role of oxidative stress and electron transfer. *Curr. Med. Chem.,* 2002, 9, 823-847.

[7] Poli, G; Cheesman, KH; Dianzani, MU; Slater, TF. Ed..; *Free Radicals in the Pathogenesis of Liver Injury.* New York: Pergmon; 1989.

[8] Kovacic, P; Thurn, LA. Cardiovascular toxins from the perspective of oxidative stress and electron transfer. *Curr. Vasc. Des.,* 2005, 3, 107-117.

[9] Kovacic, P; Somanathan, R. Neurotoxicity: The broad framework of electron transfer, oxidative stress and protection by antioxidants. *Curr. Med. Chem-CNS Agents,* 2005, 5, 249-258.

[10] Kovacic, P; Pozos, RS; Somanathan, R; Shangari, N; O'Brien, PJ. Mechanism of mitochondrial uncouplers, inhibitors, and toxins: focus on electron transfer, free radicals, and structure -activity relationships. *Curr. Med. Chem.,* 2005, 5, 2601-2623.

[11] Kovacic, P; Cooksy, AL. Unifying mechanism for toxicity and addiction by abused drugs: Electron transfer and reactive oxygen species. *Med. Hypoth.,* 2005, 64, 367-366.

[12] Halliwell, B; Gutteridge, JMC. *Free Radicals in Biology and Medicine.* New York: Oxford; 1999, pp. 1-859.

[13] Kovacic, P Novel biochemical perspectives for electron transfer mechanism in proteins: focus on iminium, hydrogen bonding, homoconjugation, amino acid side chains (redox and charged) and cell signaling. Submitted.

[14] Ben-Shaul,V; Lomnitski, L; Nyska, A; Zurovsky, Y; Bergman, M; Grossman, S. The effect of natural antioxidants, NAO and apocynin, on oxidative stress in the rat heart following LPS challenge. *Toxicol. Lett.,* 2001, 123, 1-10.

[15] Gaziano, JM, Skerrett, PJ, Buring, JE. Aspirin in the treatment and prevention of cardiovascular disease. *Haemostasis,* 2001, 30, Suppl 3:1-13.

[16] Edaravone Acute Infarction Study Group. Effect of a novel free radical scavenger, edaravone (MCI-186), on acute brain infarction. Randomized, placebo-controlled, double-blind study at multicenters. *Cerebrovasc. Dis.,* 2003, 15, 222-229.

[17] Hayashi, T; Mori, T; Sohmiya, K; Okada, Y; Inamoto, S; Okuda, N. Efficacy of edaravone, a free radical scavenger, on left ventricular function and structure in diabetes mellitus. *Cardiovasc. Pharmacol.,* 2003, 41, 923-929.

[18] Young, IS; Woodside, JV. Antioxidants in health and disease. *J. Clin. Pathol.,* 2001, 54, 176-186.

[19] Alexandrova, M L; Bochev, PG. Oxidative stress during the chronic phase after stroke. *Free Radic. Biol. Med.,* 2005, 39, 297-316.

[20] Margaill, I; Plotkine, M; Lerouet, D. Antioxidant strategies in the treatment of stroke. *Free Radic. Biol. Med.*, 2005, 39, 429-44

[21] Steinberg, FM; Mearden, MM; Keen, CL. Cocoa and chocolate flavonoids: implications for cardiovascular health. *J. Am. Diet. Assoc.,* 2003, 103, 215-223.

[22] Kwok, JC; Richardson, DR. The cardioprotective effect of the iron chelator dexrazoxane (ICRF-187) on anthracycline-mediated cardiotoxicity. *Redox. Rep.,* 2000, 5,317-24.

[23] Alul, RH; Wood, M; Longo, J; Marcotte, AL; Campione, AL; Moore, MK. Vitamin C protects low-density lipoprotein from homocysteine-mediated oxidation. *Free Radic. Biol. Med.,* 2003, 34, 881-891.

[24] Noiri, E; Yamad, S; Nakao, A; Tsuchiya, M; Masaki, I; Fujimo, K. Serum protein acrolein adducts: utility in detecting oxidant stress in hemodialysis patients and reversal using a vitamin E-bonded hemodialyzer. *Free Radic. Biol. Med.,* 2002, 33, 651-656.

[25] Pocernich, CB; Cardin, AL; Racine, CL; Lauderback, CM; Butterfield, DA. Glutathione elevation and its protective role in acrolein-induced protein damage in synaptosomal membranes: relevance to brain lipid peroxidation in neurodegenerative disease. *Neurochem. Int.,* 2001, 39, 141-149.

[26] Jo, SH; Choi, SY; Kim, KT; Lee, CO. Effects of polychlorinated biphenyl 19 (2,2',6-trichlorobiphenyl) on contraction, Ca2+ transient, and Ca2+ current of cardiac myocytes. *J. Cardiovasc. Pharmacol.,* 2001, 38, 11-20.

[27] Hennig, B; Meerarani, P; Slini, R; Toberek, M; Daugherty, A; Silverstone, AE. Proinflammatory properties of coplanar PCBs: in vitro and in vivo evidence. *Toxicol. Appl. Pharmacol.*, 2002, 181, 174-183.

[28] Kanamaru, T; Simamura, E; Koyama, J. Production of reactive oxygen and its prevention by alpha-tocopherol in the acute toxicity of dioxin. *Kanaz. Ika Daig. Zasshi,* 2002, 27, 122-130.

[29] Halliwell, B. Lipid peroxidation, antioxidants and cardiovascular disease: how should we move forward. *Caridiovasc. Res.,* 2000, 47, 410-418.

[30] Gilgun-Sherki, Y; Rosenbaum, Z; Melamed, E; Offen, D. Antioxidant therapy in acute nervous system injury: current state. *Pharmacol. Rev.,* 2002, 54, 271- 284.

[31] Engelhart, M J; Geelings, M I; Ruitenberg, A; Van Swieten, J C; Hofman, A; Witteman, JCM ; Breteler, MMB. Dietary intake of antioxidants and risk of Alzheimer's disease. *JAMA*, 2002, 287, 3223-3261.

[32] Gómez, M; Esparaza, JL; Nogués, MR; Giralt, M; Cabré, M; Domingo, JL. Pro-oxidant activity of aluminum in the rat hippocampus: gene expressin of antioxidant enzymes after melatonin administration. *Free Radic. Biol. Med.,* 2005, 38, 104-111.

[33] Geller, HM; Cheng, KY; Goldsmith, NK; Romero, AA; Zhang, AL; Morris, EG; Grandison, L. Oxidative stress mediates neuronal DNA damage and apoptosis in response to cytosine arabinoside. *J. Neurochem.*, 2001, 78, 265-275.

[34] Soderlund, DM; Clark, JM; Sheets, LP; Mullin, LS; Piccirillo, VJ; Sargent, ML; Stevens, JT; Weiner, ML. Mechanisms of pyrethroid neurotoxicity: implications for cumulative risk assessment. *Toxicology,* 2002,171, 3-59.

[35] Altuntas, I; Delibas, N; Demirci, M; Kline, I; Tamer, N. The effects of methidathion on lipid peroxidation and some liver enzymes: role of vitamins E and C. *Arch. Toxicol.*, 2002, 76, 470-473.

[36] Tariq, M; Khan, H.A; Al Moutaery, K; Al Deeb, S. Attenuation of iminodipropionitrile induced behavioral syndrome by sodium salicylate in rats. *Pharmacol. Biochem. Behav.*, 2002, 73, 647-354.

[37] Figueiredo-Pereira, ME; Li, Z; Jansen, M; Rockwell, P. N-Acetylcysteine and celecoxib lessen cadmium cytotoxicity which is associated with cyclooxygenase-2 up-regulation in mouse neuronal cells. *J. Biol Chem.*, 2002, 277, 252-283.

[38] Santamaría, A; Flores-Escartín, A; Martínez, JC; Osorio, L; Galvain-Arzate, S; Chaverrí, JP; Maldonado, PD; Medina-Campos, ON; Jiménez-Capdeville, ME; Manjarrez, J; Ríos, C. Copper blocks quinolinic acid neurotoxicity in rats: contribution of antioxidant systems. *Free Radic. Biol. Med.*, 2003, 35, 418-427.

[39] Salacinski, HJ; O'Brien, P. Evidence that the reactions of nickel in the presence of vitamin C do not produce toxic oxygen intermediates such as hydroxyl but ascorbate and carbon radicals. *Arch. Toxicol.*, 2000, 74, 5-12.

[40] Lee, KM; Muralidhara, S; White, CA; Bruckner, JV. Mechanisms of the dose-dependent kinetics of trichloroethylene: oral bolus dosing of rats. *Toxicol. Appl. Pharmacol.*, 2000, 164, 55-64.

[41] Kovacic, P; Ames, JR; Taylor, EC; Ryan, MD J. Electrochemistry of the anticancer agents methotrexate and alpha-difluoromethylornithine in iminium form. *J. Pharmaceut. Sci.*, 1988,77, 999-1002.

[42] Kovacic, P; Ames, JR; Ryan, MD. Reduction potentials of antimycobacterial agents: relationship to activity. *Bioelectrochem. Bioenerg.*, 1989, 21, 269-278.

[43] Murata, M; Kawanishi, S. Oxidative DNA damage by vitamin A and its derivative via superoxide generation. *J. Biol. Chem.*, 2000, 275, 2003-2008.

[44] Zhang, P.; Omaye, S.T. β-Carotene and protein oxidation: effects of ascorbic acid and α-tocopherol. *Toxicology*, 2000, 146, 37-47.

[45] Stehbens, WE. Oxidative stress, toxic hepatitis, and antioxidants with particular emphasis on zinc. *Exp. Mol. Pathol.*, 2003, 75, 265-276.

[46] Basu, S. Carbon tetrachloride-induced lipid peroxidation: eicosanoid formation and their regulation by antioxidant nutrients. *Toxicology*, 2003, 189, 113-127.

[47] Bagchi, D; Bagachi, M; Stohs, S; Ray, SD; Sen, CK; Preuss, HG. Cellular protection with proanthocyanidins from grape seeds. *Ann. NY. Acad. Sci.*, 2002, 957, 260-270.

[48] Matilla, B; Mauriz, JL; Culebras, JM; González-Gallego, J; González, P. Glycine: a cell-protecting anti-oxidant nutrient. *Nutr. Hosp.*, 2002, 17, 2-9.

[49] Lieber, CS. Alcohol: its metabolism and interaction with nutrients. *Ann. Rev. Nutr.*, 2000, 20, 395-430.

[50] al-Sereiti, MR; abu-Amer, KM; Sen, P. Pharmacology of rosemary (Rosmarinus offcianalis Linn.) and its therapeutic potentials. *Indian J. Exp. Biol.*, 1999, 37, 124-130.

[51] Krishnaswamy, K.; Raghuramulu, N. Bioactive phytochemicals with emphasis on dietary practices. *Indian J. Med. Res.*, 1998, 108, 167-181.

[52] Rui, YC. Advances in pharmacological studies of silymarin. *Mem. Inst. Oswaldo Cruz.*,1991, 86, 79-85.

[53] Siraki, AG; Pourahmad, J; Chan, TS; Khan, S; O'Brien, PJ. Endogenous and induced reactive oxygen species formation by isolated hepatocytes. *Free Radic. Biol. Med.*, 2002, 32, 2-10.

[54] Sharma, P; Morgan, PD. Ascorbate reduces superoxide production and improves mitochondrial respiratory chain function in human fibroblasts with electron transport chain deficiencies. *Mitochondrion.* 2001, 1,191-198.

[55] Chan, TS; Teng, S; Wilson, JX; Galati, G; Khan, S; O'Brien, PJ. Coenzyme Q cytoprotective mechanisms for mitochondrial complex 1 cytopathies involves NAD(P)H: quinone oxidoreductase 1(NQO1). *J. Free Rad. Res.*, 2002, 36, 421-427.

[56] Miquel. J. Can antioxidant diet supplementation protect against age-related mitochondrial damage?. *Ann. NY. Acad. Sci.*, 2002, 959, 508-516.

[57] Palacios, A; Piergiacomi, V; Catala, A. Antioxidant effect of conjugated linoleic acid and vitamin A during non-enzymatic lipid peroxidation of rat liver microsomes and mitochondria. *Mol. Cell Biochem.*, 2003, 250, 107-113.

[58] Lee, JH; Park, JW. Protective role of alpha-phenyl-N-t-butylnitrone against ionizing radiation in U937 cells and mice. *Canc. Res.*, 2003, 63, 6885-6893.

[59] Brookes, PS; Digerness, PS; Parks, DA; Darley-Usmar,V. Mitochondrial function in response to cardiac ischemia-reperfusion after oral treatment with quercetin. *Free Radic. Biol. Med.*, 2002, 32, 1220-1228.

[60] Tiano, L; Fedeli, D; Santoni, G; Davis, I; Wakabayashi, T; Falcioni, G. Ebselen prevents mitochondrial ageing due to oxidative stress: in vitro study of fish erythrocytes. *Mitochondrion.* 2003, 2,428-436.

[61] Eckert, A; Keil, U; Kressmann, S; Schindowski, K; Leutner, S; Leutz, S; Muller, WE. Effects of EGb 761 ginkgo biloba extract on mitochondrial function and oxidative stress. *Pharmacopsychiatry.* 2003, 36 S1,S15-23.

[62] Fernandes, MAS; Santos, MSS; Joaquim, AF; Vincente, AF; Moreno, AJM; Velena, A; Duburs, G; Oliveira, CR. Effects of 1,4-dihydropyridine derivatives (cerebrocrast, gammapyrone, glutapyrone, and diethone) on mitochondrial bioenergetics and oxidative stress: a comparative stidy. *Mitochondrion.* 2003, 3, 47-59.

[63] Kovacic, P; Edwards, W; Natale, NR; Sridhar, R; Kiser, PF. Theoretical calculations on calcium channel drugs: is electron transfer involved mechanistically?. *Chem.-Biol. Interact.*, 1990, 75, 61-70.

[64] Galati, G; O'Brien, PJ. Potential toxicity of flavonoids and other dietary phenolics: significance for their chemopreventive and anticancer properties. *J. Free Radic. Biol. Med.*, 2004, 37, 287-303.

[65] Kovacic, P; Crawford, PW; Ryan, MD; Nelson, VC. Charge-transfer mechanism for carcinogenesis by alkylating and other agents. Bioelect. Bioenerg., 1986, 15, 305-316.

[66] Norat, T.; Bingham, S; Ferrari, P; Slimani, N; Jenab, M; Mazuir, M; Overyad, K; Overvad, K; Bergmann, MM; Nieters, A; Linseisen, J; Trichopoulou, A; Trichopoulos, D; Tountas, Y; Berrino, F; Palli, D; Panicio, S; Tumino, R; Vineis, P; Bueno-de-Mesqita, HB; Peeters, PH; Engeset, D; Lund, E; Skeiè, R; Ardanz, E; Gonzalez, C; Navarro, C; Quoros, JR; Sanchez, MJ; Berglund, G; Mattisson, I; Hallmans, G; Palmqvist, R; Day, NE; Khaw, KT; Key, TJ; San Joaquin, M; Hemon, B; Saracci, R; Kaaks, R; Riboli, E. J. Meat, fish, and colorectal cancer risk: the European prospective investigation into cancer and nutrition *J. Natl. Cancer Inst.*, 2005, 97, 906-916.

[67] Barbosa, DS; Cecchini, R; El Kadri, MZ; Rodriguez, M; Bunni, RC; Dichi, I. Decreased oxidative stress in patients with ulcerative colitis supplemented with fish oil ω-3 fatty acids. *Nutrition,* 2003, 19, 837-842.

[68] Vivancos, M; Moreno, JJ. β-Sitosterol modulates antioxidant enzyme response in RAW 264.7 macrophages. *Free Radic. Biol. Med.,* 2005, 39, 91-97.

[69] Zhang, Y; Li, J; Tang, L. Cancer-preventive isothiocyantes: dichotomous modulators of oxidative stress. *Free Radic. Biol. Med.,* 2005, 38, 70-77.

[70] Kovacic, P. Role of oxidative metabolites of cocaine in toxicity and addiction: oxidative stress and electron transfer. *Med. Hypoth.*, 2005, 64, 350-356.

[71] Usal, M. The role of stimulated lipid peroxidation and impaired calcium sequestration in the enhancement of cocaine induced hepatotoxicity by ethanol. *Drug Alcohol Depend,* 2000, 58, 77-83.

[72] Diez-Fernandez, C; Zaragoza, A; Alvarez, A.M; Cascales, M. Cocaine cytotoxicity in hepatocyte cultures from phenobarbital-induced rats; involvement of reactive oxygen species and expression of antioxidant defense. *Biochem. Pharmacol.,* 1999, 58, 797-805.

[73] Sharan, N; Chong, VZ; Nair, VD; Mishra, RK; Hayes, RJ, Gardner EL. Cocaine treatment increases expression of a 40 kDa catecholamine-regulated protein in discrete brain regions. *Synapse*, 2003, 47, 33-44.

[74] Fantel, AG; Person, RE. Involvement of mitochondria and other free radical sources in normal and abnormal fetal development. *Ann. NY. Acad. Sci.* 2002; 959: 424-433.

[75] Castelli, MC; Venturini, L; Sparber, SB. Cocaine and salicylate: documentation of hydroxyl radical formation in hearts and brains of 18-day-old chick embryos and unexpected interactive toxicity. *Psychopharmacology,* 2001, 156, 23-31.

[76] Fineschi, V; Baroldi, G; Centini, F; Cerretani, D; Fiaschi, AI; Micheli, L; Parolini, M; Turillazzi, E; Giorgi, G. Markers of cardiac oxidative stress and altered morphology after intraperitoneal cocaine injection in a rat model. *Int. J. Legal Med.*, 2001, 114, 323-330.

[77] Woods, JR Jr; Plessinger, MA; Miller, RK. Vitamins C and E: missing links in preventing preterm premature rupture of membranes? *Am. J. Obstet. Gynecol.*, 2001, 185, 5-10.

[78] Zaragoza, A; Diez-Fernandez, C; Alvarez, AM; Andres, D; Cascales, M. Mitochondrial involvement in cocaine-treated rat hepatocytes: effect of N-acetylcysteine and deferoxamine. *Br. J. Pharmacol.*, 2001, 132, 1063-1070.

[79] Kovacic, P.; Cooksy, A. Iminium metabolite mechanism for nicotine toxicity and addiction: Oxidative stress and electron transfer. *Med. Hypoth.,* 2005, 64, 104-111.

[80] Kovacic, P.; Cooksy, AL. Role of diacetyl metabolite in alcohol toxicity and addiction via electron transfer and oxidative stress. *Arch. Toxicol.,* 2005, 79, 123-128.

[81] Bhat R.S.; Bhaskaran, M.; Mongia, A,; Hitosugi, N.; Singhal, P.C. Morphine-induced apoptosis: oxidative stress and strategies for modulation. *J. Leukoc. Biol.,* 2004, 75, 1131-1138.

[82] Patel, J; Manjappa, N; Bhat, R; Mehrotra, P; Bhaskaran, M; Singhal, PC. Role of oxidative stress and heme oxygenase activity in morphine-induced glomerular epithelial cell growth. *Am. J. Physiol. Renal. Physiol.,* 2003, 285:F, 861-869.

[83] Kaneto, H; Kajimoto, Y; Miyagawa, J; Matsuoka, T; Fujitani, Y; Umayahara, Y; Hanafusa, T; Matsuzawa, Y; Yamasaki, Y; Hori, M. Beneficial effects of antioxidants

in diabetes: possible protection of pancreatic beta-cells against glucose toxicity. *Diabetes*, 1999, 48, 2398-2406.

[84] Dhaunsi, GS; Bitar, MS. Antioxidants attenuate diabetes-induced activation of peroxisomal functions in the rat kidney. *J. Biomed. Sci.*, 2004, 11, 566-570.

[85] Koya, D; Hayashi, K; Kitada, M; Kashiwagi, A; Kikkawa, R; Haneda, M. Effects of antioxidants in diabetes-induced oxidative stress in the glomerulli of diabetic rats. *J. Am. Soc. Nephrol.*, 2003, 14, S250-253.

[86] Johansen, JS; Harris, AK; Rychly, DJ; Ergul, A. Oxidative stress and the use of antioxidants in diabetes: linking basic science to clinical practice. *Cardiovasc. Diabetol.*, 2005, 4, 5.

[87] Gurrero-Romero, F; Rodríguez-Morán, M. Complementary therapies for diabetes: the case for chromium, magnesium, and antioxidants. *Arch. Med. Res.*, 2005, 36, 250-257.

[88] Kovacic, P; Jacintho, JD. Systemic lupus erythematosus and other autoimmune diseases from endogenous and exogenous agents: unifying theme of oxidative stress. *Mini Rev. Med. Chem.*, 2003, 3, 568-575.

[89] Bigazzi, PE Autoimmunity caused by xenobiotics. *Toxicology*, 1997, 119, 1-121.

[90] Pelsman, A; Hoyo-Vadillo, C; Gudasheva, TA; Seredenin, SB; Ostrovskaya, RU; Busciglio, J. GVS-111 prevents oxidative damage and apoptosis in normal and Down's syndrome human cortical neurons. *Int. J. Dev. Neurosci.*, 2003, 21, 117-124.

[91] Nicotera, TM. Molecular and biochemical aspects of Bloom's syndrome. *Canc. Genet. Cytogenet.*, 1991, 53, 1-13.

[92] Rumiantsev, AG; Samochatova, EV; Afanas'ev, IB; Korkina, LG; Suslova, TB.The role of free oxygen radicals in the pathogenesis of Fanconi's anemia. *TB. Ter. Arkh.*, 1989, 61, 32-36.

[93] Polte, T; Tyrrell, RM. Involvement of lipid peroxidation and organic peroxides in UVA- induced matrix metalloproteinase-1 expressin. *Free Radic. Biol. Med.*, 2004, 36, 1566-1574.

[94] Lee, JH; Park, J-W. A manganese porphyrin complex is a novel radiation protector. *Free Radic. Biol. Med.*, 2004, 37, 272-283.

[95] Bando, N; Hayashi, H; Wakamatsu, S; Inakuma, T; Miyoshi, M; Nagao, A; Yamauchi, R; Terao, J. Participation of singlet oxygen in ultraviolet-A- induced lipid peroxidation in mouse skin and its inhibition by dietary β-carotene: an ex-vivo study. *Free Radic. Biol. Med.*, 2004, 37, 1854-1863.

[96] Manevich, Y; Fischer, A. B Peroxiredoxin 6, a 1-Cys peroxiredoxin, functions in antioxidant defense and lung phospholipids metabolism. *Free Radic. Biol. Med.*, 2005, 38, 1422-1432.

[97] Galati,G; O`Brien, PJ. Cytoprotective and anticancer properties of coenzyme Q versus capsaicin. *Biofactors*, 2003, 18, 195-205.

[98] Gorogawa, S; Kajimoto, Y; Umayahara, Y; Kaneto, H; Watada, H; Kuroda, A; Kawamori, D; Yasuda, T; Matsuhisa, M; Yamasaki, Y; Hori, M. Probucol preserves pancreatic beta-cell function through reduction of oxidative stress in type 2 diabetes. *Diabetes Res Clin. Pract.*, 2002, 57, 1-10.

[99] Hininger, I; Waters, R; Osman, M; Garrel, C; Fernholz, K; Roussel, A. M; Anderson, RA. Acute prooxidant effects of vitamin C in EDTA chelation therapy and long-term antioxidant benefits of therapy. *Free Radic. Biol. Med.*, 2005, 38, 1565-1570.

[100] Prasad, AS; Bao, B; Beck, FWJ; Kucuk, O; Sarkar, FH. Antioxidant effect of zinc in humans. *Free Radic. Biol. Med.*, 2004, 37, 1182-1190.
[101] Sha, SH; Schacht, J. Antioxidants attenuate gentamicin-induced free radical formation in vitro and ototoxicity in vivo: D-methionine is a potential protectant. *Hear Res.*, 2000, 142, 34-40.
[102] Caro, A A; Cederbaum, AI. Antioxidant properties of S-adenosyl-L-methionine in Fe2+ -intiated oxidations. *Free Radic. Biol. Med.*, 2004, 36, 1303-1316.
[103] Mursu, J; Voutilanen, S; Nurmi, T; Rissanen, TH; Virtanen, J K; Kaikkonen, J; Nyyssönen, K; Salonen, JT. Dark chocolate consumption increases HDL cholesterol concentration and chocolate fatty acids may inhibit lipid peroxidation in healthy humans. *Free Radic. Biol. Med.*, 2004, 37, 1351-1459.
[104] Miranda, C L; Stevens, J F; Ivanov, V; McCall, M; Frei, B; Deinzer, ML; Buhler, DR. Antioxidant and prooxidant actions of prenylated and nonprenylated chalcones and flavanones in vitro. *J. Agric. Food Chem.*, 2000, 48, 3876-3884.
[105] Valentová, K; Sersen, F; Ulrichová. X. Radical scavenging and anti-lipoperoxidative activities of Smallanthus sonchifolius leaf extracts. *J. Agric. Food Chem.*, 2005, 53, 5577-5582.
[106] Heo, H J; Lee, CY. Epicatechin and catechin in cocoa inhibit amyloid β protein induced apoptosis. *J. Agric. Food Chem.,* 2005, 53, 1445-1448.
[107] Gálvez, M; Martín-Cordero, C; Houghton, PJ; Ayuso, MJ. Antioxidant activity of methanol extracts obtained from Plantago species. *J. Agric. Food Chem.*, 2005, 53, 1927-1933.
[108] Heo, H. J.; Lee, C. Y. Strawberry and its anthocyanins reduce oxidative stress-induced apoptosis in PC12 cells. *J. Agric. Food Chem.*, 2005, 53, 1984-1989.
[109] Yu, J; Wang, L; Walzem, RL; Miller, EG; Pike, LM; Patil, BS. Antioxidant activity of citrus limonoids, flavonoids, and coumarins. *J. Agric. Food Chem.,* 2005, 53, 2009-2014.
[110] Auger, C; Teissedre, P-L; Gérain, P; Lequeux, N; Bornet, A; Serisier, S; Besançon, P; Caoriccio, B; Criatol, J-P; Rouanet, J-M. Dietary wine phenolics, catechin, quercetin and resveratrol efficiently protect hypercholesterolemic hamsters against aortic fatty streak accumulation. *J. Agric. Food Chem.*, 2005, 53, 2015-2021.
[111] Viljanen, K; Kylli, P; Hubbermann, E-M; Schwarz, K; Heinonen, M. Anthocyanin antioxidant active and partition behavior in whey protein emulsion. *J. Agric. Food Chem.,* 2005, 53, 2022-2027.
[112] Liyana-Pathirana, CM; Shahidi, F. Antioxidant activity of commercial soft and hard wheat (Triticum aestivum L.) as affected by gastric pH conditions. *J. Agric. Food Chem.*, 2005, 43, 2433-2440.
[113] Hassimotto, NMA; Genovese, MI; Lajolo, F. M. Antioxidant activity of dietary fruits, vegetables, and commercial frozen fruit pulps. *J. Agric. Food Chem.*; 2005, 53, 2928-2935.
[114] Gorelik, S; Lapidot, T; Shaham, I; Granit, R; Ligumsky, M; Kohen, R; Kanner, J. Lipid peroxidation and coupled vitamin oxidation in simulated and human gastric fluid inhibited by dietary polyphenols: health implications. *J. Agric. Food Chem.*, 2005, 53, 3397-3402.
[115] Heo, HJ; Lee, CY. Protective effects of quercetin and vitamin C against oxidative stress-induced neurodegeneration. *J. Agric. Food Chem.,* 2004, 52, 7514-7517.

[116] Al-Awwadi, N; Bornet, A; Azay, J; Araiz, C; Delbosc, S; Cristol, J-P; Linck, N; Cros, G; Teissedre, P-L. Red wine polyphenols alone or in association with ethanol prevent hypertension, cardiac hypertrophy, and production of reactive oxygen species in the insulin-resistant fructose-fed rat. *J. Agric. Food Chem.*, 2004, 42, 5593-5597.

[117] Singletary, KW; Stansbury, MJ; Giusti, M; Van Breemen, RB; Wallig, M; Rimando, A Inhibition of rat mammary tumorigenesis by Concord grape juice constituents. *J. Agric. Food Chem.*, 2003, 51, 7280-7286.

[118] Nùñez-Sellés, AJ Antioxidant therapy: myth or reality? *J. Braz. Chem. Soc.*, 2005, 16, 699-710.

[119] Niufar, NN; Haycock, FL; Wesemann, JL; MacStay, JA; Heasley, VL; Kovacic, P. Reduction potentials of conjugated aliphatic ketones, oximes, and imines; Correlation with structure and bioactivity. *Rev. Soc. Quim. Mex.*, 2002, 46, 307-312.

[120] Moran, LK; Gutteridge, JMC; Quinlan, GJ. Thiols in cellular redox signaling and control. *Curr. Med. Chem.*, 2001, 8, 763-772.

[121] Cotelle, N. Role of flavonoids in oxidative stress. *Curr. Top. Med. Chem.*, 2001, 1, 569-590.

In: Frontiers in Antioxidants Research
Editor: Harold V. Panglossi, pp. 39-59
ISBN 1-60021-273-5

Chapter 2

ANTIOXIDANTS AND CARDIOVASCULAR DISEASE

D. Bonnefont-Rousselot*
Laboratoire des Lipides, Hôpital de la Pitié (AP-HP), Paris Cedex 13, France
and Laboratoire de Biochimie Métabolique et Clinique (EA 3617), Faculté de Pharmacie
Paris, Paris Cedex 06, France

ABSTRACT

The results of large-scale trials on antioxidant vitamin supplementation in cardiovascular disease (CVD) have been disappointing and failed to prove any protective effect of these vitamins (especially vitamin E and beta-carotene). However, the oxidative theory of atherosclerosis has aroused much hope for more than fifteen years in these antioxidant treatments. Indeed, according to this theory, oxidative modification of lipoproteins, especially low density lipoproteins (LDL), increases their atherogenicity. Several *in vitro* and *in vivo* studies suggest that LDL oxidation promotes endothelial cell damage, foam cell accumulation and thrombosis, and interferes with normal vasomotor regulation. Antioxidant vitamins represent one of the many nonenzymatic antioxidant defense systems. Vitamin E (of which α-tocopherol is the major component) is an abundant antioxidant that is widely studied, but several other dietary antioxidants have shown a preventive role *in vitro* in limiting or inhibiting LDL oxidation, especially by scavenging free radicals; however, no prevention of experimental atherogenesis has been demonstrated in animal. In fact, basic research only provides insight into the potential mechanisms of antioxidants in limiting the development of atherosclerosis, but descriptive, analytical and intervention studies are needed to try to establish the relationship between the activity of these antioxidants and the prevention of atherogenesis. Randomized trials generally provide the best data on the benefit and risk from an intervention, and thus are required for developing preventive strategies.

In contrast with supplementation studies, many cross-sectional, case-control, and cohort studies have found an association between antioxidant consumption (especially vitamin E) and a reduced risk of coronary heart disease; moreover, people who consume a diet rich in fruits and vegetables have lower risks of CVD. This addresses the question whether the use of

* Correspondence to: Pr. Dominique BONNEFONT-ROUSSELOT, Laboratoire des Lipides, Hôpital de la Pitié, Pavillon Benjamin Delessert, 83, boulevard de l'Hôpital, 75651 Paris Cedex 13, France, Tel : (33) 1 42 17 78 03, FAX : (33) 1 42 17 78 74, e-mail : dominique.rousselot@psl.aphp.fr

antioxidant supplements to reduce cardiovascular risk is advisable. The relative inefficiency of the antioxidant vitamin supplementation probably results partly from the fact that atherosclerosis is a progressive arterial disease which develops during several years, so that an antioxidant treatment would hardly be effective on already oxidized cell targets. Besides, recent findings support the fact that oxidants may be beneficial under some conditions, for example play a role in regulating very low density lipoprotein (VLDL) secretion and also as signalling molecules. Other factors, such as the dose, the duration of treatment, the kind of vitamin E used, the association with other antioxidants, but also the initial antioxidant status of the patients included in the studies, likely play a key role in the results obtained.

As far as now, there is no sufficient data from randomized trials to justify establishment of recommendations regarding the use of vitamin E for CVD prevention. The best is to recommend a balanced diet (as proposed by the American Heart Association –AHA–) with antioxidant-rich fruits and vegetables. Anyway, even if future clinical trials could demonstrate a beneficial role of antioxidant supplementation in the reduction of CVD, the use of these supplements should be always considered as adjunct therapies, with a strict respect of the classical cardioprotective behaviors (physical activity, control of blood pressure and dyslipidemia, avoidance of obesity and smoking abstention).

Key words: antioxidants; atherosclerosis; cardiovascular disease; clinical trials; oxidative stress; oxidized lipoproteins; vitamins.

INTRODUCTION

Cardiovascular disease (CVD) is the major cause of death and disability in western countries, with coronary artery disease, hypertension, congestive heart failure and stroke. The oxidative theory of atherosclerosis (Steinberg *et al.*, 1989) claims that lipoproteins, especially low density lipoproteins (LDL) oxidized within the arterial wall are able to activate or damage endothelial cells, attract monocytes within the intima and participate to their transformation into foam cells that constitute the first step in the formation of fatty streaks (Figure 1). According to this theory, the use of antioxidants would be beneficial in human CVD (Steinberg and Lewis, 1997). However, contrary to prediction, the antioxidant supplements did not improve the clinical course of human atherosclerosis in several placebo-controlled trials, and this addresses the question of the usefulness of these antioxidants (Kuller LH, 2001; Stocker and Keaney, 2004; Zureik *et al.*, 2004). This failure of antioxidants to decrease the risk of CVD will be discussed and general recommendations will be proposed.

THE OXIDATIVE THEORY OF ATHEROSCLEROSIS: BRIEF REVIEW OF RECENT DATA AND CONSEQUENCES FOR NEW THERAPEUTIC STRATEGIES

The first step in the atherogenesis process is the LDL retention in the arterial wall (Skålén *et al.*, 2002), at the subendothelial level where they become oxidized and more generally modified by different ways (Schissel *et al.*, 1996; Tabas, 1999; Medeiros *et al.*, 2004; Stocker and Keaney 2004; Williams and Fischer, 2005). Reactive oxygen species (ROS) can be released from different sources: nicotinamide adenine dinucleotide (phosphate) oxidase

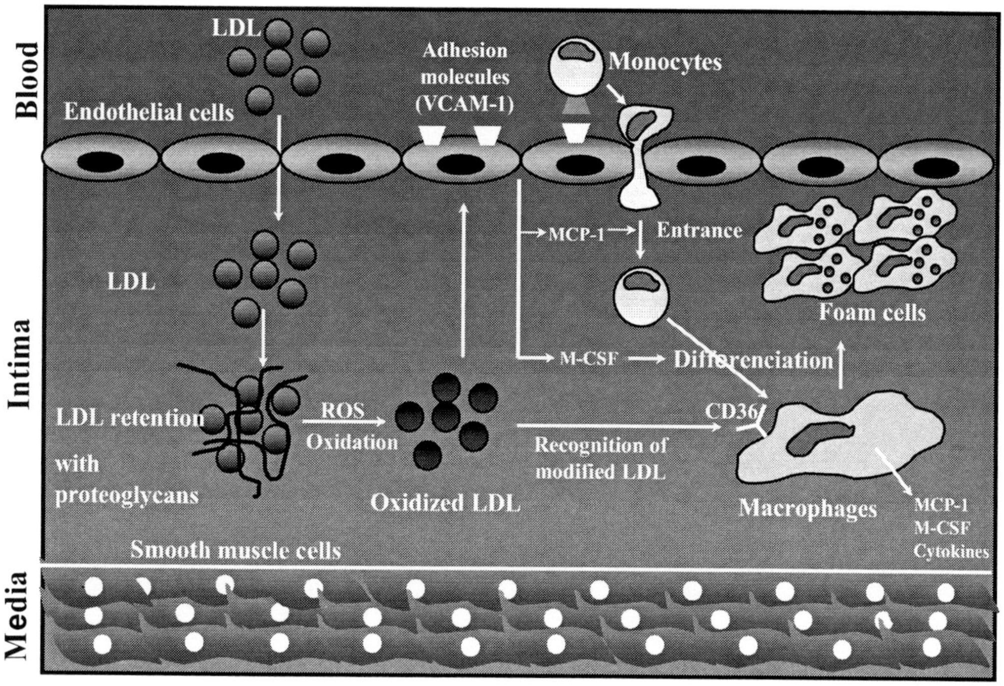

Figure 1. Oxidative modification hypothesis of atherosclerosis. LDL enters the subendothelial space when it becomes retained with proteoglycans and oxidized by vascular cells (smooth muscle cells, endothelial cells, macrophages). Oxidized LDL leads to monocyte chemotaxis and foam cell formation and vascular smooth muscle cell proliferation.

(NAD(P)H oxidase), xanthine oxidase, lipoxygenases, mitochondria, or the uncoupling of nitric oxide synthase in vascular cells (Madamanchi *et al.*, 2005); all these sources, except lipoxygenases, initially produce superoxide radicals ($O_2^{\bullet -}$) that are poorly reactive by themselves but they are able to lead to more reactive species such as hydroxyl radicals ($^{\bullet}OH$) or peroxynitrite anions ($ONOO^-$). NAD(P)H oxidase is specially involved in this ROS production in atherosclerotic human coronary arteries (Azumi *et al.*, 2002), in heart failure (Maack *et al.*, 2003) and in hypertension (Zalba *et al.*, 2001). LDL retention and modification result in the activation of endothelial cells with production of several biologically active molecules that attract monocytes and stimulate proliferation of smooth muscle cells, thereby allowing lesion growth and progression of the atherosclerotic plaques (Skålén *et al.*, 2002; Williams and Tabas, 2002; Komerup *et al.*, 2003). Oxidized lipoproteins have been immunologically found in atherosclerotic lesions (Stocker and Keaney, 2004), which supported this oxidative theory. Both vascular cells and macrophages are able to produce reactive oxygen species (ROS) and reactive nitrogen species (RNS) that have been shown to oxidize lipoproteins *in vitro* (Stocker and Keaney, 2004; Madamanchi *et al.*, 2005). Not only atherogenic LDL, but also antiatherogenic high density lipoproteins (HDL) (Bergt *et al.*, 2004) can be oxidized and this alters the function of the latter ones in a proatherogenic way.

Table 1. Summary of observational and of randomized clinical trials with vitamin E.

Studies	Population	Results
Observational studies		
Case-control studies		
• Scottish studies (Riemersma *et al.*, 1989; Riemersma *et al.*, 1991)	6,000 men, aged 35-54.	Significant inverse association between plasma lipid-standardized vitamin E concentration and CVD (angina pectoris). Vitamin C and carotene also protective but relations decreased when adjustment for cigarette smoking.
• EURAMIC (European Community Multicenter Study on Antioxidants, Myocardial Infarction, and Breast Cancer) study (Kardinaal *et al.*, 1993)	683 subjects with acute myocardial infarction (MI), vs. 727 controls.	Low vitamin E levels not associated with increased risk of MI. Supplemental vitamin E associated with low risk of MI. Protective effect of adipose levels of β-carotene.
Prospective cohort studies		
• Nurses' Health Study (NHS) (Stampfer *et al.*, 1993)	87,245 female nurses, aged 34-59.	After 8 years dietary antioxidant intake and use .of antioxidant vitamin supplements, women in highest quintile of vitamin E intake had a 34% lower risk of nonfatal MI and fatal CHD compared with those in the lowest quintile. Inverse association only for supplements.
• Health Professionals Follow-up Study (HPFS) (Rimm *et al.*, 1993)	39,310 male health professionals, aged 40-75.	The relative risk of major coronary disease for those in the highest vs. the lowest quintile of vitamin E intake was 0.60. Strongest protective association for supplements.
• Finnish Cohort Study (Knekt *et al.*, 1994)	5,133 men and women, aged 30-69.	After 14 years, significant inverse correlation between dietary intake of vitamin E and coronary mortality.
• Iowa Women's Health Study (Kushi *et al.*, 1996)	34,486 postmenopausal women, aged 55-69.	After 7 years, vitamin E intake from food but not from supplements was strongly associated with a lower risk of CHD mortality.
• Study of Middle-Age French-Canadian Men (Meyer *et al.*, 1996)	2,313 men.	After 5 years, men taking vitamin E supplements had a statistically significant lower risk of ischemic heart disease and MI.
• Multiple Risk Factor Intervention Trial (MRFIT) (Evans *et al.*, 1998)	734 men, aged 35-57, at risk for CVD	After 20 years, no association between serum vitamin E levels and risk of nonfatal MI or coronary death.
• Established Populations for Epidemiologic Studies of the Elderly (EPESE) (Losonczy *et al.*, 1996)	11,178 men and women, aged 67-105.	After 9 years, decreased risk of CHD mortality (RR = 0.53) and overall mortality (RR = 0.66) among those taking vitamin E supplements.
• Rotterdam Study (Klipstein-Grobusch *et al.*, 1999)	4,802 men and women, aged 55-95.	After 4 years, no association between vitamin E intake and MI.

Table 1. Summary of observational and of randomized clinical trials with vitamin E. (Continued)

Studies	Population	Results
Observational studies		
Randomized clinical trials		
Primary prevention		
• SU.VI.MAX Study (Supplémentation en Vitamines et Minéraux AntioXydants) (Hercberg *et al.*, 1998 ; Hercberg *et al.*, 2004)	13,017 men and women, aged 35-60.	After a median follow-up time of 7.5 years, no reduction in CVD risk among those taking a vitamin cocktail including 30 IU/day vitamin E and other antioxidants and minerals (6 mg/day β-carotene, 120 mg/day vitamin C, 0.1 mg/day selenium, 20 mg/day zinc).
• Alpha-Tocopherol, Beta-Carotene (ATBC) trial (The ATBC prevention Study Group, 1994; Rapola *et al.*, 1996; Virtamo *et al.*, 2003)	29,133 male smokers, aged 50-69.	After a median treatment period of 6.1 years, the effects of a supplementation with 50 IU/day synthetic vitamin E, 20 mg/day β-carotene, both or neither were evaluated. Supplementation with vitamin E was associated with only a minor decrease in the incidence of angina pectoris (RR = 0.91). β-carotene had no preventive effect and was associated with a slight increase of angina (RR = 1.13).
• Primary Prevention Project (PPP) (De Gaetano, 2001)	4,495 men and women with at least one risk factor for heart disease, mean age: 64.4 years.	After 3.6 years, no effect of synthetic vitamin E (300 IU/day) and/or 100 mg/day low-dose aspirin on reducing the incidence of cardiovascular events.
• Vitamin E Atherosclerosis Prevention Study (VEAPS) (Hodis *et al.*, 2002)	353 men and women ≥ 40 years old, with LDL-cholesterol higher than 130 mg/dL.	After 2 years, no difference in the progression of intima-media thickness in subjects randomized to 400 IU vitamin E (dlα-tocopherol) daily vs. placebo.
• Women's Health Study (WHS) (Lee *et al.*, 2005).	39,876 healthy women, ≥ 45 years old.	Effect of a 12-year ongoing randomized trial with 600 IU vitamin E or low-dose aspirin (100 mg) on alternate days. Primary endpoint: MI, stroke, and CVD death.
• Physicians' Health Study II (PHS II) (Christen *et al.*, 2000)	15,000 physicians recruited to date (recruiting is ongoing), ≥ 55 years old.	Evaluation of several antioxidants including 400 IU vitamin E and 50 mg β-carotene on alternate days, and 500 mg vitamin C daily for 8 years.

Table 1. Summary of observational and of randomized clinical trials with vitamin E. (Continued)

Studies	Population	Results
Observational studies		
Secondary prevention		
• Cambridge Heart Antioxidant Study (CHAOS) (Stephens *et al.*, 1996)	2,002 patients with coronary heart disease.	After a median period of 510 days, patients randomly assigned to receive vitamin E (400 or 800 IU/day) had a lower risk of nonfatal MI (relative risk=0.23) but nonsignificant increase in cardiovascular deaths (RR=1.18). Primary endpoint: combined nonfatal MI and CVD death, vitamin E reduced this risk (RR=0.53).
• Gruppo Italiano per lo Studio della Sopravvivenza nell'Infarcto miocardio (GISSI) Prevention Trial (The GISSI-Prevention Investigators, 1999)	11,324 patients with a history of acute MI within the last 3 months. No age limit.	After 3.5 years of randomization to synthetic vitamin E (300 mg daily), n-3 PUFA (1g daily), both, or neither, vitamin E did not have an effect on the combined endpoint of cardiovascular death, nonfatal MI and nonfatal stroke (RR=0.98), but had a significant effect on the secondary endpoint of cardiovascular death (RR=0.80).
• Heart Outcome Prevention Evaluation (HOPE) Study (Yusuf *et al.*, 2000)	9,541 patients (2,545 women and 6,996 men) ≥ 55 years old, with CVD or diabetes and at least one CV risk factor.	After a mean of 4.5 years of randomization to vitamin E (400 IU daily), ramipril (angiotensin-converting enzyme inhibitor), both drugs or neither, vitamin E had no effect on the primary combined endpoint of MI, stroke, or CV death (RR=1.05).
• Secondary prevention with antioxidants of CVD in endstage renal disease (SPACE) (Boaz *et al.*, 2000)	196 hemodialysis patients with preexisting CVD, aged 40-75 years.	After a median follow-up period of 519 days, treatment with 800 IU vitamin E (randomization to vitamin E or matching placebo) decreased acute MI.
• MRC/BHF Heart Protection Study (HPS) (Heart Protection Study Collaborative Group, 2002)	20,536 adults aged 40-80 with coronary disease, other occlusive arterial disease, or diabetes.	After 5 years of randomization to vitamin supplementation (600 mg synthetic vitamin E, 250 mg vitamin C, and 20 mg beta-carotene daily) or matching placebo, no significant reduction in the mortality from, or incidence of, any type of vascular disease, cancer, or other major outcome.
• Women's Antioxidant Cardiovascular Study (WACS) (Manson *et al.*, 1995)	Nearly 8,000 high-risk professionals ≥ 40 years old, with preexisting CVD or with several risk factors.	Randomization to 600 IU natural vitamin E (α-tocopherol) every other day or placebo. Ongoing study.
• Selenium and Vitamin E Cancer Prevention Trial (SELECT) (Klein *et al.*, 2001)	32,400 healthy men aged ≥ 55 years (white men) and ≥ 50 years in (black men) –since 50 55-year-old black American men have a prostate cancer incidence rate comparable to that of 55 to 60-year-old white men–.	Ongoing evaluation of any cardiovascular impact associated with taking 400 IU vitamin E every other day.

New therapeutic approaches in CVD have been developed because conventional lipid lowering treatments failed to completely inhibit cardiovascular events but only reduce them by approximately one-third (Vetter *et al.*, 2004).

Thus, as an example, trials have been conducted with artificial particles that could remove LDL, and especially oxidized LDL from the arterial wall, or improve the reverse lipid transport, with some promising results (Williams *et al.*, 1984; Rodrigueza *et al.* 1997; Nanjee *et al.*, 1999; Nissen *et al.*, 2003).

Another way was the use of antioxidant supplementation. This was based on the observation that people who consume a diet rich in fruits and vegetables had lower risk of CVD, but also of cancer and all-cause mortality; however, such an observation did not constitute an evidence for a protective effect, which required supplementation studies. Antioxidant interventions have been often reported to slow the development of atherosclerosis in animals (Carew *et al.*, 1987; Kita *et al.*, 1987; Prasad and Kalra, 1993; Pratico *et al.*, 1998; Thomas *et al.*, 2001). Moreover, studies conducted in humans have often shown a relationship between the consumption of antioxidant-rich diets and lower rates of CVD (Gey *et al.*, 1991; Riemersma *et al.*, 1991; Kushi *et al.*, 1996). The most reliable epidemiological evidence came from prospective cohort studies that have shown an inverse relationship between coronary heart disease and dietary intake of vitamin E and even β-carotene (Salonen *et al.*, 1985; Kok *et al.*, 1987; Stampfer *et al.*, 1993; Rimm *et al.*, 1993, Knekt *et al.*, 1994) (Table I). Results from randomized trials conducted to date, however, are conflicting. Antioxidant supplementation (800 IU vitamin E daily) has shown some benefit in hemodialysis patients (Boaz *et al.*, 2000), with a reduction of composite CVD endpoints and MI. Similarly, although no significant benefit of vitamin E supplementation (400 IU daily for a 4.5-year period) was detected in the entire group of Heart Outcomes Prevention (HOPE) trial (Yusuf *et al.*, 2000; Lonn *et al.*, 2002), positive results have been observed in some diabetic patients with a particular haptoglobin phenotype (Levy *et al.*, 2004); thus, in patients homozygous for the haptoglobin 2 allele, who are at high risk for CV events, there was a statistically significant reduction in the risk of CV death and nonfatal myocardial infarction (MI), but there was no statistical interaction between vitamin E use and haptoglobin type, which did not support the hypothesis that the effects of vitamin E differed by haptoglobin phenotype. Another study that revealed a positive result with antioxidant supplementation was the Transplant-Associated Atherosclerosis Study (conducted in a small number of patients, n=40) which showed that progression of the coronary intimal index (plaque area/vessel area) was inhibited with the combined supplementation of RRR-α-tocopherol (800 IU daily) and ascorbic acid (1000 mg daily) for 1 year (Fang *et al.*, 2002). A combination of RRR-α-tocopherol (272 IU daily) and slow-release ascorbic acid (500 mg daily) in the Antioxidant Supplementation in Atherosclerosis Prevention (ASAP) study (n=440) significantly decreased carotid intima-media thickness in hypercholesterolemic males (Salonen *et al.*, 2003). It must be noted that vitamin E, that is the most prevalent antioxidant in LDL (each LDL contains 5 to 9 vitamin E molecules), displays other biological effects that can be beneficial against the atherosclerotic process; for example, it inhibits protein kinase C, cell adhesion, protects nitric oxide and endothelial cell vasoactivity, inhibits proliferation of smooth muscle cells, inhibits platelet adhesion and aggregation, reduces leukotriene synthesis in neutrophils and reduces adhesion, production of oxidants and cytokine expression in monocytes (Freedman *et al.*, 1996; Keaney *et al.*, 1999; Azzi *et al.*,

2000; Pryor, 2000). Vitamin E inhibits the expression of the CD36 scavenger receptor (CD36) (Ricciarelli *et al.*, 2000). Vitamin E may also limit the progression of atherosclerosis by stabilizing the plaque and preventing its rupture and subsequent clot formation (Diaz *et al.*, 1997). Vitamin C also shows important biological properties in addition to its antioxidant effects; thus, it increases and stabilizes tetrahydrobiopterin, a cofactor involved in the synthesis of •NO by the NOS, which may enhance •NO production (Huang *et al.*, 2000) and consequently inhibit restenosis (Janero and Ewing, 2000). Conversely, other molecules than vitamin E, vitamin C or β-carotene may display beneficial effects in CVD. Thus, polyphenols that are the most abundant dietary antioxidants have also shown a positive role in various epidemiological studies, with an inverse association between the consumption of polyphenols or polyphenol-rich foods and the risk of cardiovascular disease (Manach *et al.*, 2005). A meta-analysis including seven case-control and 10 cohort studies suggested a 11% reduction of the risk of MI on consumption of 3 cups of tea per day (Peters *et al.*, 2001), and this protective effect tends to be confirmed by other studies (Hirano *et al.*, 2002; Mukamal *et al.*, 2002; Hakim *et al.*, 2003; Mennen *et al.*, 2004). These effects beside antioxidant effects should always be taken in consideration when exploring the antiatherogenic potential of antioxidants; for example, probucol (phenolic antioxidant) has several potential antiatherogenic properties in addition to inhibition of LDL oxidation, especially an anti-restenotic action in relation to a positive vascular remodeling, as shown in the follow-up study of the MultiVitamins and Probucol Trial (Côté *et al.*, 1999).

As regards hypolipidemic drugs, it is especially interesting to note that statins display beneficial cardiovascular pleiotropic effects, among them antioxidant properties (Davignon, 2004). Indeed, statins have direct antioxidant effects on LDL *in vitro* and *ex vivo* (Aviram *et al.*, 1998a; Suzumura *et al.*, 1999). Moreover, hydroxyl metabolites of atorvastatin inhibit oxidation of LDL, VLDL and HDL (Aviram *et al.*, 1998b). Statins may also lower the ability of macrophages to oxidize LDL (Giroux *et al.*, 1993) and decrease the activity of macrophage CD36 scavenger receptor that recognizes oxidized LDL (Fuhrman *et al.*, 2002). Fluvastatin has been shown to reduce the oxidation of LDL and improve endothelial function in patients with dyslipidemia (Inoue *et al.*, 2002). These antioxidant properties could act simultaneously and independently with the well-known LDL cholesterol-lowering effect of these drugs. Several mechanisms would be involved in the antioxidant effects of statins, for example reduction of NADPH-dependent superoxide formation (Delbosc *et al.*, 2002), increase of eNOS expression (Laufs *et al.*, 2002); moreover, by limiting the influx of inflammatory cells, statins may reduce the release of superoxide radicals and the oxidative modification of LDL (Rosenson, 2004).

Failure of Action of Antioxidant Supplementation in CVD

Even in some animal studies, antioxidant supplementation has been inefficient, despite an inhibition of LDL oxidation *ex vivo* or in the artery wall (Fruebis *et al.*, 1994; Witting P *et al.*, 1999; Stocker and Keaney, 2004).

In humans, several randomized clinical trials have been conducted with vitamin E (Table I). Five large-scale vitamin E supplementation trials aimed at appreciating their effect on cardiovascular events: the Cambridge Heart Antioxidant Study (CHAOS) (Stephens *et al.*,

1996), the ATBC (Alpha-Tocopherol Beta-Carotene) trial (The ATBC Prevention Study Group, 1994; Rapola *et al.*, 1996; Rapola *et al.*, 1997), the GISSI Prevention trial (The GISSI-Prevenzione Investigators, 1999), the Collaborative Group of the Primary Prevention Project (PPP) (De Gaetano, 2001) and the Heart Outcomes Protection Study (HOPE) (Yusuf *et al.*, 2000). Taken together, these trials did not show any clear evidence for benefit of vitamin E –or β-carotene–supplementation in subjects with high risk of CVD. Indeed, only the CHAOS trial displayed positive results; this trial consisted in a daily supplementation with 400 or 800 IU vitamin E or placebo and resulted in a relative risk for primary end-point of cardiovascular death and non-fatal MI of 0.53 (95% CI: 0.34 to 0.83). After exclusion of the data from the CHAOS trial, the 4 other trials yielded a relative risk for cardiovascular events of 0.97 (95% CI: 0.81 to 1.16) (Clarke and Armitage, 2002).

The MRC/BHF Heart Protection Study (HPS) trial randomized 20,536 patients at high risk of coronary heart disease, allocated to receive for a 5-year treatment period either antioxidant vitamins (600 mg vitamin E, 250 mg vitamin C and 20 mg β-carotene daily) or placebo, in order to evaluate the relevance of an association of antioxidants (Heart Protection Study Collaborative Group, 2002). Although this regimen increased blood vitamin concentrations, it did not produce any significant reductions in mortality from, or incidence of, any type of vascular disease, cancer, or other major outcome.

The Women's Health Study (WHS) is a primary prevention trial investigating the effects of vitamin E (600 IU) or aspirin (100 mg) on alternate days vs. placebo in 39,876 healthy women aged 45 years or older over a 12-year period, towards risks of CVD (Lee *et al.*, 2005). The data from this large trial indicated that 600 IU of α-tocopherol taken every other day provided no overall benefit for major CV events (nonfatal myocardial infarction, nonfatal stroke, or CV death), thereby supporting current guidelines stating that use of antioxidant vitamins is not justified for CV disease risk reduction (Mosca *et al.*, 2004; Kris-Etherton *et al.*, 2004). The WHS showed, however, a significant reduction in the secondary end point of CV deaths and a significant reduction in major CV events in the subgroup of women aged at least 65 years; this observation differs from the totality of evidence and should be explored further.

The Supplementation Vitamins Minerals and Antioxidant Trial (SU.VI.MAX) tested, in a randomized, placebo-controlled trial, a combination of antioxidant vitamins and minerals including vitamin E, vitamin C and β-carotene in 13,017 healthy men and women but the results did not provide any evidence for prevention of CVD or decrease of all-cause mortality (Hercberg *et al.*, 2004).

The worst argument against a benefit of antioxidants has been given by a comparative study of the effects of cholesterol-lowering drugs (especially simvastatin) alone or associated with antioxidants, which showed a negative effect of antioxidants (Brown *et al.*, 2001).

Ongoing studies aim at evaluating the effects of combinations of antioxidants, including vitamin E, on CVD. Indeed, antioxidants act synergistically (thus, vitamin C is able to regenerate vitamin E and vitamin E protects β-carotene), so that it seems more appropriate to treat with a combination of antioxidants rather than with a single antioxidant. The Women's Antioxidant Cardiovascular Disease Study (WACS) is a ongoing randomized, double-blind, placebo-controlled secondary prevention trial that assessed the separate effects of three antioxidants (vitamin E -600 IU/day-, vitamin C and β-carotene) vs. placebo in 8,000 women with preexisting CVD (Manson *et al.*, 1995). Each participant received either all three active agents, all three placebo agents, or a combination of active and placebo agents. Another primary prevention trial, the Physicians' Health Study II (PHS II) is an ongoing trial evaluating several antioxidants including 400 IU vitamin E every other day for 8 years (Christen *et al.*, 2000).

It must be noted that, despite the absence of clinical benefit of antioxidant supplementation in human atherosclerotic vascular disease, an increase in circulating antioxidant concentration, a decrease in the levels of circulating oxidized LDL and even a protective effect against LDL oxidation *ex vivo* are observed (Hodis *et al.*, 2002).

Possible Argumentation to Explain the Failure of Antioxidant Supplementation in CVD

The antioxidant supplementation trials are based on the oxidative theory of atherosclerosis. However, some arguments could be developed against this theory. For example, it has paradoxically been always difficult to induce foam cell formation *in vitro* with oxidized LDL, although they are recognized and internalized by scavenger receptors (Greenspan *et al.*, 1997; Tabas, 1999). Some studies even showed that scavenger receptor deficiency may accelerate atherosclerotic lesions in animal and that their overexpression retards them (de Winther *et al.*, 1999; Whitman *et al.*, 2002). Similarly, myeloperoxidase and 15-lipoxygenase, that are two sources of oxidant species involved in atherogenesis, have shown to have a potential protective role in animal (Shen *et al.*, 1996; Brennan *et al.*, 2001). It is also amazing to note that exercise and moderate alcohol consumption, that are both sources of ROS, are recommended for cardiovascular health (Meagher *et al.*, 1999; Banerjee *et al.*, 2003; Smith *et al.*, 2004). Besides, there is no consistent relationship between the titer of circulating autoantibodies against oxidized LDL and CVD (Stocker and Keaney, 2004). Moreover, a recent study trends to show that HDL would predominantly act by the reverse cholesterol transport rather than by an anti-inflammatory or antioxidant action (Choudhury *et al.*, 2004). In addition, oxidation of lipoproteins could only be a secondary event in the development of the atherosclerotic plaques, the first event being the recruitment of inflammatory cells induced by lipoprotein retention (Williams and Tabas, 2002; Stocker and Keaney, 2004).

The discrepancy observed between the results of observational and supplementation trials could have different origins. Thus, the inverse association between the dietary intake of antioxidants and the risk of CVD that has been suggested in some prospective cohort studies examining the role of antioxidants, especially vitamin E, could have limitations such as a bias in the selection of participants. Indeed, people who consume more fruits and vegetables may have more healthy lifestyles, and diets rich in antioxidants are lower in saturated fats and cholesterol, and are higher in fibers (Gaziano, 2004). This can explain that the beneficial role of diets rich in antioxidants was not always found in supplementation trials. Supplementation studies differ with the dose of antioxidant, the combination of antioxidants, the duration of treatment, the kind of antioxidant. As an example, dietary vitamin E is a mixture of tocopherols and tocotrienols, whereas vitamin E supplements generally contain only α-tocopherol, and the absence of γ-tocopherol could partly explain the disappointing trial results (Devaraj and Traber, 2003). Regarding the dose of vitamin E, the ATBS study was conducted in smokers and with a subtherapeutic dose of vitamin E (Gaziano, 2004). Efficacious threshold doses for vitamin E have been suggested at 800 IU RRR-α-tocopherol daily (Jialal and Devaraj, 2003), and the form might be important, especially for cell signaling, because most of the reported anti-inflammatory effects of α-tocopherol seem to be due to RRR-α-tocopherol (Devaraj *et al.*, 1996). Besides, antioxidants may be most effective when taken in specific associations, taken into account the synergic effect of antioxidants and the regeneration of some of them by other antioxidants (for example: regeneration of vitamin E by vitamin C (Gaziano, 2004) and some ongoing studies are designed to test this hypothesis (Table I). Also, the optimal regimen for inhibiting for example lipid peroxidation in humans needs to be determined so that test compounds can be administered in effective antioxidant regimens; higher doses of vitamin E and/or longer periods of supplementation would thus inhibit lipid peroxidation *in vivo* and perhaps be more appropriate for clinical trials (Heinecke, 2001). The bioavailability of vitamin E as a function of food intake is also to be taken into account, since plasma vitamin E concentration and plasma antioxidant activity in response to oral supplementation are markedly affected by food intake, so that vitamin E must be given with meals to obtain maximal absorption (Iuliano *et al.*, 2001).

Another point to take into account is the fact that only few studies have measured the circulating concentrations of antioxidants (especially vitamins E and C) in patients with risk factors of atherosclerosis, and these data showed a large variability in the plasma or tissue levels of antioxidants; thus, the evidence of an oxidative stress alone perhaps does not imply a low antioxidant status and justify supplementation with antioxidant vitamins (Violo *et al.*, 2004). Such indiscriminate inclusion of patients in clinical trials, without evaluating antioxidant status, could perhaps account for the negative results of antioxidant trials (Vivekananthan *et al.*, 2003). This can be related to the results obtained in the SU.VI.MAX Study (Hercberg *et al.*, 2004), where protective effects of a balanced combination of several antioxidant nutrients at nutritional doses displayed protective effect against cancer only in men; the ineffectiveness of supplementation in women may be due to their better baseline antioxidant status.

Moreover, a paradoxical increase in oxidants could be induced by antioxidants themselves; for instance, vitamin C at high doses is able to lead to DNA damage (Podmore *et al.*, 1998) and this kind of oxidative damage can be enhanced by transition metal ions (Halliwell, 2000).

Nevertheless, the classical notion that antioxidants are beneficial and oxidants deleterious should be modulated. Thus, ROS act as signaling molecules and thus oxidation should be considered not only as a deleterious phenomenon but rather with a more balanced point of view. ROS play indeed a key role in cell regulation but are also potentially toxic, this paradox being perhaps explained by dose-dependent effects (Rhee, 1999). For instance, ROS are essential for the hepatic sensitivity to insulin; indeed, deactivation of tyrosine phosphatases requires oxidation (Xu *et al.*, 2002); insulin stimulation results in an increase in H_2O_2 production that inactivates protein tyrosine phosphatases by oxidation, thus allowing insulin-stimulated tyrosine phosphorylation of its receptor and of insulin receptor substrate proteins (Mahadev *et al.*, 2001).

Similarly, ROS could be considered as beneficial in the regulation of VLDL secretion (Williams and Fischer, 2005). Indeed, the post-endoplasmic reticulum pre-secretory proteolysis is stimulated by dietary polyunsaturated fatty acids (PUFA) through the generation of ROS. Moreover, the ability of PUFA to inhibit apolipoprotein B secretion was abolished by vitamin E or by desferrioxamine, that is by two direct or indirect antioxidants (Pan *et al.*, 2004). By this way, cellular oxidants can display beneficial effects by favoring a decreased secretion of atherogenic lipoproteins. The stimulation of apolipoprotein B degradation by PUFA supports the clinical observation that dietary PUFA, especially α-linolenic acid, lower plasma cholesterol concentration (Kris-Etherton and Yu., 1997; Krauss RM, 2004). A directly related observation of the action of PUFA is that the genetic deficiency of phospholipid transfer protein (PLTP) –that is also a vitamin E transfer protein– results in mice in a relative vitamin E deficiency in the liver, thus allowing an increase in ROS formation and a decrease in hepatic apolipoprotein B secretion (Jiang *et al.*, 2005). Closely related is the fact that high PLTP activity has been associated with elevated apolipoprotein B levels and high risk of CVD (Schlitt *et al.*, 2003). It has also been recently suggested that oxidized lipids may be helpful, especially as ligands for the liver X receptor, which induces ATP-binding cassette transporters and genes involved in the reverse cholesterol transport (Brown *et al.*, 2002; Tall *et al.*, 2002; Soccio and Breslow, 2004). This could explain the previous observation (Brown *et al.*, 2001) that antioxidants may inhibit the ability of the association niacin/statins to raise HDL cholesterol plasma concentration.

More generally, to take into account the beneficial role of ROS under some circumstances, new classes of antioxidants could be developed in order to better target specific subcellular compartments such as mitochondria (Madamanchi *et al.*, 2005).

It may also be significant that animal studies of antioxidants have focused on early events in atherosclerosis, whereas the human clinical trials involved individuals with advanced disease (Heinecke, 2001) where most acute coronary events are consecutive to plaque rupture (Diaz *et al.*, 1997) whereas few is known about the effects of antioxidants on this process. Thus, it could be that atherosclerosis had progressed sufficiently for antioxidants to have little effect; further studies on younger adults with long-term follow-up may clarify whether antioxidants have a role to play in the prevention of cardiovascular disease (Rosenson, 2004). Antioxidant treatment perhaps needs to begin earlier in life to be effective. The positive results of the observational studies in opposition with the inefficiency of some clinical trials could thus reflect the difference between lifelong exposure to an antioxidant-rich diet and the limited exposure to antioxidant supplements (Kris-Etherton *et al.*, 2004).

Finally, the development of sensitive and specific markers should be required to assess the oxidative stress and its modulation by antioxidants in clinical trials (Madamanchi *et al.*, 2005). In relation with the notion of biomarkers, we used an *in vitro* model of LDL oxidation with submicromolar copper concentrations (Zarev *et al.*, 2003), closer to the physiological conditions of LDL oxidation and to the composition of atherosclerotic plaques (Upston *et al.*, 2002) than the classical model of micromolar copper oxidation (Esterbauer *et al.*, 1992). This LDL oxidation by a submicromolar copper concentration of 0.03 μM ($[Cu^{2+}]/[LDL] = 0.05$) led to oxidative modifications of the lipid and protein moieties in the presence antioxidant species (α-tocopherol and β-carotene), whose concentrations were not modified. This observation could highlight the inefficiency of antioxidants to prevent oxidation. Development of parameters of LDL oxidation that are relevant to disease progression is thus required, together with identification and characterization of suitable markers to monitor the inhibition of aortic lipoprotein oxidation and atherosclerosis (Mashima *et al.*, 2001).

Conclusion

On the basis of clinical data and on the recent recommendations of the American Heart Association, antioxidant supplementation should not be given for CVD (Brown *et al*., 2002; Kris-Etherton *et al*., 2004). Oxidation may have beneficial effects in some tissues and under some circumstances; for example, as previously noted, ROS play a role in insulin sensitivity and in the regulation of apolipoprotein B secretion; consequently, an antioxidant treatment could lead to insulin resistance and apolipoprotein B oversecretion. The beneficial effects of ROS should thus be taken into account, and a total suppression of their action by antioxidant treatment could be deleterious by eliminating some beneficial processes (Miller *et al*., 2005).

The advice to increase consumption of fruits and vegetables to reduce the risk of CVD is nevertheless maintained. Indeed, according to the American Heart Association (AHA), there is insufficient efficacy data from completed randomized trials to recommend the use of vitamin E for the prevention of CVD, and AHA recommends a balanced diet with antioxidant-rich fruits and vegetables and whole grains. Patients at risk for CVD must also carefully adhere to pharmacological regimens, especially statins and angiotensin-converting enzyme inhibitors, and to behavioural changes (eg, increasing physical activity, stopping smoking) that are known to prevent CV disease.

References

Aviram M, Hussein O, Rosenblat M, Schlezinger S, Hayek T, Keidar S. Interactions of platelets, macrophages, and lipoproteins in hypercholesterolemia: antiatherogenic effects of HMG-CoA reductase inhibitor therapy. *J Cardiovasc Pharmacol* 1998a; 31: 39-45.

Aviram M, Rosenblat M, Bisgaier CL, Newton RS. Atorvastatin and gemfibrozil metabolites, but not the parent drugs, are potent antioxidants against lipoprotein oxidation. *Atherosclerosis* 1998b; 138: 271-280.

Azumi H, Inoue N, Ohashi Y, Terashima M, Mori T, Fujita H, Awano K, Kobayashi K, Maeda K, Hata K, Shinke T, Kobayashi S, Hirata K, Kawashima S, Itabe H, Hayashi Y, Imajoh-Ohmi S, Itoh H, Yokoyama M. Superoxide generation in directional coronary atherectomy specimens of patients with angina pectoris: important role of NAD(P)H oxidase. *Arterioscler Thromb Vasc Biol* 2002; 22: 1838-1844.

Azzi A, Breyer I, Feher M, Pastori M, Ricciarelli R, Spycher S, Staffieri M, Stocker A, Zimmer S, Zingg JM. Specific cellular responses to α-tocopherol. *J Nutr* 2000; 130: 1649-1652.

Banerjee AK, Mandal A, Chanda D, Chakraborti S. Oxidant, antioxidant and physical exercise. *Mol Cell Biochem* 2003; 253: 307-312.

Bergt C, Pennathur S, Fu X, Byun J, O'Brien K, McDonald TO, Singh P, Anantharamaiah GM, Chait A, Brunzell J, Geary RL, Oram JF, Heinecke JW. The myeloperoxidase product hypochlorous acid oxidizes HDL in the human artery wall and impairs ABCA1-dependent cholesterol transport. *Proc Natl Acad Sci USA* 2004; 101: 13032-13037.

Boaz M, Smetana S, Weinstein T, Matas Z, Gafter U, Iaina A, Knecht A, Weissgarten Y, Brunner D, Fainaru M, Green MS. Secondary prevention with antioxidants of cardiovascular disease in endstage renal disease (SPACE): randomised placebo-controlled trial. *Lancet* 2000; 356: 1213-1218.

Brennan ML, Anderson MM, Shih DM, Qu XD, Wang X, Mehta AC, Lim LL, Shi W, Hazen SL, Jacob JS, Crowley JR, Heinecke JW, Lusis AJ. Increased atherosclerosis in myeloperoxidase-deficient mice. *J Clin Invest* 2001; 107: 419-430.

Brown BG, Zhao XQ, Chait A, Fisher LD, Cheung MC, Morse JS, Dowdy AA, Marino EK, Bolson EL, Alaupovic P, Frohlich J, Albers JJ. Simvastatin and niacin, antioxidant vitamins, or the combination for the prevention of coronary disease. *N Engl J Med* 2001; 345: 1583-1592.

Brown BG, Cheung MC, Lee AC, Zhao XQ, Chait A. Antioxidant vitamins and lipid therapy: end of a long romance? *Arterioscler Thromb Vasc Biol* 2002; 22: 1535-1546.

Carew TE, Schwenke DC, Steinberg D. Antiatherogenic effect of probucol unrelated to its hypocholesterolemic effect: evidence that antioxidants *in vivo* can selectively inhibit low density lipoprotein degradation in macrophage-rich fatty streaks and slow the progression of atherosclerosis in the Watanabe heritable hyperlipemic rabbit. *Proc Natl Acad Sci USA* 1987; 84: 7725-7729.

Choudhury RP, Rong JX, Trogan E, Elmalem VI, Dansky HM, Breslow JL, Witztum JL, Fallon JT, Fisher EA. High-density lipoproteins retard the progression of atherosclerosis and favorably remodel lesions without suppressing indices of inflammation or oxidation. *Arterioscler Thromb Vasc Biol* 2004; 24: 1904-1090.

Christen WG, Gaziano JM, Hennekens CH. Design of Physician's Health Study II: a randomized trial of beta-carotene, vitamins E and C, and multivitamins, in prevention of cancer, cardiovascular disease, and eye disease, and review of results of completed trials. *Ann Epidemiol* 2000; 10: 125-134.

Clarke R, Armitage J. Antioxidant vitamins and risk of cardiovascular disease. Review of large-scale randomised trials. *Cardiovasc Drugs Ther* 2002; 16: 411-415.

Côté G, Tardif JC, Lespérance J, Lambert J, Bourassa M, Bonan R, Gosselin G, Joyal M, Tanguay JF, Nattel S, Gallo R, Crépeau J. Effects of probucol on vascular remodeling after coronary angioplasty. Multivitamins and probucol Study Group. *Circulation* 1999; 99: 30-35.

Davignon J. Beneficial cardiovascular pleiotropic effects of statins. *Circulation* 2004; 109 [suppl.III]: III-39-III-43.

De Gaetano G. Collaborative Group of the Primary Prevention Project. Low-dose aspirin and vitamin E in people at cardiovascular risk: a randomised trial in general practice. *Lancet* 2001; 357: 89-95.

Delbosc S, Morena M, Djouad F, Ledoucen C, Descomps B, Cristol JP. Statins, 3-hydroxy-3-methylglutaryl coenzyme A reductase inhibitors, are able to reduce superoxide anion production by NADPH oxidase in THP-1-derived monocytes. *J Cardiovasc Pharmacol* 2002; 40: 611-617.

Devaraj S, Li D, Jialal I. The effect of alpha-tocopherol supplementation on monocyte function: decreased lipid oxidation, interleukin-1-beat secretion, and monocyte adhesion to endothelium. *J Clin Invest* 1996; 98: 756-763.

Devaraj S, Traber MG. Gamma-tocopherol, the new vitamin E? *Am J Clin Nutr* 2003; 77: 530-531.

De Winther MP, Gijbels MJ, van Dijk KW, van Gorp PJ, Suzuki H, Kodama T, Frants RR, Havekes LM, Hofker MH. Scavenger receptor deficiency leads to more complex atherosclerotic lesions in APOE3Leiden transgenic mice. *Atherosclerosis* 1999; 144: 315-321.

Diaz MN, Frei B, Vita JA, Keaney JF Jr. Antioxidants and atherosclerotic heart disease. *N Engl J Med* 1997; 337: 408-416.

Esterbauer H, Gebicki J, Puhl H, Jurgens G. The role of lipid peroxidation and antioxidants in oxidative modification of LDL. *Free Radic Biol Med* 1992; 13: 341-390.

Evans RW, Shaten BJ, Day BW, Kuller LH. Prospective association between lipid soluble antioxidants and coronary heart disease in men. The Multiple Risk Factor Intervention Trial. *Am J Epidemiol* 1998; 147: 180-186.

Fang JC, Kinlay S, Beltrame J, Hikiti H, Wainstein M, Behrendt D, Suh J, Frei B, Mudge GH, Selwyn AP, Ganz P. Effect of vitamins C and E on progression of transplant-associated arteriosclerosis: a randomised trial. *Lancet* 2002; 359: 1108-1113.

Freedman JE, Farhat JH, Loscalzo J, Keaney JF Jr. α-tocopherol inhibits aggregation of human platelets by a protein kinase C-dependent mechanism. *Circulation* 1996; 94: 2434-2440.

Fruebis J, Steinberg D, Dresel HA, Carew TE. A comparison of the antiatherogenic effects of probucol and of a structural analogue of probucol in low density lipoprotein receptor-deficient rabbits. *J Clin Invest* 1994; 94: 392-398.

Fuhrman B, Koren L, Volkova N, Keidar S, Hayek T, Aviram M. Atorvastatin therapy in hypercholesterolemic patients suppresses cellular uptake of oxidized LDL by differenciating monocytes. *Atherosclerosis* 2002; 164: 179-185.

Gaziano JM. Vitamin E and cardiovascular disease. Observational studies. *Ann NY Acad Sci* 2004; 1031: 280-291.

Gey KF, Puska P, Jordan P, Moser UK. Inverse correlation between plasma vitamin E and mortality from ischemic heart disease in cross-cultural epidemiology. *Am J Clin Nutr* 1991; 53 (suppl. 1): 326S-334S.

Giroux LM, Davignon J, Naruszewicz M. Simvastatin inhibits the oxidation of low-density lipoproteins by activated human monocyte-derived macrophages. *Biochim Biophys Acta* 1993; 1165: 335-338.

Greenspan P, Yµ H, Mao F, Gutman RL. Cholesterol deposition in macrophages: foam cell formation mediated by cholesterol-enriched oxidized low density lipoprotein. *J Lipid Res* 1997; 38: 101-109.

Hakim IA, Alsaif MA, Alduwaihy M, Al-Rubeaan K, Al-Nuaim AR, Al-Attas OS. Tea consumption and the prevalence of coronary heart disease in Saudi adults: results from a Saudi national study. *Prev Med* 2003; 36: 64-70.

Halliwell B. The antioxidant paradox. *Lancet* 2000; 355: 1179-1180.

Heart Protection Study Collaborative Group. MRC/BHF Heart Protection Study of antioxidant vitamin supplementation in 20,536 high-risk individuals: a randomised placebo-controlled trial. *Lancet* 2002; 360: 23-33.

Heinecke JW. Is the emperor wearing clothes? Clinical trials of vitamin E and the LDL oxidation hypothesis. *Arterioscler Thromb Vasc Biol* 2001; 21: 1261-1264.

Hercberg S, Preziosi P, Briancon S, Galan P, Triol I, Malvy D, Roussel AM, Favier A. A primary prevention trial using nutritional doses of antioxidant vitamins and minerals in cardiovascular diseases and cancers in a general population: the SU.VI.MAX study-design, methods, and participant characteristics. SUpplémentation en VItamines et Minéraux AntioXydants. *Control Clin Trials* 1998; 19: 336-351.

Hercberg S, Galan P, Preziosi P, Bertrais S, Mennen L, Malvy D, Roussel A-M, Favier A, Briançon S. The SU.VI.MAX Study. A randomized, placebo-controlled trial of the health effects of antioxidant vitamins and minerals. *Arch Intern Med* 2004; 164: 2335-2342.

Hirano R, Momiyama Y, Takahashi R, Taniguchi H, Kondo K, Nakamura H, Ohsuzu F. Comparison of green tea intake in Japanese patients with and without angiographic coronary artery disease. *Am J Cardiol* 2002; 90: 1150-1153.

Hodis HN, Mack WJ, LaBree L, Mahrer PR, Sevanian A, Liu CR, Liu CH, Hwang J, Selzer RH, Azen SP; VEAPS Research Group. Alpha-tocopherol supplementation in healthy individuals reduces low-density lipoprotein oxidation but not atherosclerosis: the Vitamin E Atherosclerosis Prevention Study (VEAPS). *Circulation* 2002; 106: 1453-1459.

Huang A, Vita JA, Venema RC, Keaney JF Jr. Ascorbic acid enhances endothelial nitric oxide synthase activity by increasing intracellular tetrahydrobiopterin. *J Biol Chem* 2000; 275: 17399-17406.

Inoue T, Hayashi M, Takayanagi K, Morooka S. Lipid-lowering therapy with fluvastatin inhibits oxidative modification of low density lipoprotein and improves vascular endothelial function in hypercholesterolemic patients. *Atherosclerosis* 2002; 160: 369-376.

Iuliano L, Micheletta F, Maranghi M, Frati G, Diczfalusy U, Vili F. Bioavailability of vitamin E as function of food intake in healthy subjects. Effects on plasma peroxide-scavenging activity and cholesterol-oxidation products. *Arterioscler Thromb Vasc Biol* 2001; 21: e34-e37.

Janero DR, Ewing JF. Nitric oxide and postangioplasty restenosis: pathological correlates and therapeutic potential. *Free Radic Biol Med* 2000; 29: 1199-1221.

Jialal I, Devaraj S. Antioxidants and atherosclerosis: don't throw out the baby with the bath water. *Circulation* 2003; 107: 926-928.

Jiang XC, Li Z, Liu R, Yang XP, Pan M, Lagrost L, Fisher EA, Williams KJ. Phospholipid transfer protein deficiency impairs apolipoprotein-B secretion from hepatocytes by stimulating a proteolytic pathway through a relative deficiency of vitamin E and an increase in intracellular oxidants. *J Biol Chem.* 2005; 280: 18336-18340.

Kardinaal AF, Kok FJ, Ringstad J, Gomez-Aracena J, Mazaev VP, Kohlmeier L, Martin BC, Aro A, Kark JD, Delgado-Rodriguez M, *et al.* Antioxidants in adipose tissue and risk of myocardial infarction: the EURAMIC Study. *Lancet* 1993; 342: 1379-1384.

Keaney Jr JF, Simon DI, Freedman JE. Vitamin E and vascular homeostasis: implications for atherosclerosis. *FASEB J* 1999; 13: 965-975.

Kita T, Nagano Y, Tokode M, Ishii K, Kume N, Ooshima A, Yoshida H, Kawai C. Probucol prevents the progression of atherosclerosis in Watanabe heritable hyperlipidemic rabbit, an animal model for familial hypercholesterolemia. *Proc Natl Acad Sci* 1987; 84: 5928-5931.

Klein EA, Thompson IM, Lippman SM, Goodman PJ, Albanes D, Taylor PR, Coltman C. SELECT: the next prostate cancer prevention trial. Selenium and Vitamin E Cancer Prevention Trial. *J Urol* 2001; 166: 1311-1315.

Klipstein-Grobusch K, Geleijnse JM, den Breeijen JH, Boeing H, Hofman A, Grobbee DE, Witteman JC. Dietary antioxidants and risk of myocardial infarction in the elderly: the Rotterdam Study. *Am J Clin Nutr* 1999; 69: 261-266.

Knekt P, Reunanen A, Jarvinen R, Seppanen R, Heliovaara M, Aromaa A. Antioxidant vitamin intake and coronary mortality in a longitudinal population study. *Am J Epidemiol* 1994; 139: 1180-1189.

Kok FJ, de Bruijn AM, Vermeeren R, Hofman A, van Laar A, de Bruin M, Hermus RJ, Valkenburg HA. Serum selenium, vitamin antioxidants and cardiovascular mortality: a 9-year follow-up study in the Netherlands. *Am J Clin Nutr* 1987; 45: 462-468.

Kornerup K, Nordestgaard BG, Feldt-Rasmussen B, Borch-Johnsen K, Jensen KS, Jensen JS. Increased transvascular low density lipoprotein transport in insulin dependent diabetes: a mechanistic model for development of atherosclerosis. *Atherosclerosis* 2003; 170 : 163-168.

Krauss RM. Hold the antioxidants and improve plasma lipids? *J Clin Invest* 2004; 113: 1253-1255.

Kris-Etherton PM, Yu S. Individual fatty acid effects on plasma lipids and lipoproteins: human studies. *Am J Clin Nutr* 1997; 65 (suppl. 5): 1628S-1644S.

Kris-Etherton PM, Lichtenstein AH, Howard BV, Steinberg D, Witztum JL, for the Nutrition Committee of the American Heart Association Council on Nutrition, Physical Activity, and Metabolism. Antioxidant vitamin supplements and cardiovascular disease. *Circulation* 2004; 110: 637-641.

Kuller LH. A time to stop prescribing antioxidant vitamins to prevent and treat heart diseases? *Arterioscler Thromb Vasc Biol* 2001; 21: 1253.

Kushi LH, Folsom AR, Prineas RJ, Mink PJ, Wu Y, Bostick RM. Dietary antioxidant vitamins and death from coronary heart disease in postmenoposal women. *N Engl J Med* 1996; 334: 1156-1162.

Kushi LH, Fee RM, Sellers TA, Zheng W, Folsom AR. Intake of vitamins A, C and E and postmenopusal breast cancer: the Iowa Women's Health Study. *Am J Epidemiol* 1996; 144: 165-174.

Laufs U, Gertz K, Dirnagl U, Bohm M, Nickenig G, Endres M. Rosuvastatin, a new HMG-CoA reductase inhibitor, upregulates endothelial nitric oxide synthase and protects from ischemic stroke in mice: *Brain Res* 2002; 942: 23-30.

Lee I-M, Cook NR, Gaziano JM, Gordon M, Rodker PM, Manson JAE, Hennekens CH, Buring JE. Vitamin E in the Primary prevention of Cradiovascular Disease and Cancer. The Women's Health Study: a randomized controlled trial. *J Am Med Assoc* 2005; 294: 56-65.

Levy AP, Gerstein HC, Miller-Lotan R, Ratner R, McQueen M, Lonn E, Pogue J. The effect of vitamin E supplementation on cardiovascular risk in diabetic individuals with different haptoglobin phenotypes. *Diabetes Care* 2004; 27: 2767.

Lonn E, Yusuf S, Hoogwerf B, Pogue J, Yi Q, Zinman B, Bosch J, Dagenais G, Mann JF, Gerstein HC ; HOPE Study ; MICRO-HOPE Study. Effects of vitamin E on cardiovascular and microvascular outcomes in high-risk patients with diabetes : results of the HOPE study and MICRO-HOPE substudy. *Diabetes Care* 2002; 25: 1919-1927.

Losonczy KG, Harris TB, Havlik RJ. Vitamin E and vitamin C supplement use and risk of all-cause and coronary heart disease mortality in older persons : the Established Populations for Epidemiologic Studies of the Elderly. *Am J Clin Nutr* 1996; 64: 190-196.

Maack C, Kartes T, Kilter H, Schafers HJ, Nickenig G, Bohm M, Laufs U. Oxygen free radical release in human failing myocardium is associated with increased activity of rac1-GTPase and represents a target for statin treatment. *Circulation* 2003; 108: 1567-1574.

Madamanchi NR, Vendrov A, Runge MS. Oxidative stress and vascular disease. *Arterioscler Thromb Vasc Biol* 2005; 25: 29-36.

Mahadev K, Zibering A, Zhu I, Goldstein BJ. Insulin-stimulated hydrogen peroxide reversibly inhibits protein-tyrosine phosphatase 1b *in vivo* and enhances the early insulin action cascade. *J Biol Chem* 2001 ; 276 : 21938-21942.

Manach C, Mazur A, Scalbert A. Polyphenols and prevention of cardiovascular diseases. *Curr Opin Lipidol* 2005; 16: 77-84.

Manson JE, Gaziano JM, Spelsberg A, Ridker PM, Cook NR, Buring JE, Willett WC, Hennekens CH. A secondary prevention trial of antioxidants vitamins and cardiovascular disease in women: rationale, design, and methods. *Ann Epidemiol* 1995; 5: 261-269.

Mashima R, Witting PK, Stocker R. Oxidants and antioxidants in atherosclerosis. *Curr Opin Lipidol* 2001; 12: 411-418.

Meagher EA, Barry OP, Burke A, Lucey MR, Lawson JA, Rokach J, FitzGerald GA. Alcohol-induced generation of lipid peroxidation products in humans. *J Clin Invest* 1999; 104: 805-813.

Medeiros LA, Khan T, El Khoury JB, Pham CL, Hatters DM, Howlett GJ, Lopez R, O'Brien KD, Moore KJ. Fibrillar amyloid protein present in atheroma activates CD36 signal transduction. *J Biol Chem* 2004; 279: 10643-10648.

Mennen LI, Sapinho D, de Bree A, Arnault N, Bertrais S, Galan P, Hercberg S. Consumption of foods rich in flavonoids is related to a decrease cardiovascular risk in apparently healthy French women. *J Nutr* 2004; 134: 923-926.

Meyer F, Bairati I, Dagenais GR. Lower ischemic heart disease incidence and mortality among vitamin supplement users. *Can J Cardiol* 1996; 12: 930-934.

Miller ER III, Pastor-Barriuso R, Dalal D, Riemersma RA, Appel LJ, Guallar E. Meta-analysis: high-dosage vitamin E supplementation may increase all-cause mortality. *Ann Intern Med* 2005; 42: 37-46.

Mosca L, Appel LJ, Benjamin EJ, Berra K, Chandra-Strobos N, Fabunmi RP, Grady D, Haan CK, Hayes SN, Judelson DR, Keenan NL, McBride P, Oparil S, Ouyang P, Oz MC, Mendelsohn ME, Pasternak RC, Pinn VW, Robertson RM, Schenck-Gustafsson K, Sila CA, Smith SC Jr, Sopko G, Taylor AL, Walsh BW, Wenger NK, Williams CL; American Heart Association. Evidence-based guidelines for cardiovascular disease prevention in women. *Circulation.* 2004; 109 :672-93.

Mukamal KJ, Maclure M, Muller JE, Sherwood JB, Mittleman MA. Tea consumption and mortality after acute myocardial infarction. *Circulation* 2002; 105: 2476-2481.

Nanjee MN, Doran JE, Lerch PG, Miller NE. Acute effects of intravenous infusion of ApoA1/phosphatidylcholine discs on plasma lipoproteins in humans. *Arterioscler Thromb Vasc Biol* 1999; 19: 979-989.

Nissen SE, Tsunoda T, Tuzcu EM, Schoenhagen P, Cooper CJ, Yasin M, Eaton GM, Lauer MA, Sheldon WS, Grines CL, Halpern S, Crowe T, Blankenship JC, Kerensky R. Effect of recombinant ApoA-I Milano on coronary atherosclerosis in patients with acute coronary syndromes: a randomized controlled trial. *J Am Med Assoc* 2003; 290: 2292-2300.

Pan M, Cederbaum AI, Zhang YL, Ginsberg HN, Williams KJ, Fisher EA. Lipid peroxidation and oxidant stress regulate hepatic apolipoprotein B degradation and VLDL production. *J Clin Invest* 2004; 113: 1277-1287.

Peters U, Poole C, Arab L. Does tea affect cardiovascular disease? A meta-analysis. *Am J Epidemiol* 2001; 154: 495-503.

Podmore ID, Griffiths HR, Herbert KE, Mistry N, Mistry P, Lunec J. Vitamin C exhibits pro-oxidant properties. *Nature* 1998; 392: 559.

Prasad K, Kalra J. Oxygen free radicals and hypercholesterolemic atherosclerosis: effect of vitamin E. *Am Heart J* 1993; 125: 958-973.

Pratico D, Tangirala RK, Rader DJ, Rokach J, FitzGerald GA.. Vitamin E suppresses isoprostane generation in vivo and reduces atherosclerosis in ApoE-deficient mice. *Nat Med* 1998; 4: 1189-1192.

Pryor WA. Vitamin E and heart disease: basic science to clinical intervention trials. *Free Radic Biol Med* 2000; 28: 141-164.

Rapola JM, Virtamo J, Haukka JK, Heinonen OP, Albanes D, Taylor PR, Huttunen JK. Effect of vitamin E and beta-carotene on the incidence of angina pectoris: a randomized, double-blind, controlled trial. *J Am Med Assoc* 1996; 275: 693-698.

Rapola JM, Virtamo J, Ripatti S, Huttunen JK, Albanes D, Taylor PR, Heinonen OP. Randomised trial of alpha-tocopherol and beta-carotene supplements on incidence of major coronary events in men with previous myocardial infarction. *Lancet* 1997; 349: 1715-1720.

Rhee SG. Redox signalling: hydrogen peroxide as intracellular messenger. Exp Mol Med 1999 31: 53-59.

Ricciarelli R, Zingg JM, Azzi A. Vitamin E reduces the uptake of oxidized LDL by inhibiting CD36 scavenger receptor expression in cultured aortic smooth muscle cells. *Circulation* 2000; 102: 82-87.

Riemersma RA, Wood DA, Macintyre CC, Elton R, Gey KF, Oliver MF. Low plasma vitamins E and C: increased risk of angina in Scottish men. *Ann NY Acad Sci* 1989; 570: 291-295.

Riemersma RA, Wood DA, Macintyre CC, Elton RA, Gey KF, Oliver MF. Risk of angina pectoris and plasma concentrations of vitamins A, C and E and carotene. *Lancet* 1991; 337: 1-5.

Rimm EB, Stampfer MJ, Ascherio A, Giovannucci E, Colditz GA, Willett WC. Vitamin E consumption and the risk of coronary heart disease in men. *N Engl J Med* 1993; 328: 1450-1456.

Rodrigueza WV, Mazany KD, Essenburg AD, Pape ME, Rea TJ, Bisgaier CL, Williams KJ. Large versus small unilamellar vesicles mediate reverse cholesterol transport in vivo into two distinct hepatic metabolic pools. Implications for the treatment of atherosclerosis. *Arterioscler Thromb Vasc Biol* 1997; 17: 2132-2139.

Rosenson RS. Statins in atherosclerosis: lipid-lowering agents with antioxidant capabilities. *Atherosclerosis* 2004; 173: 1-12.

Salonen RM, Nyyssönen K, Kaikkonen J, Porkkala-Sarataho E, Voutilainen S, Rissanen TH, Tuomainen T-P, Valkonen V-P, Ristonmaa U, Lakka H-M, Vanharanta M, Salonen JT, Poulsen HE. Six-year effect of combined vitamin C and E supplementation on atherosclerotic progression: The Antioxidant Supplementation in Atherosclerosis Prevention (ASAP) study. *Circulation* 2003; 107: 947-953.

Schissel SL, Tweedie-Hardman J, Rapp JH, Graham G, Williams KJ, Tabas I. Rabbit aorta and human atherosclerotic lesions hydrolyze the sphingomyelin of retained low-density lipoprotein. Proposed role for arterial-wall sphingomyelinase in subendothelial retention and aggregation of atherogenic lipoproteins. *J Clin Invest* 1996; 98: 1455-1464.

Schlitt A, Bickel C, Thumma P, Blankenberg S, Rupprecht HJ, Meyer J, Jiang XC. High plasma phospholipids transfer protein levels as a risk factor for coronary artery disease. *Arterioscler Thromb Vasc Biol* 2003; 23: 1857-1862.

Shen J, Herderick E, Cornhill JF, Zsigmond E, Kim HS, Kuhn H, Guevara NV, Chan L. Macrophage-mediated 15-lipoxygenase expression protects against atherosclerosis development. *J Clin Invest* 1996; 98: 2201-2208.

Skålén K, Gustafsson M, Rydberg EK, Hulten LM, Wiklund O, Innerarity TL, Boren J. Subendothelial retention of atherogenic lipoproteins in early atherosclerosis. *Nature* 2002; 417: 750-754.

Smith SC Jr, Jackson R, Pearson TA, Fuster V, Yusuf S, Faergeman O, Wood DA, Alderman M, Horgan J, Home P, Hunn M, Grundy SM. Principles for national and regional guidelines on cardiovascular disease prevention: a scientific statement from the World Heart and Stroke Forum. *Circulation* 2004; 109: 3112-3121.

Soccio RE, Breslow JL. Intracellular cholesterol transport. *Arterioscler Thromb Vasc Biol* 2004; 24: 1150-1160.

Stampfer MJ, Hennekens CH, Manson JE, Colditz GA, Rosner B, Willett WC. Vitamin E consumption and the risk of coronary disease in women. *N Engl J Med* 1993; 328: 1444-1449.

Steinberg D, Parthasarathy S, Carew TE, Khoo JC, Witztum JL. Beyond cholesterol. Modification of low-density lipoprotein that increases its atherogenicity. *N Engl J Med* 1989; 320: 915-924.

Steinberg D, Lewis A. Conner memorial lecture. Oxidative modification of LDL and atherogenesis. Circulation and atherogenesis. *Circulation* 1997; 95: 1062-1071.

Stephens NG, Parsons A, Schofield PM, Kelly F, Cheeseman K, Mitchinson MJ. Randomised controlled trial of vitamin E in patients with coronary disease: Cambridge Heart Antioxidant Study (CHAOS). *Lancet* 1996; 347: 781-786.

Stocker R, Keaney JF Jr. Role of oxidative modifications in atherosclerosis. *Physiol Rev* 2004; 84: 1381-1478.

Suzumura K, Yasuhara M, Tanaka K, Suzuki T. Protective effect of fluvastatin sodium (XU-62-320), a 3-hydroxy-3-methylglutaryl coenzyme A (HMG-CoA) reductase inhibitor, on oxidative modification of human low-density lipoprotein *in vitro*. *Biochem Pharmacol* 1999; 57: 697-703.

Tabas I. Nonoxidative modifications of lipoproteins in atherogenesis. Annu Rev Nutr 1999; 19: 123-139.

Tall AR, Costet P, Wang N. Regulation and mechanisms of macrophage cholesterol efflux. *J Clin Invest* 2002; 110: 899-904.

The Alpha-Tocopherol Beta-Carotene Cancer Prevention Study Group. The effect of vitamin E and beta-carotene on the incidence of lung cancer and other cancers in male smokers: the Alpha-Tocopherol, Beta-Carotene Cancer Prevention Study Group. *N Engl J Med* 1994; 330: 1029-1035.

The GISSI-Prevenzione Investigators. Dietary supplementation with n-3 polyunsaturated fatty acids and vitamin E after myocardial infarction: results of the GISSI-Prevenzione trial. Gruppo Italiano per lo Studio della Sopravvivenza nell'Infarto miocardico. *Lancet* 1999; 354: 447-455.

Thomas SR, Leichtweis SB, Pettersson K, Croft KD, Mori TA, Brown AJ, Stocker R. Dietary cosupplementation with vitamin E and coenzyme Q(10) inhibits atherosclerosis in apolipoprotein E gene knockout mice. *Arterioscler Thromb Vasc Biol* 2001; 21: 585-593.

Upston JM, Terentis AC, Morris K, Keaney Jr JF, Stocker R. Oxidized lipid accumulates in the presence of alpha-tocopherol in atherosclerosis. *Biochem J* 2002; 363: 753-760.

Vetter S, Ruf G, Regourd E, Marz W. The use of atorvastatin treatment in usual care environments: pooled analysis of six prospective, observational studies in 90,535 patients. *Int J Clin Pharmacol Ther* 2004; 42: 423-433.

Violi F, Loffredo L, Musella L, Marcoccia A. Should antioxidant status be considered in interventional trials with antioxidants? *Heart* 2004; 90: 598-602.

Virtamo J, Rapola JM, Ripatti S, Heinonen OP, Taylor PR, Albanes D, Huttunen JK. Effect of vitamin E and beta-carotene on the incidence of primary nonfatal myocardial infarction and fatal coronary heart disease. *Arch Intern Med* 1998; 158: 668-675.

Virtamo J, Pietinen P, Huttunen JK, Korhonen P, Malila N, Virtanen MJ, Albanes D, Taylor PR, Albert P; ATBC Study Group. Incidence of cancer and mortality following alpha-tocopherol and beta-carotene supplementation: a postintervention follow-up. *J Am Med Assoc* 2003; 290: 476-485.

Vivekananthan DP, Penn MS, Sapp SK, Hsu A, Topol EJ. Use of antioxidant vitamins for the prevention of cardiovascular disease: meta-analysis of randomised trials. *Lancet* 2003; 361: 2017-2023.

Whitman SC, Rateri DL, Szilvassy SJ, Cornicelli JA, Daugherty A. Macrophage-specific expression of class A scavenger receptors in LDL receptor(-/-) mice decreases atherosclerosis and changes spleen morphology. *J Lipid Res* 2002; 43: 1201-1208.

Williams KJ, Fischer EA. Oxidation, lipoproteins, and atherosclerosis: which is wrong, the antioxidants or the theory? *Curr Opin Clin Nutr Care* 2005; 8: 139-146.

Williams KJ, Tabas I. Atherosclerosis and inflammation. *Science* 2002; 297: 521-522.

Williams KJ, Werth VP, Wolff JA. Itravenously administered lecithin liposomes: a synthetic antiatherogenic lipid particle. *Perspect Biol Med* 1984; 27: 417-431.

Witting P, Pettersson K, Ostlund-Lindqvist AM, Westerlund C, Wagberg M, Stocker R. Dissociation of atherogenesis from aortic accumulation in lipid hydro(pero)xides in Watanabe heritable hyperlipidemic rabbits. *J Clin Invest* 1999; 104: 213-220.

Xu D, Rovira II, Finkel T. Oxidants painting the cysteine chapel: redox regulation of PTPs. *Dev Cell* 2002; 2: 251-252.

Yusuf S, Dagenais G, Pogue J, Bosch J, Sleight P. Vitamin E supplementation and cardiovascular events in high-risk patients: the Heart Outcomes Prevention Evaluation Study Investigators. *N Engl J Med* 2000; 342: 154-160.

Zalba G, San Jose G, Moreno M, Fortuno M, Fortuno A, Beaumont F, Diez J. Oxidative stress in arterial hypertension: role of NAD(P)H oxidase. *Hypertension* 2001; 38: 1395-1399.

Zarev S, Bonnefont-Rousselot D, Jedidi I, Cosson C, Couturier M, Legrand A, Beaudeux J-L, Thérond P. Extents of copper LDL oxidation depends on oxidation time and copper/LDL ratio: chemical characterization. *Arch Biochem Biophys* 2003; 420: 68-78.

Zureik M, Galan P, Bertrais S, Mennen L, Czernichow S, Blacher J, Ducimetiere P, Hercberg S. Effects of long-term daily low-dose supplementation with antioxidant vitamins and minerals on structure and function of large arteries. *Arterioscler Thromb Vasc Biol* 2004; 24: 1485-1491.

In: Frontiers in Antioxidants Research
Editor: Harold V. Panglossi, pp. 61-76
ISBN 1-60021-273-5

Chapter 3

ERYTHROCYTE MEMBRANE ELECTRON TRANSFER, OXIDATIVE STRESS, BODY MASS AND LIFESTYLE IN HEALTHY AND IN TYPE 1 DIABETIC FAMILIES

E. Matteucci and O. Giampietro
Department of Internal Medicine, University of Pisa, Italy

ABSTRACT

Erythrocytes export electrons across the cell membrane to external oxidants (such as ferryicyanide) through a redox system that remains still unknown. The rate of ferricyanide reduction varies as a function of cytoplasmic electron donor concentration. Indeed, the pathway is linked to a set of intracellular redox couples including $NADH/NAD^+$, GSSG/SGSH, and ascorbate/vitamin C.

Since the activity of membrane electron transport systems appears to be closely related to the redox homeostasis and the metabolic state of the cell, our aim was to characterise the membrane reducing system in healthy and in type 1 diabetes (T1DM) families and its relationship with nutritional indicators and oxidative biomarkers. Particularly, present research work aimed at evaluating in healthy and T1DM families: (a) the rate of erythrocyte electron transport in relation with body mass and metabolic efficiency, (b) modulating effects of diet and lifestyle on erythrocyte electron transfer system.

We measured the erythrocyte electron transport to extracellular ferricyanide (RBC vfcy) in 100 healthy controls and 99 non-diabetic relatives of type 1 diabetics. Erythrocyte Na/H exchange (RBC NHE), RBC glutathione (GSH), plasma thiols, plasma and RBC malondialdheyde were also determined, in addition to plasma glucose, insulin, lipids, HbA1c, creatinine clearance, and urinary albumin. Moreover, we assessed dietary habits and lifestyle of 76 relatives and 95 healthy subjects by using the European Prospective Investigation of Cancer and Nutrition questionnaires.

a. Among healthy controls, individuals with BMI≤25 kg/m^2 had lower rates of electron transport in comparison with age-gender-matched subjects who were overweight or obese. Indeed, RBC vfcy correlated positively with two indices of fat body mass (BMI and circulating triglycerides), and negatively with an index of lean body mass (24-hour urinary creatinine excretion). Moreover, RBC vfcy showed a negative association with RBC NHE and plasma MDA. On the contrary, among relatives, RBC vfcy did not change significantly with BMI. It showed a positive association with RBC MDA, negative with RBC GSH.
b. Both Spearman's rank correlation and stepwise multiple regression analyses including lifestyle information found different independent variables to be positively associated with RBC vfcy: daily dietary intake of vitamin C among healthy controls, whereas time spent in regular exercise among relatives.

In conclusion, (a) electron transfer catalysed by the transmembrane ferricyanide reductase activity may reflect the functional state of membrane proton pumps that modulate cellular metabolism by regulating the intracellular redox levels. In the case we should have a useful tool to indirectly evaluate some aspects of energy balance in human metabolic diseases by using easily accessible cells and simple laboratory procedure. Moreover, the transport system, that seems functionally normal, contributes to oxidation in T1DM families, whereas in healthy people it protects from oxidation. Furthermore, (b) dietary intake of vitamin C and sporting activities modulate erythrocyte electron transfer efficiency. In the cytosol, ascorbic acid or vitamin C can donate electrons to trans-plasma membrane electron transfer activity in erythrocytes. Thus, intracellular electron donors available from dietary sources can be very important in maintaining the redox environment of a cell, i.e. the summation of the products of the reduction potential and reducing capacity of the linked redox couples present. Our data also support indirect evidence suggesting that regular exercise may improve electron transport efficiency. However, the reason why independent lifestyle variables associated with RBC vfcy markedly differed among population subgroups remains unknown.

ABBREVIATIONS

AFR	ascorbate free radical
BMI	body mass index
DHAA	dehydro-L-ascorbic acid
EPIC	European Prospective Investigation of Cancer and Nutrition
FPG	fasting plasma glucose
FPI	fasting plasma insulin
HDL-C	HDL cholesterol
MBP	mean blood pressure
MDA	malondialdehyde
NEFA	non-esterified fatty acid
RBC GSH	erythrocyte glutathione
RBC NHE	erythrocyte Na/H exchange
RBC vfcy	erythrocyte rate of extracellular ferricyanide reduction
ROS	reactive oxygen species

SH groups	Plasma sulfhydryl groups
Tchol	total cholesterol
UAER	urinary albumin excretion rate

DEGENERATIVE DISEASES AND REDOX CYCLING

The worldwide prevalence of obesity and its associated metabolic and cardiovascular disorders has risen dramatically the past two decades. The aetiology of obesity represents a complex interaction of genetics, nutrition, metabolism, and physical activity. White adipose tissue is no longer considered only an energy storage tissue but a critical endocrine organ, at the heart of a complex network influencing energy homeostasis, glucose and lipid metabolism, vascular homeostasis, immune response, and even reproduction [1]. The inflammatory state that is associated with obesity suggested that obesity could be a low-grade systemic inflammatory disease [2].

Diabetes is a collection of genetic diseases with the common phenotype of glucose intolerance. Since the prevalence of diabetes genotypes is much greater than that of diabetes phenotypes, factors in addition to genetics probably influence the phenotypic expression of the diabetes genotype [3].

Diabetes mellitus and diabetic chronic complications have been considered linked to damage from reactive oxygen species, ROS [4] as a result of an imbalance between radical-generating and radical-scavenging systems (oxidative stress). They could arise as a response to an unfavourable interaction among diet, lifestyle and the genetic background of the individual. Nutrition (high calorie diet, dietary fat, antioxidant insufficiencies) and lifestyle (sedentary life, smoking, toxins) seem to determine whether the phenotype would be expressed. Indeed, nutrients and micronutrients can influence: genome stability, expression of nuclear and mitochondrial genes, cell apoptosis, metabolic regulation, mitochondrial function, immune response. ROS modify both structure and function of biological macromolecules: lipids (lipid peroxidation), proteins (carbonyl formation, covalent modifications, nitration and glycation), nucleic acids (8-hydroxydeoxyguanosine formation, mutations and single/double strand breaks). The inseparable relationship of oxidative stress to inflammation has become well known along with the recognition that ROS at low levels can function as signaling intermediates in regulation of cell activities [5]. Moreover, calorie restriction may stabilise redox balance and protect redox-sensitive transcription factors from activation [6].

Mitochondria are the main site of ROS generation in the cell and their primary target [7]. Mitochondrial dysfunction is the major pathogenic determinant in degenerative processes associated with increased levels of cellular oxidative stress. Complexes I, III, IV of the respiratory chain are redox-linked proton pumps which convert redox energy into electrical work, potential energy, and heat. The electron transfers through the enzyme are coupled to an increase in the potential energy of the protein, so that the associated conformational changes drive the unidirectional flow of protons across the membrane. Efficient proton translocation requires redox linkage, electron gating, and proton gating. Deviations from this pathway constitute electron leaks/proton slips and correlate to metabolic efficiency. In these conditions, electron transfer and proton transfer are decoupled and the protein is removed from the proton-pumping reaction pathway. Electrons are transferred to final O_2. ROS production increases when proton electrochemical gradient is high.

Transplasma Membrane Electron Transport Systems

Although members of electron transport systems are considered predominantly expressed in the mitochondrial membrane, they have been demonstrated to be also expressed in the plasma membrane [8].

Plasma membranes of eukaryotic cells have enzymes that transfer electrons from internal NADH to external electron acceptors. In fact, human erythrocytes export electrons across the membrane to external oxidants or acceptors, many non-physiological, such as ferricyanide [9]. Erythrocyte electron transfer has usually been measured spectrophotometrically as the rate of extracellular ferricyanide reduction. Neither the molecular structure of the putative trans-plasma membrane oxidoreductase nor the identity of the natural cytoplasmic electron donors (ascorbate, NADH, GSH) have been established [10]. Proposed functions for this electron transport activity include signal transduction, cell growth, protection from oxidative stress, and "controlled" generation of ROS [8]. The activity of membrane electron transport systems closely relates to the metabolic state of the cell. In order for glycolysis to remain operative, NAD^+ must continuously be regenerated. One source for NAD^+ supply is mitochondrial respiration. However, other compensatory enzyme systems, such as the plasma membrane NADH-oxidoreductase, may play a major role in the survival of cells by maintaining homeostasis of intracellular NADH/NAD^+ levels. Maintenance of high aerobic glycolytic fluxes by up-regulating of plasma membrane redox systems in cells deficient of mitochondrial electron transport chain (as observed in ageing or diabetes mellitus) may explain why energy-deficient cells may still survive [11].

Electron Transfer across the Red Cell Membrane

The erythrocyte contains the largest store of iron in any cell and, being the body's oxygen and carbon dioxide transporter, is under constant exposure to possible sources of ROS. The cell is equipped with different types of enzymatic and non-enzymatic defences. Sparing or recycling of alpha-tocopherol by ascorbate in the erythrocyte tends to stabilise the erythrocyte membrane and thus prevent haemolysis. The mobility, number, and antioxidant capacity of the red blood cell makes it an ideal antioxidant for its own local environment, but also an oxidant scavenger throughout blood-accessible parts of the body [10]. Protection against ROS may be the role of RBC membrane transport systems. In fact the redox environment of a linked set of redox couples in a biological fluid (plasma), cell (erythrocyte), or tissue (blood) is the summation of the products of the reduction potential and reducing capacity of the linked redox couples present. In turn, redox couples are responsive to electron flow, that is, changes in the reducing/oxidising environment. Erythrocyte transmembrane electron transfer systems provide a crucial link between ascorbate and the blood antioxidant reserve. Ascorbate is an outstandingly effective scavenger of aqueous peroxyl radicals in plasma and within cells; its oxidation is a two-step reaction that yields the ascorbate free radical (AFR) in the first step and dehydro-L-ascorbic acid (DHAA) in the second step. DHAA is an unstable compound at neutral pH and 37°C that undergoes an irreversible hydrolysis reaction to form 2,3-diketogulonic acid. Erythrocytes, whose ascorbate concentration is the same as that in plasma, are able to reduce AFR and DHAA extracellularly by redox enzymes in the plasma membrane [12-13].

Even though a transplasma membrane electron transport system is expressed in every living cell and there is increasing experimental evidence for its direct involvement in vital biological functions (bioenergetics and homeostasis, defence, hormone signal transduction, cell growth and differentiation), the importance of such systems is often under-rated [8]. Limited success in the identification of the different electron transport processes present in erythrocyte membrane has been achieved.

So far the activity of erythrocyte plasma membrane electron systems in disease states has not been systematically investigated. Apart our recent observation in type 1 diabetes nephropathy [14], the only precedent study related to erythrocyte electron transfer in haemodialysis dates back to 1979 [15].

DIET, LIFESTYLE AND CELL ANTIOXIDANT CAPACITY

Clinical data and in vitro observations confirm that inflammation and oxidative stress are involved in the pathogenesis of numerous chronic diseases, such as obesity, diabetes, and cardiovascular disease. Whether known factors of increased risk for chronic diseases are directly modifiable through the diet is an intense area of research. Understanding the biological basis of diet-health relationship is complicated by the multifactorial nature of chronic diseases, the polygenic inheritance of different modes of gene expression and responsiveness to a variety of specific dietary factors, and the long lag time between risk exposure and expression of the disease. Additionally, a main methodological drawback for carrying out survey studies to assess the impact of lifestyle on health is the lack of standardisation of the dietary assessment methods.

Although observational epidemiological studies have shown an inverse relationship between intakes of antioxidants and disease risk, supplementation studies show inconsistent results [16]. Diet seems to impact on all relevant pathways determining genome stability [17]. Epidemiological data link low levels of the acute-phase C-reactive protein to high fruit, vegetable, fibre and to moderate alcohol consumption. Fruits and vegetables contain antioxidant vitamins, but also a variety of bioactive compounds with antioxidant properties. Thus, total antioxidant capacity of the diet, which summarises the capacity of the different food antioxidants in scavenging preformed free radicals, could exert a substantial and independent effect on inflammation [18].

An active lifestyle is also being promoted as a protective factor for chronic diseases. Recent epidemiological studies suggest that regular exercise in advanced age can reduce morbility and mortality. However, there remains a paucity of information regarding the benefits of exercise on the cellular redox status in aging humans. Antioxidant capacity is a key variable in determining cellular redox status and survival. Oxidative damage increases in an age-dependent manner in the meanwhile antioxidant enzyme capacity increases in order to adapt to an increase in oxidant production. The age-related increased production of oxidants is thought to be a result of inefficiencies in the electron transport chain secondary to aberrations in mtDNA. Evidence suggests that exercise training may increase plasma levels of vitamin C and vitamin E, up-regulate antioxidant enzyme and improve electron transport chain efficiency [19-21]. Vitamin C supplementation maintains reduced glutathione concentrations in blood [22] and improves the overall antioxidant protection capacity of blood during exercise [23].

Cellular defence against stress is another key function in which the plasma membrane redox system is involved. The human erythrocyte membrane contains a number of electron transfer systems whose activity appears to be closely related to the metabolic state of the cell and could be modifiable by lifestyle. Multiple electron donors have been identified. Ascorbic acid, or vitamin C, is the primary antioxidant in plasma and cannot be synthesised by human cells. The two-electron oxidation product of ascorbate, DHAA, undergoes irreversible ring-opening, unless reduced back to ascorbate. The erythrocyte is the most likely cell to fulfil this function in blood. The intracellular conversion of DHAA to ascorbate is largely dependent on alpha-tocopherol and GSH [24]. In turn, NADPH is considered the primary source of reducing equivalents for the GSH, which is considered the major thiol-disulfide redox buffer of the cell. The three redox systems (nicotinamide adenine dinucleotide phosphate, glutathione, and thioredoxin) are thermodynamically connected to each other. The concentration of sulfhydryl groups in cells and tissues plays a role in the antioxidant network and thereby influences the redox environment also in the erythrocyte. For example, during adaptation to decreasing amount of dietary protein, there are changes in the concentration and kinetics of erythrocyte glutathione that suggest a reduced antioxidant capacity and increased susceptibility to oxidant stress [25].

Our Previous Observations

We have previously observed in T1DM families that:

- markers of inflammation and oxidative stress are abnormal in non-diabetic relatives of type 1 diabetics supporting the view that familial elements precede diabetes [26];
- the activity of erythrocyte Na/H exchange (RBC NHE, secondary countertransport regulating cell pH, volume and proliferation) is increased both in type 1 diabetics and in non-diabetic relatives. NHE up-regulation, secondary to chronic oxidative stress, further points to familiar redox disequilibrium [27];
- the redox imbalance observed in T1DM families is also related to immunologic hallmarks suggesting the involvement of immunoregulatory mechanisms [28];
- erythrocyte electron transfer, as the rate of extracellular ferricyanide reduction, is selectively increased in diabetic nephropathy [14]. The abnormality is not contributed by familial or hereditary components, as the electron flow was normal in siblings. Changes in the transfer matrix (irreversible chemical protein modifications or water molecule reorientation) could account for the finding;
- on the basis of a primary school health program, anthropometric and anamnestic data on child and family seem to yield more accurate estimates of family risk profile [29];

- a detailed assessment of nutrient intake levels and lifestyle using standardised European Prospective Investigation of Cancer and Nutrition (EPIC) questionnaires provides evidence indicating unhealthy dietary behaviours, which could even predispose to the development of diabetes and cardiovascular complications, in subjects living in Pisa [30]. Indeed, the combination of vitamin B9 and vitamin E deprivation could be deleterious for endothelial function, since these dietary antioxidants have been implicated in the modulation of nitric oxide and eicosanoid signaling.

OBJECTIVES OF THE STUDY

The present research work aimed at evaluating in healthy and T1DM families:

a. The rate of erythrocyte electron transports in relation with body mass and metabolic efficiency.
b. Modulating effects of diet and lifestyle on erythrocyte electron transfer.

The study was undertaken to elucidate the biological correlates of oxidant-induced erythrocyte electron transfer in well-characterised clinical settings. Anthropometric indices and nutritional biomarkers (such as plasma levels of albumin, iron, lipids, homocysteine, and urinary outputs of nitrogen, sodium and potassium), erythrocyte rate of extracellular ferricyanide reduction (RBC vfcy), biomarkers of lipid peroxidation (erythrocyte and plasma malondialdehyde), protein peroxidation (protein thios), and antioxidant consumption (erythrocyte glutathione) were measured. Using the European Prospective Investigation of Cancer and Nutrition questionnaires were also assessed lifestyle, dietary intake of energy and selected nutrients. The data in this paper provide first in vivo evidence that: 1) RBC vfcy activity reflects the functional state of cellular membrane redox systems that are involved in the regulation of body metabolism. 2) It can serve to protect from oxidant stress in healthy people, whereas it contributes to oxidation in T1DM families. 3) Concerning lifestyle, different independent variables were positively associated with RBC vfcy: daily dietary intake of vitamin C among healthy controls, whereas time spent in regular exercise among relatives.

An understanding of the origin of oxidative stress in diabetic families, and the role of diet and lifestyle choices in modulating electron transfer and oxidative damage is critical for developing preventive strategies.

Method

We measured erythrocyte electron transport rate in 100 healthy subjects (53F/47M, mean age 44±14 years) and 99 non-diabetic relatives (52 parents and 47 siblings, 55F/44M, 49±16 years) of 37 T1DM patients. Diabetic probands, whose mean disease duration was 19±9 years, included 12 patients with diabetic retinopathy (determined by fluorescent angiography) and 12 with nephropathy. Among patients with nephropathy, one was on dialysis (serum creatinine levels > 133 μmol/l), 6 had persistent macroalbuminuria (urinary albumin excretion rate, UAER > 200 μg/min and serum creatinine levels < 133 μmol/l), and 5 had persistent microalbuminuria (UAER > 20 μg/min in 2 of 3 consecutive 24-hour urine collections within 6 months in the absence of a urinary tract infection or hearth failure). None of the relatives had clinical evidence of illness or was taking any drugs. If fasting plasma glucose levels were ≥ 7 mmol/l, a 75-g oral glucose tolerance test was performed to exclude diabetes. All subjects gave the informed consent. The clinical and biochemical parameters evaluated were the same as previously reported [14, 26-30]. These were body mass index (BMI), mean blood pressure (MBP), fasting plasma glucose (FPG), fasting plasma insulin (FPI), HbA1c, total and HDL cholesterol (TChol and HDL-C), triglycerides, creatinine clearance, urinary albumin excretion rate (UAER). RBC vfcy was measured as the rate of ferrocyanide production [9, 14]. RBC NHE was quantified as amiloride-sensitive H^+ efflux from acid-loaded cells [31]. Erythrocyte glutathione (RBC GSH) was determined by the method of Beutler [32]. The peroxidation of plasma (plasma malondialdehyde, MDA) and membrane (RBC MDA) lipids was measured according to Esterbauer and Cheeseman [33]. Plasma sulfhydryl groups (SH groups) were measured using the colorimetric assay described by Ellman [34] and fresh plasma.

Seventy-six T1DM relatives and 95 control subjects also participated nutritional screening survey, as described in detail elsewhere [30]. To assess dietary intake the country-specific questionnaire designed to capture local dietary habits in the prospective collaborative study European Prospective Investigation of Cancer and Nutrition (EPIC) was administered. EPIC study has been a large multicenter prospective cohort study conducted by the International Agency for Research on Cancer. Study aim was to investigate the relationship between nutrition and lifestyle factors and the etiology of cancer and other chronic diseases [35]. The EPIC questionnaire is a scanner-readable food frequency questionnaire (146 food items) whose development, reproducibility, and relative validity were described in detail previously [36]. It is capable of assessing the complete diet of subjects over the past year, including total caloric intake, as well as selected macro-nutrient and micro-nutrient intake. After the questionnaire was optically read, a software program is used to check the questionnaire data for completeness and plausibility. Energy and nutrient intakes from dietary assessment were calculated by using data from the country-specific food code [37]. Finally, the questionnaire provides daily intakes of the following nutrients: water, total protein, total fat, saturated fat, oleic acid, monounsaturated fat, linoleic acid, linolenic acid, polyunsaturated fat, cholesterol, total carbohydrate, monosaccharide, disaccharides, polysaccharides, dietary fiber, alcohol, energy, iron, calcium, sodium, potassium, phosphorus, zink, thiamin, riboflavin, niacin, vitamin C, vitamin B6, folic acid, retinol equivalents, retinol, beta-carotene, vitamin E, and vitamin D.

Demographic, socio-economic and lifestyle information was obtained by Lifestyle EPIC questionnaire (including questions on history of previous illness and disorders of surgical operations, lifetime history of consumption of tobacco and alcoholic beverages, and physical activity) [38]. Subjects reported the daily number of hours they engaged in housework as well as the weekly number of hours they engaged in physical activities during leisure (walking, cycling, gardening, repairing, exercise; through the year or seasonally) and during work (sedentary; standing; manual work; heavy manual work). Exercise (or sporting activities) included gymnastics, running, playing tennis, swimming, etc.

The reported values are means±SD. Differences were tested by the unpaired t test. In the evaluation of differences in means between groups differentiated on the basis of BMI, some of the healthy subjects (Table 2) and relatives (Table 3) were excluded for the best age matching. The Chi-squared test was used to compare categorical variables between groups. The two-way analysis of variance (ANOVA) was used to test the main effect and the interaction effect of the two independent factors (BMI ≤ or > 25 kg/m^2, and grouping category as control or relative) versus the dependent variable RBC vfcy. Systematic relations between variables were sought in each whole sample by exploratory data analysis. Multiple regression analysis was performed using as independent variables those selected by stepwise method. Statistical significance was defined as $p<0.05$.

Table 1. Comparison (unpaired t test) between age-gender-matched control subjects and type 1 diabetic patients

Characteristic	Controls	Type 1	p<
F/M	22/15	22/15	
Age (years)	33±9	35±11	
BMI (kg/m^2)	25±4	24±2	
MBP (mmHg)	91±10	92±13	
FPG (mmol/l)	4.8±0.5	15.1±6.7	0.001
HbA1c (%)	5.3±0.3	8.3±1.4	0.001
TChol (mmol/l)	5.1±1.0	5.1±0.9	
HDL-C (mmol/l)	1.5±0.4	1.5±0.4	
Triglycerides (mmol/l)	1.1±0.6	0.9±0.5	
RBC vfcy (mmol/ml h)	12.3±4.3	14.2±5.3	
RBC NHE (mmol/l h)	5.2±1.9	6.8±2.0	0.001
RBC GSH (mg/ml)	0.87±0.11	0.75±0.13	0.001
SH groups (μmol/l)	444±63	399±68	0.01
Plasma MDA (nmol/ml)	0.33±0.19	0.66±0.42	0.001
RBC MDA (nmol/ml)	0.28±0.16	0.36±0.18	0.05

Table 2. Comparison (unpaired t test) between healthy control subjects gathered on the basis of BMI

Characteristic	BMI≤25 kg/m^2	BMI>25 kg/m^2	p<
F/M	30/19	19/28	
Age (years)	42±14	47±13	
BMI (kg/m^2)	23±2	28±3	0.001
MBP (mmHg)	90±10	96±10	0.01
FPG (mmol/l)	4.9±0.6	5.2±0.6	0.01
FPI (μU/ml)	8.2±3.6	11.8±5.5	0.01
TChol (mmol/l)	5.2±1.1	5.4±1.0	
HDL-C (mmol/l)	1.5±0.3	1.3±0.3	0.001
Triglycerides (mmol/l)	0.9±0.4	1.4±0.7	0.001
RBC vfcy (mmol/ml h)	11.9±3.9	13.8±4.4	0.05
RBC NHE (mmol/l h)	5.4±2.3	5.6±1.8	
SH groups (μmol/l)	447±63	417±61	0.05
Plasma MDA (nmol/ml)	0.40±0.20	0.52±0.30	0.05
RBC MDA (nmol/ml)	0.27±0.10	0.32±0.19	

Table 3. Comparison (unpaired t test) between age-matched relatives of type 1 diabetic patients gathered on the basis of BMI

Characteristic	BMI≤25 kg/m^2	BMI>25 kg/m^2	p<
F/M	24/16	22/19	
Age (years)	46±14	51±11	
BMI (kg/m^2)	23±2	29±3	0.001
MBP (mmHg)	93±11	98±13	
FPG (mmol/l)	5.3±1.3	5.6±0.9	
FPI (μU/ml)	9.9±3.7	13.1±6.2	0.01
TChol (mmol/l)	5.5±1.2	5.6±1.2	
HDL-C (mmol/l)	1.6±0.4	1.2±0.3	0.001
Triglycerides (mmol/l)	1.1±0.5	1.9±2.2	0.05
RBC vfcy (mmol/ml h)	13.1±5.9	14.6±4.9	
RBC NHE (mmol/l h)	8.2±2.5	8.2±2.6	
SH groups (μmol/l)	416±59	398±71	
Plasma MDA (nmol/ml)	0.40±0.20	0.52±0.30	0.05
RBC MDA (nmol/ml)	0.36±0.18	0.40±0.18	

Result

As previously reported [27], T1DM patients differed from matched healthy controls in having a higher FPG, HbA1c, RBC NHE activity, plasma and RBC MDA levels, while lower RBC GSH and SH groups (Table 1). Erythrocyte electron transport capacity still gave positive correlation with UAER and plasma creatinine and negative correlation with plasma SH groups (multiple $r = 0.6$, $p<0.01$), as previously observed [14].

Among 100 healthy control subjects, body mass was confirmed to increase with RBC vfcy. Indeed, 49 individuals with BMI≤25 kg/m^2 differed from the other 47 age-gender-matched subjects, who were overweight or obese, in the lower rate of electron transport (Table 2). In addition, they showed lower mean blood pressure, fasting plasma levels of glucose, insulin, triglycerides, and MDA, while higher circulating HDL cholesterol and SH groups. HbA1c did not change (data not shown). BMI was correlated with RBC vfcy, plasma MDA concentration, and age (multiple R 0.4, $p<0.001$; coefficient 0.2, 3, 0.1; t-value 2, 3, and 3, respectively). According to stepwise and multiple regression analysis, RBC vfcy was significantly correlated (multiple R 0.5, $p<0.001$) with 24 hour urinary creatinine excretion (coefficient -0.5, t-value 3), RBC NHE (-0.01, 3), BMI (0.3, 2), plasma MDA (-2.5, 2) and triglycerides (1.3, 2).

Among relatives of T1DM patients, neither RBC vfcy nor MBP, FPG, SH groups changed significantly with BMI. Forty individuals with BMI≤25 kg/m^2 had similar rates of electron transport to 41 overweight relatives (Table 3). Furthermore, they showed lower fasting plasma insulin, triglycerides, and MDA, higher levels of plasma HDL cholesterol and erythrocyte GSH. HbA1c was unchanged. In the multiple regression analysis (R 0.3, $p<0.05$), RBC vfcy showed a positive association with RBC MDA (coefficient 3, t-value 1), whereas negative with RBC GSH (-6.8, 2). The two-way ANOVA confirmed that RBC vfcy changes significantly only with BMI (p 0.01) with no significant interaction between BMI and grouping category.

The results of our assessment of nutrient intake levels and lifestyle of healthy subjects and T1DM families in Pisa using EPIC questionnaires have been published [30]. Emerging health issues were:

- 45% of controls were overweight. Increasing age was associated with increasing body mass and decreasing activity in sport in front of an unchanged intake of total calories.
- The distribution of energy sources was incorrect. The proportion of caloric intake derived from total fat and cholesterol did not match general guidelines. Total dietary fiber consumption was above 25 g/d only in 27% of all participants.
- Estimated daily intakes of water-soluble vitamin B9 and fat-soluble vitamin D and vitamin E were deficient in comparison with dietary reference intakes.
- The prevalence of adoption and maintenance of healthful eating and physical activity habits was higher in women and T1DM patients (probably as a consequence of the medical educational intervention). On the contrary, supportiveness of the family in term of changing the undesirable behaviors at home seemed to fail.

Hence and herein, we sought any relationship between nutritional and lifestyle individual characteristics obtained by using the EPIC food frequency questionnaires and the values of RBC vfcy that had been contextually measured. Both Spearman's rank correlation and stepwise multiple regression analyses including lifestyle information found the following independent variables to be positively associated with RBC vfcy: daily dietary intake of vitamin C among healthy controls (Rho 0.23, Z-value 2.22, p 0.03), whereas time spent in regular exercise among relatives (0.36, 3.05, 0.002). Daily intake of vitamin C was 121±47 mg in 95 healthy controls and 131±64 in 76 T1DM relatives; regular exercise was 2.4±1.8 hour/week and 2.1±1.9, respectively.

CONCLUSION

So far, a number of electron transport systems have been suggested to be involved in erythrocyte membrane redox activity [10]. Many in vitro studies have engaged in the identification of membrane components involved in electron trasport, intracellular electron donors, and physiological extracellular acceptors [10]. In contrast, very few clinical studies have given evidence of links of electron transport activity to disease states [10, 14]. Our previous study reported first evidence about erythrocyte electron transfer rate in T1DM patients and their siblings [14]. Type 1 diabetes per se seemed not to affect RBC vfcy, which was similar in the diabetic group compared with the control group. The rate of ferrocyanide generation by erythrocytes was peculiarly elevated only in those patients who had diabetic nephropathy. The abnormality did not appear to originate from familiar or hereditary components (electron flow was normal in siblings) and was suggested to be attributable to chemical changes in the intervening medium.

In vitro evidence supports a direct interplay at the bioenergetic level between the plasma membrane NADH-ferricyanide reductase activity and the mitochondrial respiratory chain function [11]. Both systems, together with the glycolytic pathways, regulate and maintain an appropriate $NADH/NAD^+$ ratio. In turn, changes in intracellular redox state may be a major factor that contributes to the regulation of glucose and fat metabolic pathway because it impacts on the activity of NAD-linked dehydrogenases. Cytosolic free $NADH/NAD^+$ is a sensor of the redox state of mitochondria, cytosol and extracellular milieu. An increased rate of glycolysis, even under aerobic conditions and at constant glucose levels, is associated with an increased cytosolic $NADH/NAD^+$. NADH must be oxidised to NAD^+, or the glycolysis will be blocked. In the cytosol NADH is oxidised by lactate dehydrogenase and glyceraldehyde 3-phosphate dehydrogenase. Otherwise reducing equivalents can be transported into mitochondria for oxidation by the electron transport chain, or members of the membrane electron transport system may extrude them.

The present study gains some new insights into electron movements across human erythrocyte cell membranes in humans. First of all, in healthy controls RBC vfcy correlates positively with two indices of fat body mass (BMI and circulating triglycerides) and negatively with an index of lean body mass (24 hour urinary creatinine excretion). In the light of data in literature, it is rather difficult to address precisely this issue. Central to metabolic regulation is the provision of the high-energy compound ATP in the mitochondria, where the respiratory chain and the ATPase work together. Among the controllers is the availability of reducing equivalents transported by several shuttle mechanisms. When the phosphorylation state is high, lipogenesis is active. Different consequences on the efficiency of the respiratory chain have been observed in vitro, depending on the mechanism of flux modulation [39]. In contrast, the consequences in vivo remain unknown. In physiological conditions, we ignore the mechanisms of energy expenditure and adaptive thermogenesis in humans, whose skeletal muscle mass largely exceeds that of brown fat [40]. Body compositional differences considerably influence bioenergetic scaling [41]. An increased electron flow drives a greater membrane potential as more protons are pumped out. Substantially, energy fate (either storage or wastage) depends on proton fate (coupled respiration or leak back). The greater membrane potential alone increases both proton leak and uncoupled respiration as thermogenic mechanisms. Moreover, depending on the close relation demonstrated between nonesterified fatty acids (NEFA) and triglyceride concentrations [42], the positive association of RBC vfcy with plasma triglycerides might seem to contrast with the uncoupling effect of NEFA in isolated mitochondria [43]. However, the activity of fatty acids in vivo is still disputed, being confounded by their dual role as oxidation substrates and as uncouplers.

Secondly, RBC vfcy correlates negatively with RBC NHE activity. Perhaps, the unknown erythrocyte membrane complex involved in the process of electron transfer is influenced by changes in protonation state of the enzyme. Alternatively, the reduction of ferricyanide could be a non-electrogenic process, unlike the reduction of AFR [44]. In the case, NHE activity may prevent the electron shuttle in the plasma membrane to bind a proton when accepting an electron. A more plausible explanation, however, could be suggested on the basis of the next and final point.

Thirdly, in the healthy control group, RBC vfcy is negatively associated with at least two markers of oxidative damage, plasma MDA and RBC NHE activity, inasmuch as NHE has been suggested to represent a common mediator of the different effects induced by oxidative stress on cells [45]. Erythrocytes supply electrons to reduce extracellular oxidants, thus neutralising their noxious potential. On the contrary, in the relatives of T1DM patients, RBC vfcy is either positively associated with erythrocyte MDA, i.e. the product of the damaging effect exerted by radicals upon the cell membrane, and negatively associated with the intracellular electron donor GSH. It is plausible that, under conditions of increased ROS generation as observed in T1DM families, the rate of erythrocyte electron transfer is up regulated as a function of the oxidative stimulus. In the same process of transmembrane transport, electrons may leak and, in turn, reduce O_2 to $O^{\cdot -}_2$ radical and H_2O_2. Furthermore, it was proposed that uncoupling, perhaps as a feed back response to the overproduction of radicals by the electron transport chain, could represent a mechanism for the auto-regulation of ROS production, beyond its role in regulating thermogenesis. Recent observation that superoxide increases mitochondrial proton conductance and induces uncoupling [46] supports the hypothesis. The dissipation of the protonmotive force by uncouplers might explain why relatives of T1DM patients show no relation between RBC vfcy and fat body mass indices.

Lastly, we sought any relationship between nutritional and lifestyle individual characteristics and the values of RBC vfcy that had been contextually measured, having previously analysed extensively and compared data from EPIC food frequency questionnaire in healthy adults and T1DM families [30].

From investigating the influence of dietary habits and lifestyle on erythrocyte electron transport emerged interesting observations in support of a role of dietary intake of vitamin C and sporting activities in modulating erythrocyte electron transfer efficiency. Indeed, in the cytosol, ascorbic acid or vitamin C can donate electrons to trans-plasma membrane electron transfer activity in erythrocytes. In vitro, ascorbate may become the major electron donor, when erythrocyte ascorbate concentrations are increased by loading the cells with ascorbate, as well as a selective depletion of erythrocyte ascorbate decreases the capacity for ferricyanide reduction [12]. In vivo, intracellular electron donors available from dietary sources can be important in maintaining the redox environment of a cell, i.e. the summation of the products of the reduction potential and reducing capacity of the linked redox couples present [18, 22-23]. In this work, we show for the first time that daily vitamin C intake influences in particular RBC vfcy capacity.

Additionally, our data also extend to RBC vfcy previous indirect evidence suggesting that regular exercise may improve electron transport efficiency [47-49]. Physical exercise has been associated with an increase in the activities of key enzymes of the electron transport chain [47]; functional improvement should be the principal mechanism of the observed enhanced electron transport activity [48]. The reduction in oxidative damage, the lack of an increase in antioxidant enzyme protein content, and the increase in electron transport activity following training have suggested that an up-regulation of electron transport activity may be responsible for indirect antioxidant effects.

The reason why the independent lifestyle variables associated with RBC vfcy markedly differed among population subgroups (healthy control subjects and T1DM relatives) remains unknown.

Our data suggest that erythrocyte electron transport, whose activity seemingly reflects the functional state of cellular membrane redox systems, behaves differently in diabetes than in healthy. Electron carriers are involved in the maintenance of redox state and reactive oxygen species concentration. A precise understanding of the origin of oxidative stress in diabetic families is critical for developing preventive strategies: a transport system, that seems to be functionally normal, contributes to oxidation in T1DM families whereas in healthy people it protects from oxidation.

ACKNOWLEDGEMENTS

We wish to acknowledge the superb technical assistance of Francesca Fagnani and Ilaria Evangelista. We are obliged to Prof. Giuliano Mariani for the radioimmunoassay of plasma insulin and to our patients for encouragement and support.

REFERENCES

[1] Havel, PJ. Peripheral signals conveying metabolic information to the brain: short-term and long-term regulation of food intake and energy homeostasis. *Exp Biol Med,* 2001, 226, 963-977.

[2] Das, UN. Is obesity an inflammatory condition? *Nutrition,* 2001, 17, 953-966.

[3] McIntyre, EA; Walker M. Genetics of type 2 diabetes and insulin resistance: knowledge from human studies. *Clin Endocrinol,* 2002, 57, 303-311.

[4] Droge, W. Free radicals in the physiological control of cell function. Physiol Rev, 2002, 82: 47-95.

[5] Hensley, K; Robinson, KA; Gabbita, SP; Salsman, S; Floyd RA. Reactive oxygen species, cell signaling, and cell injury. *Free Radic Biol Med,* 2000, 28, 1456-1462.

[6] Kim, HJ; Jung, KJ; Yu, BP; Cho, CG; Choi, JS; Chung, HY. Modulation of redox-sensitive transcription factors by calorie restriction during aging. *Mech Ageing Dev,* 2002, 123, 1589-1595.

[7] Schultz, BE; Chan, SI. Structures and proton-pumping strategies of mitochondrial respiratory enzymes. *Annu. Rev. Biophys Biomol Struct,* 2001, 30, 23-65.

[8] Ly, JD; Lawen, A. Transplasma membrane electron transport: enzymes involved and biological function. *Redox Report,* 2003, 8, 3-21.

[9] May, JM; Qu, Z; Cobb, CE. Recycling of the ascorbate free radical by human erythrocyte membranes. *Free Radic Biol Med,* 2001, 31, 117-124.

[10] Kennett, EC; Kuchel, PW. Redox reactions and electron transfer across the red cell membrane. *IUBMB Life,* 2003, 55, 375-385.

[11] Larm, JA; Vaillant, F; Linnane, AW; Lawen, A. Up-regulation of the plasma membrane oxidoreductase as a prerequisite for the viability of human Namalwa ρ^0 cells. *J Biol Chem,* 1994, 269, 30097-30100.

[12] May, JM; Qu, ZC; Whitesell, RR. Ascorbate is the major electron donor for a transmembrane oxidoreductase of human erythrocytes. *Biochim Biophys Acta,* 1995, 1238, 127-136.

[13] Himmelreich, U; Drew, KN; Serianni, AS; Kuchel, PW. 13C NMR studies of vitamin C transport and its redox cycling in human erythrocytes. *Biochemistry* 1998, 37, 7578-7588.

[14] Matteucci, E; Giampietro, O. Transmembrane electron transfer in diabetic nephropathy. *Diab Care,* 2000, 23, 994-999.

[15] Orringer, EP; Roer, MES. An ascorbate-mediated transmembrane-reducing system of the human erythrocyte. *J Clin Invest,* 1979, 63, 53-58.

[16] Morris, CD; Carson, S. Routine vitamin supplementation to prevent cardiovascular disease: a summary of the evidence for the U.S. Preventive Service Task Force. *Ann Intern Med,* 2003, 139, 56-70.

[17] Fenech, M; Ferguson, LR. Vitamins/minerals and genome stability in humans. *Mutation research,* 2001, 475, 1-6.

[18] Brighenti, F; Valtuena, S; Pellegrini, N; Ardigò, D; Del Rio, D; Salvatore, S; Piatti, PM; Serafini, M; Zavaroni, I. Total antioxidant capacity of the diet is inversely and independently related to plasma concentration of high-sensitive C-reactive protein in adult Italian subjects. *British J Nutr,* 2005, 93, 619-625.

[19] Svensson, MB; Ekblom, B; Cotgreave, IA; Norman, B; Sjoberg, B; Ekblom, O; Sjodin, B; Sjodin, A. Adaptive stress response of glutathione and uric acid metabolism in man following controlled exercise and diet. *Acta Physiol Scand,* 2002, 176, 43-56.

[20] Aguilo, A; Tauler, P; Pilar Guix, M; Villa, G; Cordova, A; Tur, JA; Pons, A. Effect of exercise intensity and training on antioxidants and cholesterol profile in cyclists. *J Nutr Biochem,* 2003, 14, 319-325.

[21] Parise, G; Phillips, SM; Kaczor, JJ; Tarnopolsky, MA. Antioxidant enzyme activity is up-regulated after unilateral resistance exercise training in older adults. *Free Rad Biol Med,* 2005, 39, 289-295.

[22] Johnston, CS; Meyer, CG; Srilakshmi, JC. Vitamin C elevates red blood cell glutathione in healthy adults. *Am J Clin Nutr,* 1993, 58, 103-105.

[23] Tauler, P; Aguilo, A; Gimeno, I; Fuentespina, E; Tur, JA; Pons, A. Influence of vitamin C supplementation on endogenous antioxidant defences during exhaustive exercise. *Pflugers Arch,* 2003, 446, 658-664.

[24] Schafer, FQ; Buettner, GR. Redox environment of the cell as viewed through the redox state of the glutathione disulfide/glutathione couple. *Free Rad Biol Med,* 2001, 11, 1191-1212.

[25] Jackson, AA; Gibson, NR; Lu, Y, Jahoor, F. Synthesis of erythrocyte glutathione in healthy adults consuming the safe amount of dietary protein. *Am J Clin Nutr,* 2004, 80, 101-107.

[26] Matteucci, E; Giampietro, O. Oxidative stress in families of type 1 diabetic patients. *Diab Care,* 2000, 23, 1182-1186.

[27] Matteucci, E; Giampietro, O. Oxidative stress in families of type 1 diabetic patients: further evidence. *Diab Care,* 2001, 24, 167-168.

[28] Matteucci, E; Malvaldi, G; Fagnani, F; Evangelista, I; Giampietro, O. Redox status and immune function in type 1 diabetes families. *Clin Exp Immunol,* 2004, 136, 549-554.

[29] Giampietro, O; Virgone, E; Carneglia, L; Griesi, E; Calvi, D; Matteucci, E. Anthropometric indices of school children and familiar risk factors. *Prev Med,* 2002, 35, 492-498.

[30] Matteucci, E; Passerai, S; Mariotti, M; Fagnani, F; Evangelista, I; Rossi, L; Giampietro, O. Dietary habits and nutritional biomarkers in italian type 1 diabetes families. Evidence of unhealthy diet and combined-vitamin deficient intakes. *Eur J Clin Nutr* 2005, 59, 114-122.

[31] Giampietro, O; Matteucci, E; Pedrinelli, R. Erythrocyte sodium-hydrogen exchange and microalbuminuria in type 1 diabetes. *Diab Care,* 1996, 19, 995-997.

[32] Beutler, E; Duron, O; Kelly BM. Improved method for the determination of blood glutathione. *J Lab Clin Med,* 1963, 61, 882-888.

[33] Esterbauer, H; Cheeseman, KH. Determination of aldehydic lipid peroxidation products: malonaldehyde and 4-hydroxynonenal. *Methods Enzymol,* 1990, 186, 407-413.

[34] Ellman, GL. Tissue sulfhydryl groups. *Arch Biochem Biophys,* 1959, 82, 70-77.

[35] Riboli, E; Kaaks, R. The EPIC project: rationale and study design. *Int J Epidemiol,* 1997, 26, S6-14.

[36] Pasanisi, P; Berrino, F; Bellati, C; Sieri, S; Krogh, V. (2002) Validity of the Italian EPIC questionnaire to assess past diet. *IARC Sci Publ,* 2002, 156, 41-44.

[37] Salvini, S; Parpinel, M; Gnagnarella, P; Maisonneuve, P; Turrini, A. Banca dati di composizione degli alimenti per studi epidemiologici in Italia. Edited by: Istituto Europeo di Oncologia, 1998.

[38] Salvini, S; Saieva, C; Sieri, S; Vineis, P; Panico, S; Tumino, R; Palli, D. Physical activity in the EPIC cohort in Italy. *IARC Sci Publ,* 2002, 156, 267-269.

[39] Nogueira, V; Rigoulet, M; Piquet, M-A; Devin, A; Fontaine, E; Leverve, XM. Mitochondrial respiratory chain adjustment to cellular energy demand. *J Biol Chem,* 2001, 276, 46104-46110.

[40] Spiegelman, BM; Flier, JS. Obesity and regulation of energy balance. *Cell,* 2001, 104, 531-543.

[41] Dobson, GP; Headrick, JP. Bioenergetic scaling: metabolic design and body-size constraints in mammals. *Proc Natl Acad Sci* USA, 1995, 92, 7317-7321.

[42] Reaven, GM. The fourth Musketeer-from Alexander Dumas to Claude Bernard. *Diabetologia,* 1995, 38: 3-13.

[43] Hermesh, O; Kalredon, B; Bar-Tana, J. Mitochondria uncoupling by a long chain fatty acyl analogue. *J Biol Chem,* 1998, 273, 3937-3942.

[44] VanDuijn, MN; Van der Zee, J; Van den Broek, PJA. The ascorbate-driven reduction of extracellular ascorbate free radical by the erythrocyte is an electrogenic process. *FEBS Lett,* 2001, 491, 67-70.

[45] Svegliati-Baroni, G; Di Sario, A; Casini, A; Ferretti, G; D'Ambrosio, L; Ridolfi, F; Bolognini, L; Salzano, R; Orlandi, F; Benedetti, A. The Na+/H+ exchanger modulates the fibrogenic effect of oxidative stress in rat hepatic stellate cells. *J Hepatol,* 1999, 30, 868-875.

[46] Echtay, KS; Roussel, D; St-Pierre, J; Jekabsons, MB; Cadenas, S; Stuart, JA; Harper, JA; Roebuck, SJ; Morrison, A; Pickering, S; Clapham, JC; Brand, MD. Superoxide activates mitochondrial uncoupling proteins. *Nature*, 2002, 415, 96-99.

[47] Hawley, JA. Adaptations of skeletal muscle to prolonged, intense endurance training. *Clin Exp Pharmacol Physiol,* 2002, 29: 218-222.

[48] Menshikova, EV; Ritov, VB; Toledo, FG; Ferrell, RE; Goodpaster, BH; Kelley, DE. Effects of weight loss and physical activity on skeletal muscle and mitochondrial function in obesity. *Am J Physiol Endocrinol Metab,* 2005, 288, E818-825.

[49] Parise, G; Brose, AN; Rarnopolsky, MA. Resistance exercise training decreases oxidative damage to DNA and increases cytochrome oxidase activity in older adults. *Exp Gerontol*, 2005, 40, 173-180.

In: Frontiers in Antioxidants Research
Editor: Harold V. Panglossi, pp. 77-102

ISBN 1-60021-273-5

Chapter 4

Ascorbic Acid, Nitric Oxide and the Autonomic Nervous System

Gianfranco Piccirillo**, Damiano Magrì and Erika Schifano
Policlinico Umberto I, Università "La Sapienza", Rome, Italy

Abstract

High sympathetic and low vagal activity have a determinant role in the genesis of sudden cardiac death (SCD). Particularly in chronic heart failure (CHF), low baroreflex sensitivity and heart rate variability are risk factors for SCD. Recent investigations show that in normal subjects nitric oxide (NO) modulates cardiovascular autonomic control. Conversely, in various conditions including aging, CHF, hypertension, metabolic syndrome, and diabetes, NO synthesis is altered. Three different isoforms of NO synthase (NOS) produce NO: endothelial NOS (eNOS), neuronal NOS (nNOS), and cytokine-inducible NOS (iNOS). Many studies showed that eNOS and nNOS are both expressed in cardiomyocytes, while nNOS is widely distributed in central and peripheral sites of the autonomic nervous system. In vitro studies show that eNOS and nNOS attenuate sympathetic and increase parasympathetic sinus responses. Human studies confirmed this behavior, but failed to clarify the underlying mechanism and the cell types stimulated. In healthy subjects, during NOS inhibition, high-frequency power, a sinus spectral marker of vagal modulation, decreases, and in patients with CHF, during infusion of the NO substrate L-arginine, the same spectral component increases. Ample evidence indicates that ascorbic acid improves endothelial function by increasing NO. The numerous mechanisms involved in preserving NO are largely hypothetical. For example, an open question is whether ascorbic acid acts as an antioxidant, diminishing oxidative stress, or whether it acts directly on NOS. Recent data indicate that in patients with CHF, who typically have low baroreflex sensitivity and decreased heart rate variability, acute administration of L-arginine and ascorbic acid improves sympathovagal control. Furthermore, in elderly subjects, infusion of ascorbic acid at high doses increases baroreflex sensitivity. Although all these results suggest that ascorbic acid might improve the age-related and

* Correspondence to: Dr Gianfranco Piccirillo, Dipartimento di Scienze dell'Invecchiamento, I Clinica Medica, Policlinico Umberto I, 00161 Rome, Italy, Tel. 39-064463301-2-3, Fax 39-064940594, e-mail: gianfranco.piccirillo@uniroma1.it

disease-related imbalance of autonomic control, studies using chronic oral administration have so far yielded disappointing results. Our aim in this review is to consider possible interactions between NO and ascorbic acid and to examine their influence on autonomic control and the possible benefits of administering ascorbic acid.

ABBREVIATIONS

ACE:	Angiotensin-converting enzyme
ACH:	Acetylcholine
ADMA:	Asymmetric dimethylarginine
BH_4:	Tetrahydrobiopterin
BRS:	Baroreflex sensitivity
CVLM:	Caudal ventro-lateral medulla
DDAH:	Dimethylarginine dimethylaminohydrolase
DMV:	Dorsal motor nucleus of the vagus
EDRF:	Endothelium-derived relaxing factor
eNOS:	Endothelial nitric oxide synthase
FAD:	Flavin-adenine dinucleotide
FGF:	Fibroblast growth factor
FMN:	Flavin mononucleotide
G3PDH:	Glyceraldehyde 3-phosphate dehydrogenase
GABA:	γ-aminobutyric acid
Gi:	Inhibitory G-protein
Gs:	Stimulatory G-protein
GTP:	Guanosine triphosphate
IFN-γ:	Interferon γ
iNOS:	Inducible nitric oxide synthase
LDL:	Low-density lipoprotein
L- NAME:	N^G-nitro-L-arginine methylester
L- NNA:	N^G-nitro-L-arginine
L-NMMA:	N^G-monomethyl-L-arginine
MR:	Muscarinic receptor
NA:	Noradrenaline
NADPH:	Nicotinamide adenine dinucleotide phosphate
NANC:	Non-adrenergic, non-cholinergic
nNOS:	Neuronal nitric oxide synthase
NO:	Nitric oxide
NTS:	Nucleus tractus solitarius
PKA :	Protein kinase A
PKG :	Protein kinase G
PNN50:	Number of pairs of adjacent RR intervals differing by more than 50 ms divided by the total number of all RR intervals in the entire recording.
PVN:	Paraventricular nucleus

RMSSD: The square root of the mean of the sum of the squares of differences between adjacent RR intervals
RSNA: Renal sympathetic nerve activity
RVLM: Rostral ventro-lateral medulla
SOD: Superoxide dismutase
TGF-β1: Transforming growth factor β1
TNFα: Tumor necrosis factor α

INTRODUCTION

The autonomic nervous system plays a central role in the pathophysiology of chronic heart failure (CHF), sudden cardiac death (SCD), myocardial ischemia, arterial hypertension, ventricular hypertrophy and atherosclerosis [1,2]. These clinical conditions almost invariably lead to altered autonomic cardiovascular control with increased sympathetic activity and reduced parasympathetic activity. In CHF, indexes of autonomic nervous control, including increased catecholamine concentrations, [3] reduced baroreflex sensitivity [4] and reduced heart rate variability are associated with a poor prognosis [5,6]. Evidence confirming the crucial importance of a sympathovagal imbalance in generating fatal and non-fatal cardiac events is that when β-blocker therapy in CHF and post-infarction [7] restores autonomic cardiovascular control [8], mortality and morbidity improve.

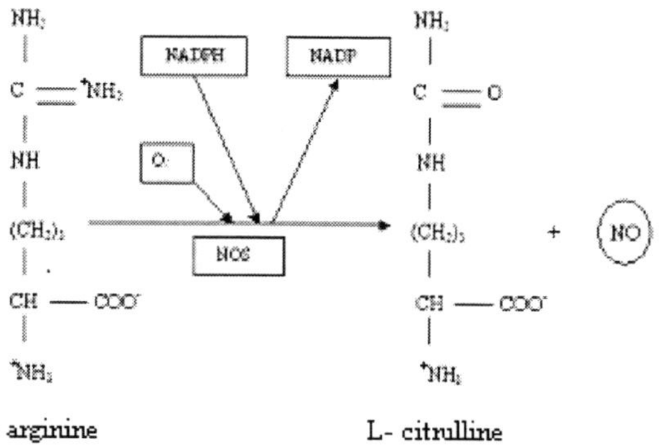

Figure 1. Biosynthesis of nitric oxide
Nitric oxide (NO) is generated together with citrulline by nitric oxide synthase (NOS), an enzyme that uses as a substrate the amino acid L-arginine, oxidizing its terminal guanidino-nitrogen (Figure 1) [13]. Nicotinamide-adenine dinucleotide phosphate (NADPH) is a NOS cofactor and acts as an electron donor.

In all the aforementioned clinical conditions, altered autonomic control is accompanied by endothelial dysfunction [9]. This condition is characterized by a reduced endothelial ability to produce nitric oxide (NO), a mediator that regulates vascular tone. This vasodilator, produced at various levels (in the endothelium, cardiomyocytes, and neurons in the central and peripheral autonomic nervous systems), modulates autonomic control of the heart. At physiological concentrations NO can reduce sympathetic modulation and increase vagal modulation [10,11]. Hence NO could intervene in various ways also in the autonomic dysregulation present in the aforementioned clinical conditions.

NITRIC OXIDE

Research from the late 1980s onwards led to the discovery of an endothelium-derived relaxing factor (EDRF) able to mediate endothelial-dependent vasodilation [12]. This factor later proved to be the nitric oxide (NO) molecule, generated together with L-citrulline from nitric oxide synthase (NOS), an enzyme that acts by oxidation of the terminal guanidino-nitrogen of the amino acid L-arginine (Figure 1) [13].

NOS exists in three isoforms [13]: neuronal NOS (nNOS or NOS I), inducible NOS (iNOS or NOS II) and endothelial NOS (eNOS or NOS III). The genes coding for nNOS, iNOS and eNOS reside respectively in chromosomes 12, 17 and 7 [13]. Whereas iNOS is mainly expressed during inflammation, the other two NOS isoforms are constitutively expressed in various tissues and their activity requires binding of the calcium-calmodulin complex [13].

eNOS has two domains [14,15]: a reductase domain and an oxygenase domain; moreover a flexible protein strand serves as a link between these two domains (Figure 2). The reductase domain links the reduced form of the nicotinamide adenine dinucleotide phosphate (NADPH) cofactor and catalyzes NADPH dehydrogenation. The electrons donated by NADPH are transported by the cofactors flavin mononucleotide (FMN) and flavin adenine dinucleotide (FAD) and transferred through the flexible protein strand to the oxygenase domain. This electron transfer is activated by calcium-calmodulin binding to a specific site in the flexible strand protein. The oxygenase domain catalyzes the conversion of L-arginine into L-citrulline and NO. This domain binds heme, L-arginine and tetrahydrobiopterin (BH_4), another cofactor essential for the activity of all NOS isoforms [13].

Among the factors essential for eNOS activity are post-transcriptional myristoylation and palmitoylation [13,14], modifications through which the enzyme binds to specific plasma membrane domains, termed caveolae. In the caveolae, eNOS interacts with the coat protein caveolin-1, which inhibits the enzyme. Binding of calcium to calmodulin shifts caveolin-1 thereby activating eNOS (Figure 2).

eNOS activity is regulated also by phosphorylation induced by the protein kinase AKT of a serine residue at position 1177 and a threonine residue at position 495 in the enzyme molecule. Phosphorylation of serine activates eNOS whereas phosphorylation of threonine inhibits eNOS. Contact between eNOS and the protein kinase AKT is guaranteed by heat-shock protein 90 (HSP90), a stress protein that forms a scaffold between the two components (Figure 2).

eNOS activity can be inhibited by the presence of L-arginine analogues that act as competitive antagonists [15] including N^G-monomethyl-L-arginine (L-NMMA), N^G-nitro-L-arginine (L-NNA) and its methyl ester (L-NAME), non-isoform-specific inhibitors [10]. L-NNA nevertheless exhibits poor selectivity for nNOS and is more potent against this isoform than against L-NMMA; L-NAME and L-NNA have lower potency against iNOS and higher potency against the constitutive isoforms; L-NMMA is equipotent against all NOS isoforms [10]. Last, also 7-nitroindazole, a non amino acidic compound, is an nNOS inhibitor [10]. Other factors necessary for eNOS activity are the substrate and cofactors [14]. If the substrate is absent, eNOS continues to receive electrons from donors and donates them to its second substrate for affinity, oxygen, thereby producing anion superoxide (O_2^-) [13]. This reaction takes place also in the absence of BH_4, insofar as BH_4 increases eNOS affinity for its substrate and participates in directing electron flow towards L- arginine [13].

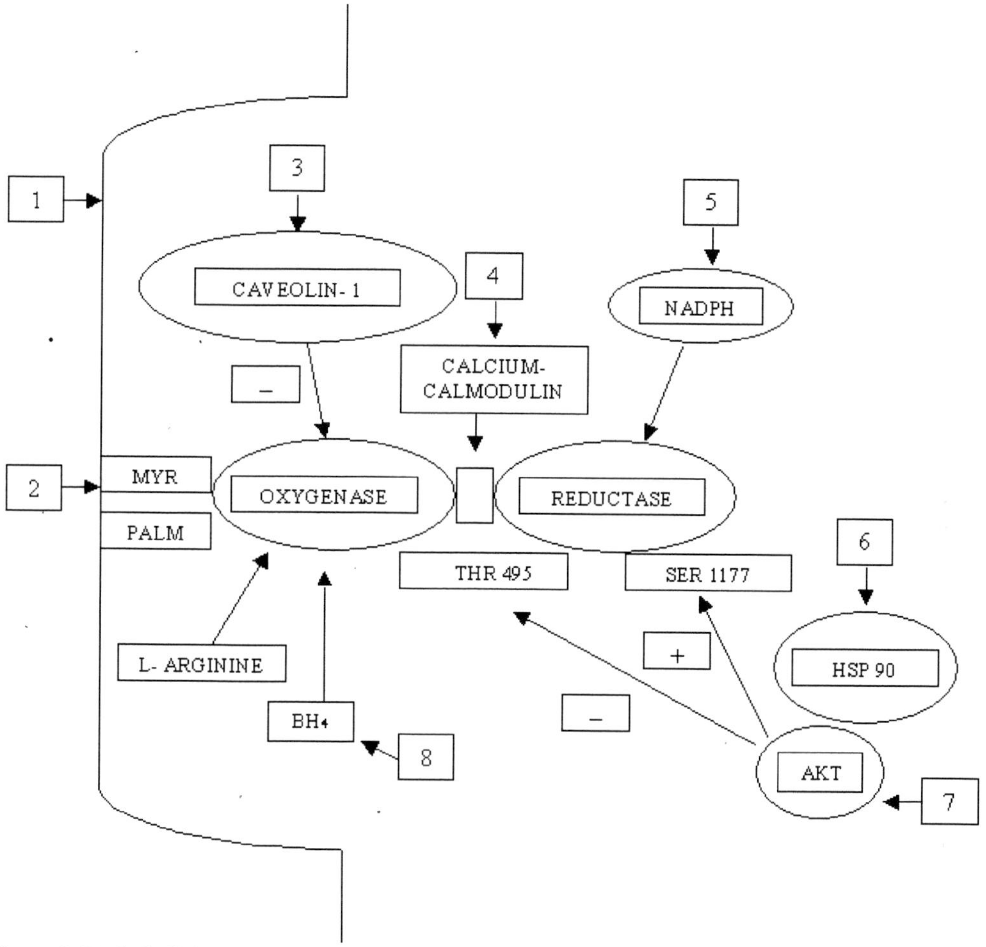

Figure 2. Endothelial nitric oxide synthase (eNOS)

1. caveola: the plasma membrane invagination containing eNOS.
2. myr and palm: myristate (C_{14}) and palmitate (C_{16}) favor anchorage of eNOS to the caveola.
3. caveolin-1: the major caveola coat protein that inhibits eNOS.
4. calcium-calmodulin: the complex that activates electron transfer from the reductase domain to the catalytic domain.
5. NADPH: nicotinamide-adenine dinucleotide phosphate is a cofactor that donates electrons to endothelial nitric oxide synthase (eNOS).
6. HSP90: the heat-shock protein that favors contact between eNOS and the protein kinase AKT.
7. AKT: a kinase that modulates eNOS activity by phosphorylating the serine residue at position 1177 thus activating the enzyme, and the threonine residue at position 495, inhibiting the enzyme.
8. BH_4: tetrahydrobiopterin is one of the NOS cofactors.

As a gas, NO can rapidly diffuse into nearby cells, regulating cellular metabolism, stimulating the synthesis of cyclic guanylic acid (GMP), an intermediary molecule that acts as second messenger, and reducing cellular concentrations of calcium. NO is a reactive molecule with unpaired electrons (i.e., free radical) and as such has an extremely short half-life (3-5 sec) [13]. Among its various actions NO causes endothelial-dependent vasodilation, reduces platelet aggregation and adhesion, reduces leukocyte adhesion and migration and reduces smooth-muscle cell proliferation and migration. Hence NO possesses antiinflammatory, antithrombotic, anticoagulant and profibrinolytic actions [16]. NO also acts not only as an endothelial-cell released paracrine mediator but also as an autonomic nervous system and central nervous system neurotransmitter and an autonomic nervous system modulator [17,11]. NO interacts with the autonomic nervous system at central and peripheral levels. The principal action of NO is that of reducing basal sympathetic tone [11]. NO produced by eNOS present in heart muscle cells attenuates the positive inotropic response to catecholamines and potentiates the negative chronotropic response to acetylcholine. Hence NO reinforces vagal activity but reduces sympathetic activity [17,18]. Infusion of L -arginine in healthy subjects increases vagal control of the heart [19, 20].

NO production is stimulated by shear stress [13], namely stress generated by blood flow on the endothelial surface, by physical exercise, by estrogens, by some growth factors including transforming growth factor (TGFβ1) and fibroblast growth factor (FGF) [13] and by endothelial agonists including acetylcholine, bradykinin, serotonin and substance P [14] (Figure 3). Conversely, NO production is negatively regulated by hypoxia, by tumor necrosis factor-α (TNF-α) [13] and by cardiovascular risk factors [21].

Endothelial function can be assessed as the vasomotor response to pharmacologic stimuli such as acetylcholine. The endothelium-dependent vasodilatory response serves to estimate the bioavailability of NO [14]. Vasodilation can be measured by assessing changes in arterial diameter in the coronary artery district with angiography or with noninvasive techniques such as Doppler ultrasonography. Vasodilation can also be measured with venous occlusion plethysmography or high-resolution ultrasonography to evaluate increased brachial-artery blood flow [15]. When the endothelium is no longer able to produce sufficient NO, the vasodilatory response to endothelial agonists diminishes. Vascular endothelial dysfunction is an early marker of atherosclerosis, because it manifests before the endothelial lesions typical of this disease develop [14]. Coronary-artery and peripheral endothelial dysfunction is a predictor of cardiovascular events [14]. Endothelial dysfunction is typical of all cardiovascular risk factors [21]. The vasodilatory response to acetylcholine diminishes also with aging [21]. Specifically, in healthy subjects younger than 60, endothelial dysfunction seems to be caused by an alteration in the biosynthetic pathways of L-arginine whereas in subjects older than 60 a crucial role is played by oxidative stress [21]. The term oxidative stress refers to a pathologic condition characterized by an over-production of oxygen-derived free radicals that has a damaging effect on the cellular microenvironment. Hypertension therefore anticipates the onset of these typically age-related alterations, and together with age has an additive effect on endothelial dysfunction [21]. Other conditions associated with endothelial dysfunction are diabetes, hypercholesterolemia, cigarette smoking and CHF [13, 15, 16, 22].

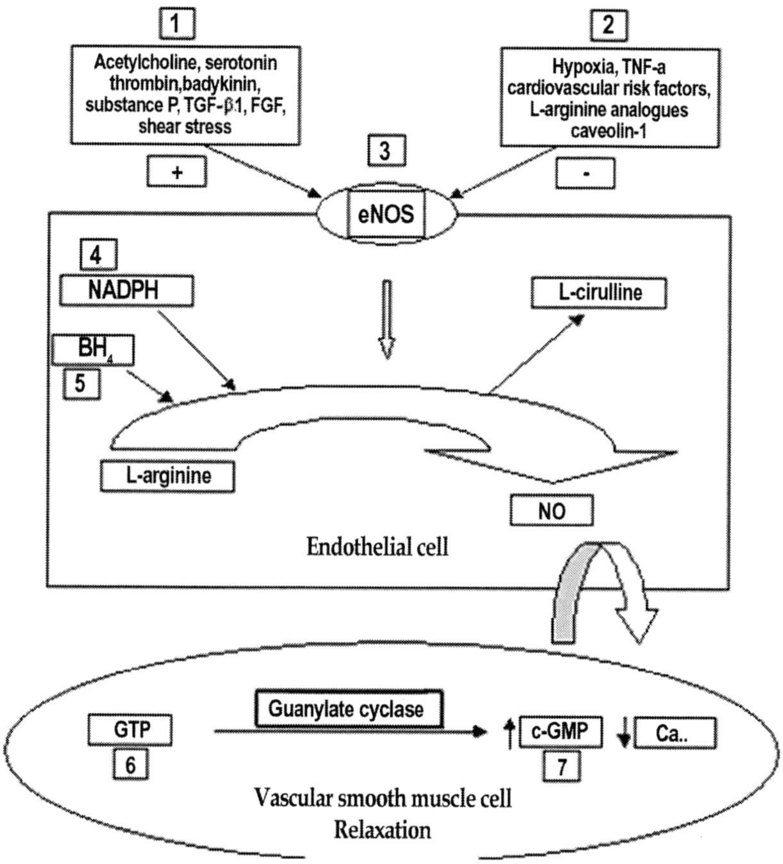

Figure 3. Production of nitric oxide by endothelial cells

1. Acetylcholine, serotonin, thrombin, bradykinin, substance P, transforming growth factor-β1(TGF-β1), fibroblast growth factor (FGF) and shear stress are eNOS activators.
2. Hypoxia, tumor necrosis factor–α (TNF-α), cardiovascular risk factors, L-arginine analogues and caveolin-1 are eNOS inhibitors.
3. eNOS: endothelial nitric oxide synthase.
4. NADPH: nicotinamide-adenine dinucleotide phosphate is an eNOS cofactor.
5. BH_4: tetrahydrobiopterin, is another eNOS cofactor.
6. GTP: guanosine triphosphate is hydrolyzed to cyclic guanosine monophosphate (cGMP) by guanylate cyclase activated by NO.
7. cGMP and Ca^{++}: cyclic guanosine monophosphate and calcium; NO increases guanosine monophosphate levels and reduces calcium thus inducing vascular smooth muscle cell relaxation.

Under all these pathologic conditions, endothelial dysfunction arises mainly through the following mechanisms: increased NO degradation caused by an increase in free radicals and reduced NO formation owing to a reduction in eNOS cofactors, an increase in inhibitors or changes in the microenvironment where NOS resides [14]. For example, hypercholesterolemia increases the cholesterol-rich membrane domains; this change increases membrane rigidity and alters active arginine transport and ion channel function [22]. At the same time, the increased number of caveolae and amount of oxidized LDL facilitate eNOS binding to CD36, a protein that dislocates the enzyme from the caveolae, reducing its activity. Besides, lipids increase levels of the NOS inhibitor, caveolin-1 [15,22].

The well-known beneficial effect of statins and ACE-inhibitors on endothelial dysfunction goes beyond their respective roles in reducing cholesterol levels and arterial pressures [15]. Specifically, both drugs reduce oxidative stress and increase eNOS activity [15,22]. Another pharmacological approach under study is that of improving endothelial function by reducing concentrations of oxygen reactive species with the antioxidants vitamin C and E [16].

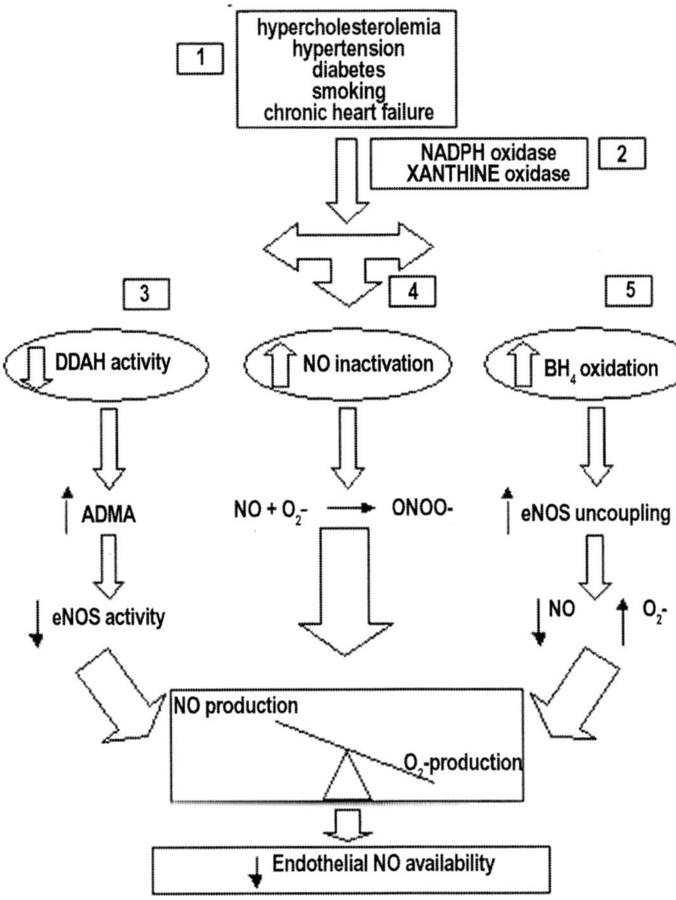

Figure 4. Mechanisms reducing NO availability

1. Hypercholesterolemia, hypertension, diabetes, cigarette smoking and chronic heart failure increase activation of enzymes that produce oxygen reactive species.
2. NADPH oxidase (nicotinamide adenine dinucleotide phosphate oxidase) and xanthine oxidase release oxygen electrons, thus producing anion superoxide, a highly reactive oxygen species.
3. Reactive oxygen species reduce dimethylaminohydrolase (DDAH) activity. The reduction increases levels of asymmetric dimethylarginine (ADMA), an eNOS inhibitor.
4. Superoxide anions inactivate NO thus forming peroxynitrite ($ONOO^-$), another reactive species.
5. Oxygen reactive species oxidize tetrahydrobiopterin (BH_4). This reaction uncouples eNOS so that it begins to produce superoxide anions instead of NO.

All these reactions reduce endothelial NO availability.

ASCORBIC ACID AND NITRIC OXIDE

Age, cardiovascular risk factors and heart failure favor production of oxygen reactive species thus reducing NO bioavailability in three ways [17] (Figure 4):

a) anion superoxide directly inactivates NO;
b) oxygen reactive species reduce the activity of dimethylaminohydrolase (DDAH), thereby increasing asymmetric dimethylarginine (ADMA), which in turn reduces eNOS activity;
c) oxygen reactive species oxidize BH_4 thus uncoupling eNOS to produce anion superoxide.

The major source of superoxide is NADPH oxydase, which catalyzes oxygen reduction in superoxide using NADPH as the electron donor [17] (Figure 5). Another potential source of superoxide is xanthine oxidase [17] (Figure 5).

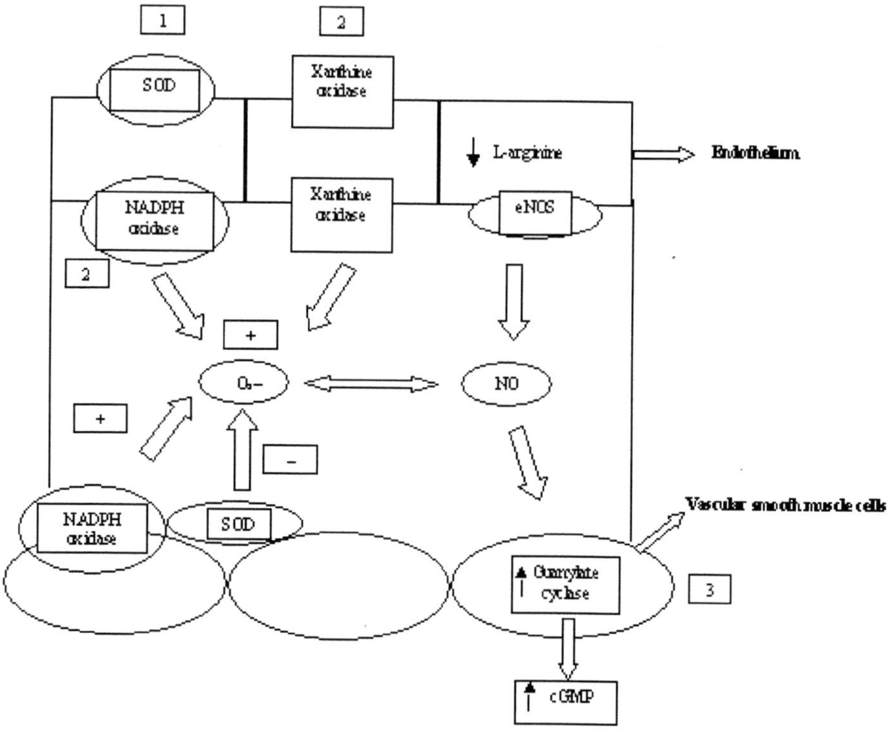

Figure 5. Balance between endothelial NO and O_2^- production
1) SOD: superoxide dismutase is an enzyme located between the endothelium and the vascular smooth-muscle cells whose rôle is to inactivate superoxide anion. SOD expression is induced by NO.
2) NADPH oxidase and xanthine dehydrogenase are two enzymes that produce oxygen reactive species. NOS activity is regulated by the balance between superoxide anion produced and superoxide anion inactivated by superoxide dismutase.
3) Guanylate cyclase activated by NO produces cyclic guanosine monophosphate (cGMP), a signaling molecule that acts as a second messenger inducing vascular smooth-muscle cell relaxation.

Oxidization of BH_4 leads to the production of superoxide by eNOS (Figure 4). This sets up a vicious circle, worsened by the fact that NO normally induces superoxide dismutase (SOD) expression between the endothelium and smooth muscle cells. Hence reduced levels of NO reduce the activity of SOD [17] (Figure 5).

Oxygen reactive species induce oxidative stress by oxidizing protein, structurally disrupting DNA and inducing lipid peroxidation and LDL oxidation [23].

Recent studies [23] have reported that the antioxidant properties of vitamin C and vitamin E are associated with reduced activation of NADPH oxidase and increased activity of eNOS. Whereas vitamin C at all concentrations has a beneficial effect on endothelial function, vitamin E only at high concentrations improves the endothelial-dependent vasodilatory response [23].

Besides, infusion of vitamin C in subjects younger than 60 years leaves the endothelial response unchanged, whereas in those older than 60 it increases the endothelial response to agonists [21]. In the same way, vitamin C improves endothelial function in hypertensive subjects younger than 30 years [21]. These findings indicate that in healthy subjects, oxidative stress intervenes in endothelial dysfunction from 60 years onward and in hypertensive subjects from 30 years onwards. Hypertension therefore accelerates the age-related changes in endothelial function [21].

Administration of vitamin C in subjects with coronary artery disease restores normal endothelial function [24], and improves endothelium-dependent vasodilation in chronic smokers [25], humans with hypercholesterolemia [26], essential hypertension [27] and coronary artery disease [28]. Vitamin C could act through various mechanisms [29,30]:

a) by preventing endothelial dysfunction induced by oxidized LDL through the reduction of oxygen reactive species;
b) by increasing plasma NO release towards the arterial wall by detaching NO from its plasma carriers, namely albumin (S-nitrosoalbumin) and free cysteine (S-nitrosothiol);
c) by reducing nitrites (NO_2^-) to NO in a low environmental pH, thus maintaining local NO concentrations constant;
d) by protecting the thiol groups necessary for eNOS enzymatic activity;
e) by facilitating the activation of NO-dependent guanylate cyclase, conserving iron in the reduced state;
f) by increasing the availability of BH_4.

The hypothesis of increased BH_4 availability was confirmed in a recent study [29] investigating the effects of long-term vitamin C treatment in rats. Yet whereas vitamin C increased BH_4 levels vitamin E had no effect. Vitamin C induces a chemical stabilization of BH_4. The major pathway of BH_4 degradation is oxidation to quinonoid 6,7-[8H]-dihydrobiopterin. Vitamin C acts to reduce this quinonoid. Vitamin C could also increase affinity of BH_4 for eNOS preserving on the enzyme the thiol groups required for binding to the cofactor [29]. Furthermore, plasma vitamin C concentrations are inversely proportional to the increased risk of atherosclerosis [29]. Indeed, the inflammatory cytokines involved in atherogenesis such as TNF-α, IFN-γ and interleukin1-β (IL1-β), stimulate BH_4 synthesis by increasing the expression and activity of GTP cyclohydrolase I [29,31]. Prolonged iNOS activity can be harmful to the endothelium through enzymatic uncoupling and in turn superoxide production. By conserving BH_4 levels, vitamin C therefore has an antiatherogenic effect.

Another beneficial effect of vitamin C is to improve NO production in the presence of native, glycosylated and oxidized LDL [32]. LDLs, especially the oxidized forms, can inhibit the high-affinity transporter CAT-1, responsible for transporting arginine into the endothelial cells, thus contributing to endothelial dysfunction. The effects of vitamin C and L-arginine combined are no greater than those of L- arginine alone [32] either with or without LDL. Hence although oxidative stress plays an important role in LDL-induced endothelial dysfunction, its importance diminishes and even disappears when endothelial cells contain high levels of the NOS substrate, L -arginine [32].

Finally, vitamin C reduces NO oxidization products such as N_2O_3 and N_2O_4, but tends to preserve intracellular concentrations of NO [33]. High NO concentrations can be toxic for cells by virtue of protein and enzyme iron nitrosylation but especially owing to its reactive species, including peroxynitrite and nitrosoperoxocarbonate [33]. If the oxygen reactive species is absent, NO is a reducing agent, but if added to an oxygenated medium its actions can be potentially harmful for cells. Specifically, high concentrations of NO inhibit the activity of eNOS as well as of glyceraldehyde 3-phosphate dehydrogenase (G3PDH) owing to nitrosylation of iron in eNOS and of the G3PDH sulfhydryl groups [33].

Vitamin C protects these two enzymes from inhibition induced by reactive NO species reconverting them into NO [33].

In conclusion, convincing evidence shows that vitamin C benefits NO production and endothelial function even though the underlying mechanisms remain to be determined.

Nitric Oxide and the Autonomic Nervous System

Among the multiple actions of NO is its role as a neurotransmitter and modulator of autonomic nervous system [10,11,18]. NOS activity is present in central and peripheral autonomic nervous system sites [10]. In the central nervous system, NOS is found in the nucleus tractus solitarius (NTS), in the rostral ventrolateral medulla (RVLM) and caudal ventrolateral medulla (CVLM), in the dorsal motor nucleus of the vagus (DMV) and nucleus ambiguous. In the periphery, NOS is found in the carotid sinuses, in the vagal and intrinsic cardiac neurons, in the preganglionic neurons and sympathetic ganglions, and at the level of the sinoatrial and atrioventricular nodes and perivascular nerves [10]. The nervous system pathways using NO as a transmitter, previously known as non-adrenergic non-cholinergic (NANC) nerves, are now described as nitrergic nerves [10].

Effects of Nitric Oxide on Sympathetic and Parasympathetic Cardiovascular Control

The role of NO in regulating sympathetic and parasympathetic activity at cardiovascular level has been determined using non-isoform-specific NOS inhibition after systemic administration of L-arginine analogues such as L-NMMA [10,11,18]. The results of these studies indicate that if NO synthesis is inhibited the ability to increment vagal activity is reduced both directly and during baroreflex stimulation [18,19,20].

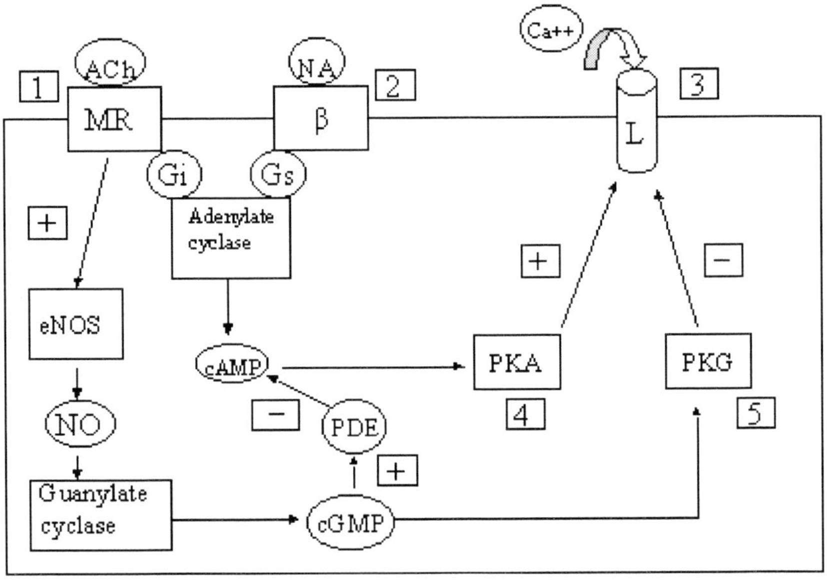

Figure 6. Possible mechanisms of NO-dependent control of accentuated antagonism

1) Ach: Acetylcholine; MR: muscarinic receptor. Ligand-receptor coupling activates an inhibitory G protein (Gi), which inhibits adenylate cyclase, thus reducing production of cyclic AMP while activation of the muscarinic receptor stimulates eNOS to produce NO.
2) NA: noradrenaline; β: β-adrenergic receptor. Ligand-receptor coupling activates a stimulatory G protein (Gs), which activates adenylate cyclase, thereby increasing production of cyclic AMP.
3) Type L calcium channels are responsible for the entry of calcium ions into cardiomyocytes and undergo functional modulation by second-messenger-dependent kinases.
4) PKA: protein kinase A is a kinase activated by cyclic AMP and therefore by adrenergic stimulation. It increases the entry of calcium ions into cells by acting on L type calcium channels.
5) PKG: protein kinase G, a kinase activated by cyclic GMP, inhibits opening of L type calcium channels.

NO seems to modulate direct parasympathetic activity, by activating muscarinic receptors, and indirect parasympathetic activity, also termed accentuated antagonism, namely muscarinic inhibition of adrenergic activity [10, 34, 35]. NO therefore facilitates vagal activity directly through a post-synaptic mechanism or a mechanism distal to the muscarinic receptor, whereas it could control vagal activity directly through a presynaptic mechanism [34]. Presynaptic vagal control receives confirmation from evidence in animal studies that nNOS gene transfer into atrial cardiomyocytes triggers increased release of acetylcholine from vagal nerve terminals in response to electrical stimulation [36]. The NO-induced facilitation of accentuated antagonism could reflect inhibition of calcium ion influx through phosphorylation of the L-type calcium channels in the cardiomyocytes and the sinoatrial node, by a cGMP-dependent protein kinase (PKG); or cGMP could activate a phosphodiesterase that hydrolyzes cAMP, reducing the activity of a cAMP-dependent protein kinase (PKA), which also serves to modulate calcium channels (Figure 6) [10].

NO also modulates baroreflex-mediated vagal activity [37]. Specifically, NO regulates baroreflex sensitivity (BRS) at brainstem level [38]; its bioavailability at carotid and aortic artery level could alter BRS through its effect on arterial distensibility or baroreceptor discharge [38]. Vitamin C could improve BRS by increasing NO bioavailability [20,38,39].

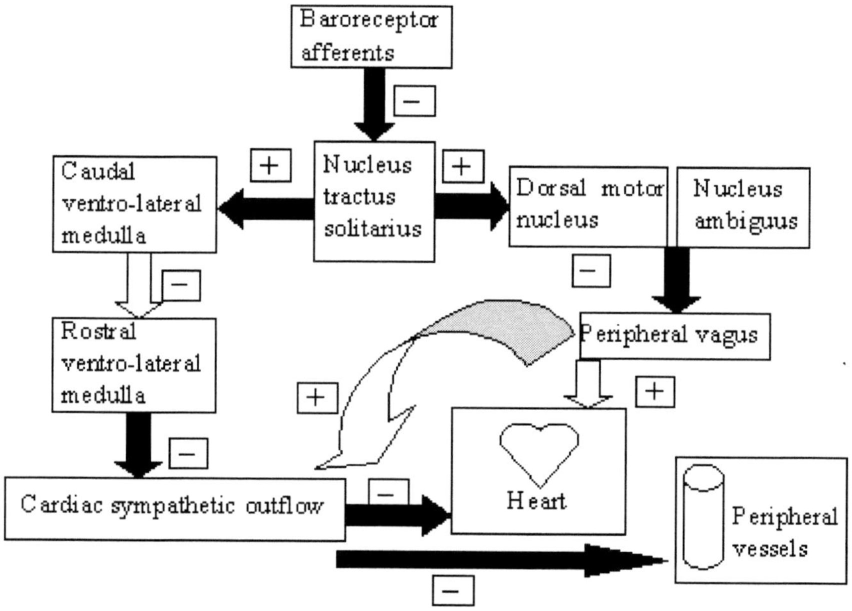

Figure 7. Actions of NO at central sites of cardiovascular autonomic control.
The white arrows in the figure indicate the inhibitory pathways and the black arrows the excitatory pathways of NO. The symbol + indicates the NO action potential and the – sign the attenuating action. NO inhibits the discharge rates of the afferent baroreceptor fibers, which terminate in the nucleus tractus solitarius (NTS). NO increases the activity of neurons located in this nucleus, which activate the caudal ventrolateral medulla (CVLM), the dorsal motor nucleus of the vagus (DMV) and the nucleus ambiguus. The CVLM is a sympathoinhibitory site and NO acts by reducing its activity. The CVLM nerve fibers reach the rostral ventro-lateral medulla, a site involved in sympathetic system activation. NO reduces activity at this site thus reducing sympathetic outflow. Conversely, NO increases the activity of DMVoutflow, whose role is to stimulate the peripheral vagal nerve. The final effect is therefore to reduce sympathetic activity and reduce vagal activity.

Besides exerting a facilitatory role on vagal cardiovascular control, NO has a sympathicolytic action [10,11,18]. The vasoconstrictor response to systemic inhibition of NOS could be explained by removal of the tonic vasodilation exerted by endothelial NO, or by removal of the tonic inhibition exerted by neuronal NO on sympathetic nervous activity [10]. NO inhibits sympathetic cardiovascular activity at both central and peripheral levels [35]. Support for its central and peripheral actions comes from experiments in animals showing that sympathectomy, a pharmacological block of the sympathetic ganglia and acute administration of β-blockers, substantially reduces the hypertensive response to chronic NOS inhibition [40,41]. In anesthetized rats, systemic administration of L-NMMA induces a biphasic response in renal sympathetic nerve activity (RSNA) [42]. After an initial decrease, owing to sympathetic baroreflex-mediated sympathetic inhibition, RSNA then increases; the increase is abolished by cervical spinal cord section, showing that NO acts centrally [42]. In reality, NO has a more complex action. Besides having a dual role in regulating autonomic control of the cardiovascular system, it also has sympathoinhibitory and depressor effects and under some circumstances sympathoexcitatory effects [11].

Nitric Oxide Control of Sympathetic Activity Mediated by Central Nervous System

Evidence that L-NMMA acts centrally comes from experiments in rats showing that a dose inducing no effects when given systemically, induced effects when administered intraventricularly [11]. Hence NO also acts centrally. A possible site for nitrergic modulation of sympathetic activity is the NTS, the central area where primary baroreceptor afferent fibers mainly terminate. L-arginine injected into this nucleus reduces arterial pressure and sympathetic activity (Figure 6) [43,44]. Another central site of action is the RVLM, the brainstem zone where sympathetic afferent inflow is processed. L -arginine injected into this zone also reduces arterial pressure and sympathetic activity (Figure 7) [44]. Another brain area involved in modulating NO is the CVLM. NO donors injected into this zone increase RSNA [45]. This finding indicates that the CVLM is a sympathoinhibitory site and NO inhibits its action (Figure 7) [10]. Insofar as the action of NO on these two bulbar sites gives rise to antagonist effects on sympathetic activity, NO seems to act preferentially on the RVLM, thus giving rise to central inhibition of sympathetic outflow (Figure 7) [10]. This central mechanism could be important in limiting sympathetic activation during stress, because in rats undergoing stress, NO-producing neurons in these two bulbar sites increase in number [46]. NO could act as a sympathetic modulator also at the paraventricular nucleus (PVN) in the hypothalamus, an important site for sympathetic regulation of blood-volume homeostasis [35]. At this level, NO seems to inhibit sympathetic outflow through a GABA-like mechanism [35]. Among its nitrergic effects on reflex control of sympathetic activity, NO reduces central adaptation [10,35]. This process has been studied in animals in vivo by applying sustained pressure to the vascularly isolated rabbit carotid sinus [47]. This experimental condition brings about rapid inhibition of RSNA followed by a gradual return to baseline values. NO, reducing the amplitude and velocity of these changes maintains reflex inhibition of sympathetic activity during each increase in arterial pressure [10,35].

Last, NO could also act at RVLM level by attenuating the reflex sympathoexcitatory response to muscle stimulation [10].

Nitric Oxide Control of Parasympathetic Activity Mediated by the Central Nervous System

Administration of NOS inhibitors increases baroreceptor-heart-rate reflex [10]. NO is thought to reduce reflex vagal cardiac control through its central action probably mediated by nNOS [10]. The precise central site through which NO acts to inhibit the baroreflex remains controversial. Notwithstanding ample evidence that the NTS contains NO-sensitive neurons,

L-glutamate-induced NO release in these sites stimulates rather than inhibits neuronal activity in response to baroreceptor afferent stimulation [48]. The NTS therefore seems an unlikely site for nitrergic inhibition of the baroreflex. Conversely, NO seems to increase neuronal activity in the DMV. This nucleus contains the cardiac vagal C fiber motoneurons. These motoneurons are insensitive to modulation by baroreceptor afferents and thus produce a tonic, slow influence on heart rate [10]. In contrast, the nucleus ambiguus is the source of the cardiac vagal B fiber motoneurons which are sensitive to the baroreflex, and exert a rapid, phasic influence on heart rate [10]. Hence NO might increase tonic activity by acting on C fibers but inhibit baroreflex control by acting on B fibers [10]. This difference could explain why even though NO increases neuronal activity in the NTS and DMV, it reduces baroreflex sensitivity for heart rate [10].

Effects of Nitric Oxide in Cardiomyocytes

Cardiac muscle cells express eNOS and nNOS [17]. Both enzymes modulate cardiac excitation-contraction coupling and the cardiac muscle response to autonomic nervous system regulation. Efficient modulation of the muscarinic response requires eNOS and muscarinic receptors to colocalize in the cardiomyocytes caveolae [17]. Cardiomyocyte production of endothelial NO potentiates the chronotropic muscarinic response and attenuates the inotropic and chronotropic effects of catecholamines, increasing accentuated antagonism [17]. nNOS resides in the sarcoplasmic reticulum of the cardiomyocytes and like eNOS, is involved in regulating cardiac contractility [49]. nNOS inhibition increases baseline cardiac contractions and augments the contractile response to β-adrenergic stimulation [49]. NO could act on cardiomyocytes through various mechanisms (Figure 6):

a) by inhibiting calcium ATPases (SERCA2a) in the sarcoplasmic reticulum;
b) by inhibiting influx of calcium ions through L-type calcium channels (Figure 6);
c) by exerting lusitropic effects on cardiomyocytes, by reducing myofilament sensitivity to calcium secondary to PKG-induced phosphorylation of troponin I.

The second hypothesis, inhibiting calcium flow, seems the most probable [49]. NO therefore inhibits voltage-dependent calcium channels thereby reducing the influx of calcium ions in response to adrenergic stimulation [10]. Neuronal NO acts also through presynaptic inhibition of adrenaline release from sympathetic nerve endings [10,35].

Effects of Nitric Oxide on Vascular Resistance

NO inhibits the peripheral vascular response to sympathetic activation not only by acting as a vasodilator but also by inhibiting presynaptic and post-synaptic noradrenergic transmission [10]. NO acts on both central and peripheral vascular resistances [11]. Specifically, NO, generated by eNOS and by nNOS located near neurons within the brainstem vasomotor centers, reduces sympathetic outflow towards preganglionic and postganglionic neurons whereas it reduces vascular α-adrenergic receptor activation (Figure

8) [11]. Hence the central and peripheral actions of NO contribute to vasodilation. Systemically infused L-NMMA provokes vasoconstriction through two actions, namely, by facilitating central sympathetic outflow and by directly increasing vascular tone (Figure 9) [11]. The cholinergic block potentiates L-NMMA-induced vasoconstriction indicating that cholinergic vasodilation counterbalances the pressure changes caused by inhibition of NOS [11].

NO also modulates the vasodilatory actions of insulin [11]. Insulin increases blood flow and reduces resistance in skeletal muscle vessels; it also activates L-arginine transport and stimulates NO release. Insulin-induced vasodilation is therefore mediated by endothelial NO and reduced by sympathetic vasoconstrictor tone [11].

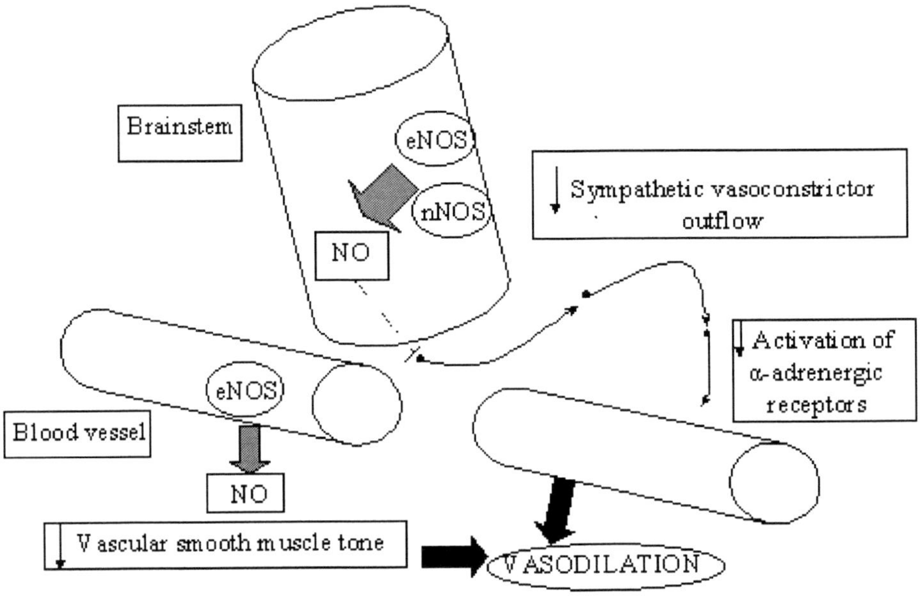

Figure 8. Interaction between NO and the sympathetic nervous system in the regulation of peripheral vascular tone

In the brainstem, NO is produced by endothelial cells and neurons. Centrally-produced NO diminishes sympathetic vasoconstrictor outflow and thereby reduces vascular α-adrenergic receptor activation. In blood vessels, eNOS produces NO that acts directly on vascular smooth-muscle cells to reduce their tone. The central and peripheral actions of NO lead to vasodilation.

Besides being regulated by endothelial NO, muscle flow is regulated also by neuronal NO produced by skeletal muscle cells [11]. During muscular exercise skeletal muscle cell NO mediates functional sympatholysis, namely the reduction of sympathetic vasoconstriction. In Duchenne muscular dystrophy a dystrophin deficiency causes a loss of NO; as a result in patients with this disorder during muscular exercise functional sympatholysis is absent and ischemia develops [11].

NOS-induced inhibition of sympathetic vasoconstriction has been observed also in rat mesenteric arteries [50]. In normotensive rats, neuronal NO modulates the sympathetic response, obtained by electrically stimulating the perivascular nerves, through a presynaptic mechanism. Conversely, in hypertensive rats, the activity of neuronal NO is suppressed and endothelial NO prevails but at reduced concentrations [50]. Hypertension is associated with sympathetic hyperactivity and reduced production of NO, especially of neuronal NO [35,50,51]. Yet NO does not always induce vasodilation through its sympatholytic action. A recent study detected at coronary artery endothelial cell level the presence of a β_3 adrenergic receptor able to exert NO-mediated vasodilation. This receptor type was studied with β-blockers such as nebivolol, drug that apart from its intense β_1 antagonist actions, also exhibits β_3 agonist activity. Hence nebivolol induces NO-mediated coronary artery vasodilation [52].

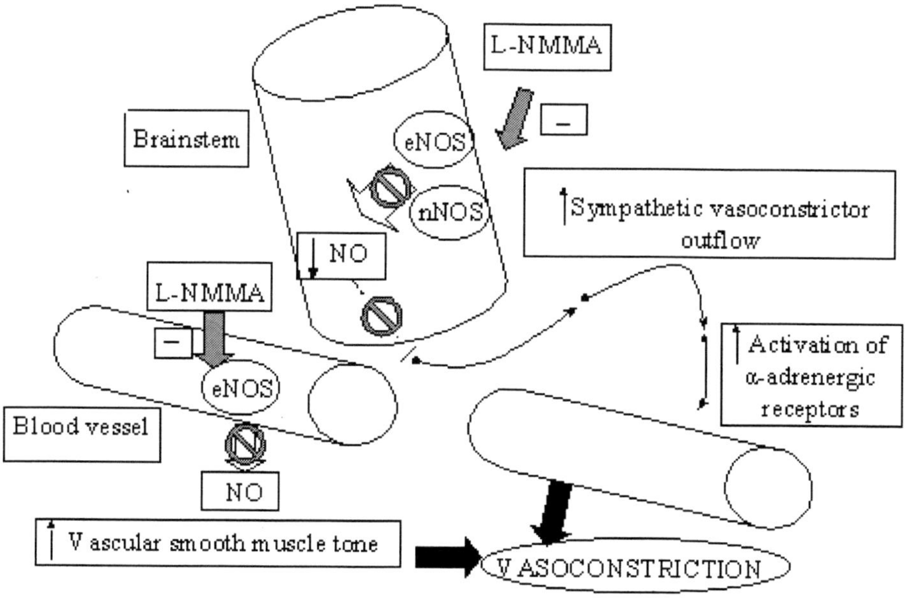

Figure 9. Effects of NOS inhibition on the regulation of vascular tone
Systemic inhibition of NOS by L-arginine analogues such as L-NMMA takes place at central and peripheral levels. At brainstem level L-NMMA blocks production of NO by eNOS and nNOS. The NO reduction increases vasoconstrictor sympathetic outflow and activates vascular α-adrenergic receptors. L-NMMA also inhibits the activity of blood-vessel eNOS thus increasing vascular smooth-muscle cell tone.

EFFECTS OF NITRIC OXIDE AND ASCORBIC ACID ON AUTONOMIC CONTROL IN HUMANS

As we have underlined in the preceding chapters, infusion of NOS inhibitors such as L-NMMA in experimental animals and humans results in vasoconstriction and hence increases arterial blood pressure. In subjects with a normal baroreflex infusion of vasoconstrictor drugs determines a reflex reduction in heart rate. The slope between the variations in heart rate and arterial pressure during infusion of a vasoconstrictor (generally phenylephrine) is used to measure vagal activity and is termed baroreflex sensitivity (BRS) [4,53-54]. Infusion of L-NMMA, conversely, induces an increase in arterial pressure unaccompanied by a marked reduction in heart rate. This datum was obtained by comparing variations in the vagal response during infusion of phenylephrine, an α agonist that has no action on NOS, with variations during infusion of L-NMMA. During infusion of the NOS inhibitor, pressure increases induced by infusing phenylephrine being equal, normal subjects had a smaller increase in vagal markers after L-NMMA infusion than after phenylephrine [18] both in the frequency domain (high-frequency power, α- high frequency) and in the time domain (RMSSD, the square root of the mean of the sum of the squares of differences between adjacent RR intervals, and pNN50, i.e. the number of pairs of adjacent RR intervals differing by more than 50 ms divided by the total number of all RR intervals in the entire recording) [56]. Furthermore, infusion of exogenous NO donor vasodilators (nitroprusside), vasodilation being equal, induced higher levels of the same vagal markers and of baroreflex sensitivity than hydralazine [18]. This experiment indirectly shows that in healthy humans NO increases vagal modulation of the sinus node. Because L-NMMA is not selective for nNOS or eNOS, whether one or both enzymatic systems are implicated remains unknown [10]. Other studies provided complementary information showing that L-arginine infused in normal subjects induces vasodilation and bradycardia [19,20]. Other direct vasodilators, such as hydralazine, vasodilatation being equal, induce tachycardia. Again, comparison of markers in the frequency and in the time domains showed that L-arginine infusion induced vagal stimulation [19]. This response is meaningful because it is stereospecific [19] and was obtained with L-arginine at low doses (10 g). These low doses yield plasma L-arginine levels of ≈ 2 mmol/L, which induce selective NO-dependent vasodilation [19,20].

Among the many open questions an exceptionally interesting one is the precise post-receptor mechanism underlying the cardiac vagal effect of NO. What remains unknown is whether NO acts directly on muscarinic receptors or indirectly through an antiadrenergic mechanism, for example accentuated antagonism (Figure 6). A complex yet elegant study conducted by Chowdhary et al. to investigate the influence of NO on the cardiac response to parasympathetic stimulation seems to throw some light on the question [34]. In healthy subjects, these investigators infused edrophonium, a muscarinic agonist that acts by inhibiting cholinesterase, during NOS inhibition with L-NMMA, placebo or phenylephrine [34]. They obtained an almost overlapping reduction in heart rate in the three types of NOS inhibition. Hence they concluded that NO does not act directly on muscarinic receptors. Conversely, compared with phenylephrine and placebo, L-NMMA induced notable accentuated antagonism. More than 50% of the reduction in heart rate took place through an antiadrenergic mechanism, that is when subjects underwent edrophonium-induced cholinergic stimulation during adrenergic stimulation with isoproterenol [34]. These data confirm the hypothesis that activation of cardiac NOS induces cGMP-dependent inhibition of type L calcium influx channels (Figure 6) rather than a muscarinic-receptor-mediated increase in potassium outflow. What remains unclear is whether a central nitrergic mechanism of vagal modulation is active in humans or whether NO influences synaptic release of acetylcholine, or whether both mechanisms act in concert.

If ascorbic acid improves NO production only under conditions of oxidative stress (aging, hypercholesterolemia, smoking, diabetes, hypertension and heart failure) as we saw in the foregoing paragraphs, vitamin C infusion should have no effect on the cardiovascular autonomic nervous system under normal conditions. Three studies conducted almost simultaneously and published between January 2003 and March 2004 investigated this matter with various techniques but reached the same conclusion [38,39,57]: acute infusion of ascorbic acid does not improve cardiovascular autonomic nervous system in young or middle-aged subjects. The three studies differed in design: two were designed to evaluate the influence of vitamin C on the autonomic nervous system in CHF [38,57] and the data for normal subjects as a control group; the third study aimed to compare ascorbic acid-dependent changes in BRS (phenylephrine method) in young adults and elderly subjects [39]. The first study, published by our group, studied the autonomic nervous system in greater detail because it compared more than one technique: spectral analysis of RR and arterial pressure variability, α index (spectral analysis of BRS), time domain analyses (RMSSD) and BRS measured with the phenylephrine method [57]. The second study used only the sequential method for BRS [38] and the third used the phenylephrine method. All three studies concluded that vitamin C has no effect in subjects younger than about 60 years. Its effect in older persons and in patients with chronic heart failure could arise from the typical improvement in oxidative stress in these subjects after infusion of vitamin C [21]. In the elderly, by suppressing the formation of oxygen reactive species, ascorbic acid could improve NO availability, in turn implicated in modulating the increase in parasympathetic or antiadrenergic activity. In the elderly, the reduction in autonomic cardiovascular control nevertheless follows a logarithmic pattern, takes place chiefly between 40 and 60 years [54,55,58-62] and correlates with an increase in cardiovascular risk factors (hypertension, diabetes, and hypercholesterolemia) [54], all conditions that can themselves increase oxidative stress. The age-related reduction in autonomic function is probably not a physiological phenomenon but arises from increased oxidative stress.

Last, for the sake of completeness, we wish to mention a study conducted before the three aforementioned studies yet seems out of line with the more recent observations. This earlier study reported that L-NMMA infused in normal subjects reduced reflex tachycardia in response to head-up tilt [63], a typical maneuver that stimulates sympathetic activation and inhibits vagal activation, The investigators suggested that L-NMMA diminished the ability to increase heart rate in response to tilt because it reduced sympathetic activity or increased vagal activity or induced both changes [63]. They provided no time domain or frequency domain markers to support their observation. Why NOS inhibition should cause sympathetic activation to decrease or vagal activation to increase or both events to happen when we would expect the contrary is hard to explain. Presumably NO-induced modulation of baroreflex sensitivity is a far more complex matter than current knowledge leads us to expect. Hence further studies are warranted to deepen our knowledge.

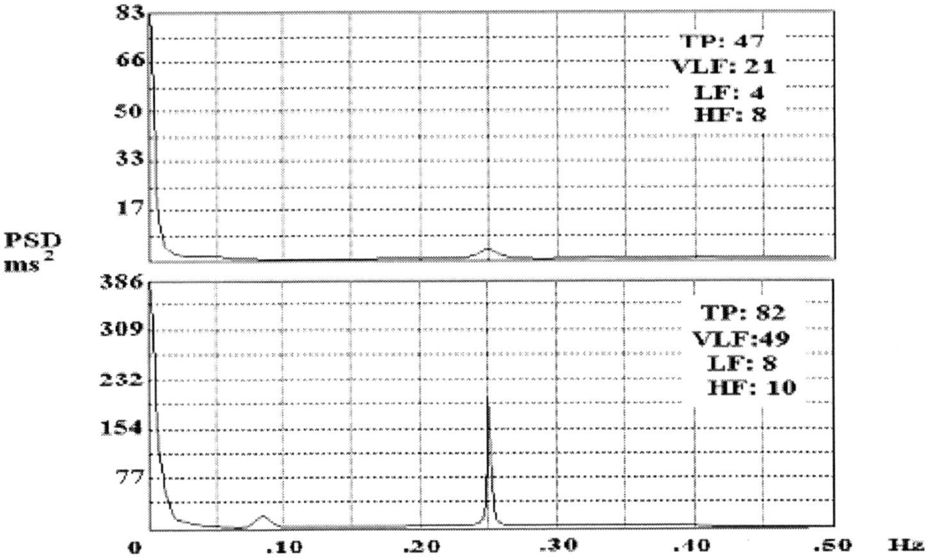

Figure 10. Changes in RR spectral variables during L-arginine and vitamin C infusion in subjects with chronic heart failure. The upper panel shows the RR variability spectrum for a representative patient with chronic heart failure (CHF) in NYHA class IV during infusion of placebo, and the lower panel during infusion of L -arginine and vitamin C in combination. In the lower panel, note the increased total area or total power (TP), low-frequency power (LF) and high-frequency (HF) power [20].

Influence of Ascorbic Acid on Autonomic Modulation in Chronic Heart Failure

A typical disorder associated with severe oxidative stress and endothelial dysfunction is chronic heart failure (CHF). High levels of angiotensin II and of cytokines such as TNF-α, can increase oxidative stress and reduce NO [64]. As we explain in the preceding chapters NO could have notable antiadrenergic or vagomimetic activity or both. Hence also a decrease in this vasodilator in CHF could help to shift the sympathovagal balance towards sympathetic hypertone and reduce vagal activation. This autonomic imbalance is *per se* able to worsen CHF clinically and favor the onset of sudden death from malignant ventricular arrhythmias.

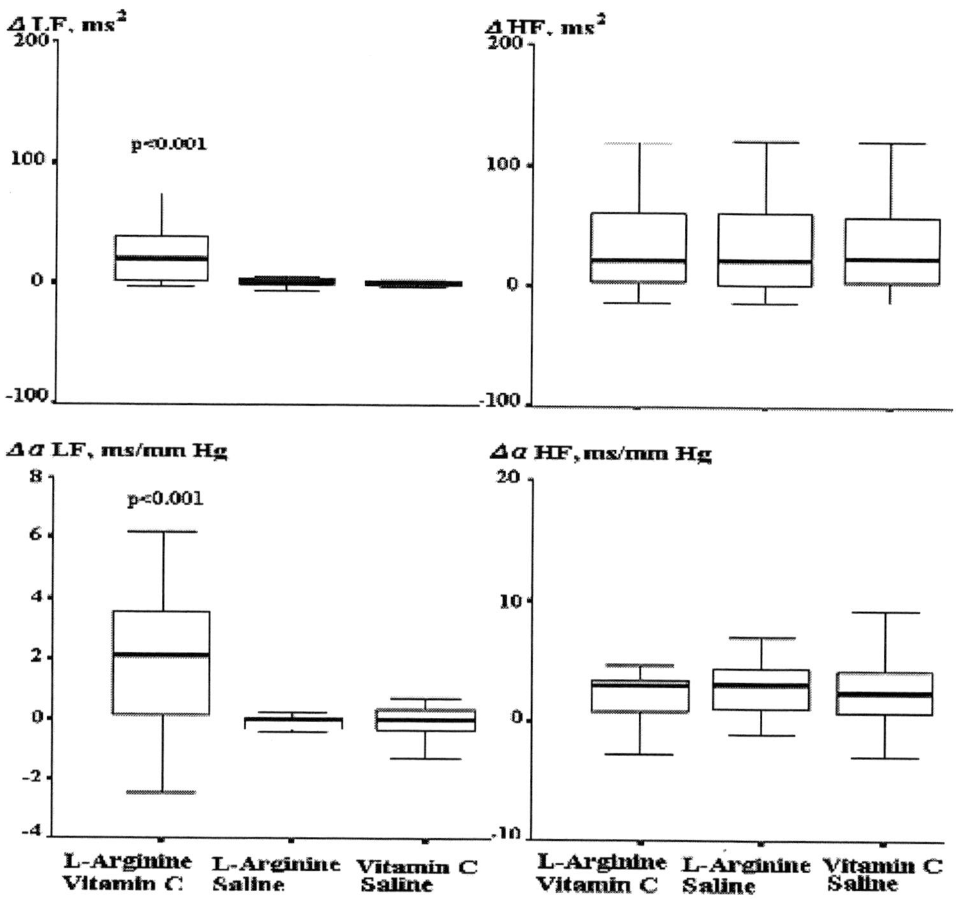

Figure 11. Effects of L-arginine and vitamin C infusion in subjects with chronic heart failure. Differences in low-frequency (LF) of RR variability (upper panel, left), in high-frequency (HF) of RR (upper panel, right), in α LF (lower panel, left) and α HF (lower panel, right) between placebo and the three study conditions (L-arginine and vitamin C combined, L-arginine alone, and vitamin C alone) in subjects with chronic heart failure (CHF). In this and the subsequent box plots, the central line represents the median distribution; each box spans from 25 to 75 percentile points, and error bars extend from 10 to 90 percentile points (one-way ANOVA). Note that LF and α LF powers increase significantly only during infusion of L-arginine and vitamin C in combination, whereas HF and α HF powers increase significantly during infusion of L-arginine and vitamin C singly and combined [20].

In patients with CHF, compared with healthy subjects, the pressure increase induced by the α-agonist phenylephrine being equal, NOS inhibition induced by L-NMMA leads to a smaller increase than phenylephrine in HF power, α-HF and RMSSD [37]. Because the HF power increase during phenylephrine infusion is thirteen times higher than the increase during L-NMMA, NO production in CHF is presumably a determinant mechanism opposing the sympathovagal imbalance [37]. In another series of experiments our group showed that L-arginine infusion doubles the vagal marker, HF power (figure 10) [20]. This datum acquires even greater importance insofar as vagal activity improves even when the hemodynamic status remains unchanged. The next question was whether ascorbic acid infusion could improve autonomic control during CHF. Two studies conducted as almost the same time clarified this question. In the first, we found that endovenous infusion of vitamin C at high doses (from 2.5 to 3 g) acutely increased vagal activity measured in various ways: RMSSD, HF power and baroreflex sensitivity induced spontaneously (α-HF) and with the phenylephrine method [57]. These data were confirmed in the second study by others who observed an increase in BRS assessed with the sequential method [38]. This latter study failed, however, to provide evidence that chronic oral administration of vitamin C (4 g/day) in subjects with CHF improves autonomic control. Oral doses are probably unable to guarantee sufficiently high plasma vitamin C levels owing to an autonomic effect. Oral administration yields plasma vitamin C concentrations of around 100 μmol/L, whereas an endovenous bolus gives concentrations exceeding 1000 μmol/L [38]. Because these high concentrations result in a scavenging effect of superoxide anions the same mechanism probably underlies the actions of vitamin C on the autonomic system. Although some evidence suggested that the improvement in BRS might reflect the vitamin-C induced increase in vascular distensibility, measurement of this variable during vitamin C infusion tended to exclude this possibility [38].

In subjects with CHF, infusion of vitamin C and NO combined brings about a greater improvement in cardiovascular autonomic modulation than both agents infused singly (figure 10-11) [20]. From a spectral viewpoint, combined administration brings about larger increases not only in the vagal spectral component, HF power, but also more efficiently increases LF power. The LF component measured in normal subjects is an index of sympathetic modulation of the sinus node. In CHF this index undergoes a paradoxic reduction: the more severe the symptoms of CHF the more depressed is LF power [65,67]. A reduction in LF power below the threshold of 13 ms^2 is a risk factor for sudden cardiac death [4]. Acute administration of ascorbic acid and NO improves LF power (figure 11) [20,57]. If we could find a way of obtaining sufficient, long-lasting plasma levels of ascorbic acid and NO this therapy could be used in preventing sudden death in subjects with a low ejection fraction.

The underlying mechanism and the level (central or peripheral) at which vitamin C improves cardiovascular autonomic control clearly remain unknown. An extremely likely mechanism is one that involves a vitamin-C-induced improvement in NO bioavailability.

References

[1] Willich SN, Maclure M, Mittleman M, Arntz HR, Muller JE. Sudden cardiac death. Support for a role of triggering in causation. *Circulation.* 1993;87(5):1442-50.

[2] Airaksinen KE Autonomic mechanisms and sudden death after abrupt coronary occlusion. *Ann Med.* 1999;31(4):240-5.

[3] Cohn JN, Levine TB, Olivari MT, Garberg V, Lura D, Francis GS, Simon AB, Rector T. Plasma norepinephrine as a guide to prognosis in patients with chronic congestive heart failure. *N Eng J Med* 1984;311(13):819-823.

[4] La Rovere MT, Bigger JT Jr, Marcus FI, Mortara A, Schwartz PJ. Baroreflex sensitivity and heart-rate variability in prediction of total cardiac mortality after myocardial infarction. ATRAMI (Autonomic Tone and Reflexes After Myocardial Infarction) Investigators. *Lancet* 1998; 351(9101):478-84.

[5] Guzzetti S, La Rovere MT, Pinna GD, Maestri R, Borroni E, Porta A, Mortara A, Malliani A. Different spectral components of 24 h heart rate variability are related to different modes of death in chronic heart failure. *Eur Heart J* 2005; 26(4):357-62.

[6] La Rovere MT, Pinna GD, Maestri R, Mortara A, Capomolla S, Febo O, Ferrari R, Franchini M, Gemmi M, Opasich C, Riccardi PG, Traversi E, Corbelli F. Short-term heart rate variability strongly predicts sudden cardiac death in chronic heart failure patients. *Circulation* 2003;107:565-570.

[7] Ellison KE, Gandhi G. Optimising the use of beta-adrenoceptor antagonists in coronary artery disease. *Drugs.* 2005;65(6):787-97

[8] Piccirillo G, Leonetti Luparini R, Celli V, Moisè A, Lionetti M, Marigliano V, Cacciafesta M. Effects of Carvedilol on heart rate and blood pressure variability in subjects with chronic heart failure. *Am J Cardiol* 2000;86:1392-1395.

[9] Drexler E. Endotelial dysfunction: clinical implication. *Prog Cardiovasc Dis.* 1997; 39(4):287-324.

[10] Chowdhary S, Townend JN. Role of nitric oxide in the regulation of cardiovascular autonomic control. *Clin Sci* 1999 Jul;97(1):5-17.

[11] Sartori C, Lepori M, Scherrer U. Interaction between nitric oxide and the cholinergic and sympathetic nervous system in cardiovascular control in humans. *Pharmacol Ther.* 2005; 106(2):209-20.

[12] Furchgott R.F, Zawadzki J.V. The obligatory role of endothelial cells in the relaxation of arterial smooth muscle by acetylcholine. *Nature* 1980;288:373-376.

[13] Società italiana di cardiologia. L'endotelio, fisiopatologia e valore clinico. Cap 1, pag. 5-19: Delli Gatti C, Cosentino F, Luscher T. Il monossido di azoto. Ed: Salvetti A, Taddei S. 2002.

[14] Behrendt D, Ganz P. Endothelial function: from vascular biology to clinical applications. *Am J Cardiol* 2002; 90: 40L-48L.

[15] Davignon J, Ganz P. Role of endothelial dysfunction in atherosclerosis. *Circulation* 2004;109(suppl. III):27-32.

[16] Landmesser U, Hornig B, Drexler H. Endothelial function: a critical determinant in atherosclerosis? *Circulation* 2004; 109(suppl.II): 27-33.

[17] Massion P.B, Dessy C, Desjardins F, Pelat M et al. Cardiomyocyte-restricted overexpression of endothelial NOS (NOS3) attenuates β adrenergic stimulation and reinforces vagal inhibition of cardiac contraction. *Circulation* 2004; 110(17):2666-2672.

[18] Chowdhary S, Vaile C.J, Fletcher J. et al. Nitric oxide and cardiac autonomic control in humans. *Hypertension* 2000;36:264-269.

[19] Chowdhary S, Nuttall S.L, Coote J.H. et al. L-Arginine augments cardiac vagal control in healthy human subjects. *Hypertension* 2002,39:51-56.

[20] Piccirillo G, Lionetti M, Naso C. et al. Influence of L-arginine and vitamin C on autonomic nervous system in chronic heart failure secondary to ischemic cardiomyopathy. *Am J Cardiol.*2004; 93: 650-654.

[21] Taddei S, Virdis A, Ghiadoni L. et al. Age-related reduction of NO availability and oxidative stress in humans. *Hypertension* 2001,38:274-279.

[22] Mason R.P, Walter M.F, Jacob R.F. Effects of HMG-CoA reductase inhibitors on endothelial function, role of microdomains and oxidative stress. *Circulation* 2004; 109:34-41.

[23] Ulker S, Mc Keown P.P. et al. Vitamins reverse endothelial dysfunction through regulation of eNOS and NADPH oxidase activities. *Hypertension* 2003; 41:534-539.

[24] Erbs S, Gielen S, Linke A et al. Improvement of peripheral endothelial dysfunction by acute vitamin C application: different effects in patients with coronary artery disease, ischemic and dilated cardiomyopathy. *Am Heart J* 2003; 146(2):280-285.

[25] Takase B, Etsuda H, Matsushima Y. et al. Effect of chronic oral supplementation with vitamins on the endothelial function in chronic smokers. *Angiology* 2004; 55(6):653-660.

[26] Ting HH, Timimi FK, Haley EA, Roddy MA. Et al. Vitamin C improves endothelium-dependent vasodilation in forearm resistance vessels of humans with hypercholesterolemia. *Circulation* 1997;95:2617-2622.

[27] Taddei S, Virdis A, Ghiadoni L. et al. Vitamin C improves endothelium-dependent vasodilation by restoring nitric oxide activity in essential hypertension. *Circulation* 1998;97:2222-2229.

[28] Gokce N, Keaney JF Jr, Frei B. et al. Long-term ascorbic acid administration reverses endothelial vasomotor dysfunction in patients with coronary artery disease. *Circulation* 1999;99:3234-3240.

[29] D'Uscio L.V., Milstien S, Richardson D. et al. Long-term vitamin C treatment increases vascular tetrahydrobiopterin levels and nitric oxide synthase activity. *Circ. Res.* 2003;92:88-95.

[30] May J.M. How does ascorbic acid prevent endothelial dysfunction? *Free Radical Biol. And Med.* 2000; 28(9):1421-1429

[31] Heller R, Unbehaun A, Schellenberg B. L-Ascorbic acid potentiates endothelial nitric oxide synthesis via a chemical stabilization of tetrahydrobiopterin. *Journal of biological chemistry* 2002;276:40-47.

[32] Ji Y. Han Y.et al. Inhibition of endothelial nitric oxide generation by LDL is partially prevented by L- -arginine and L--ascorbate. *Atherosclerosis* 2004; 176:345-353.

[33] May J.M, Qu Z. Nitric oxide-induced oxidant stress in endothelial cells: amelioration by ascorbic acid. *Archives of Biochemistry and Biophysics* 2004;429:106-113.

[34] Chowdary S, Marsh A.M, Coote J.H, Townend J.N. Nitric oxide and cardiac muscarinic control in humans. *Hypertension* 2004; 43:1023-1028.

[35] Chowdary S, Townend J.N. Nitric oxide and hypertension: not just an endothelium derived relaxing factor! *J Hum Hypertens* 2001; 15:219-227.

[36] Moham RM, Heaton DA, Danson EJ, Krishnam SP, Channon KM, Paterson DJ. Neuronal nitric oxide synthase gene transfer promotes cardiac gain of function. *Circ Res* 2002;91:1089-1091

[37] Chowdary S, Nuttall S.L, Coote J.H. et al. Nitric oxide and cardiac parasympathetic control in human heart failure. *Cli Sci* 2002; 102:397-402.

[38] Nightingale A.K, Blackman D.J, Field R, Glover N.J. et al. Role of nitric oxide and oxidative stress in baroreceptor dysfunction in patients with chronic heart failure. *Cli Sci* 2003; 104:529-535.

[39] Monahan K.D, Eskurza I, Seals D.R. Ascorbic acid increases cardiovagal baroreflex sensitivity in healthy older men. Am J Physiol 2004; 286: H2113-H2117.

[40] Sander M, Hansen P.G, Victor R.G. Sympathetically mediated hypertension caused by chronic inhibition of nitric oxide. *Hypertension* 1995;26:691-695.

[41] Cunha R.S, Cabral A.M, Vasquez E.C. Evidence that the autonomic nervous system plays a major role in the L-NAME-induced hypertension in conscious rats. *Am J Hypertens* 1993;6:806-809.

[42] Sakuma I, Togashi H, Yoshioka M. et al. N^G-methyl-L-arginine, an inhibitor of L-arginine-derived nitric oxide synthesis, stimulates renal sympathetic nerve activity in vivo. A role for nitric oxide in the central regulation of sympathetic tone? *Circ Res* 1992;70:607-611.

[43] Harada S, Tokunaga S, Momohara M. et al. Inhibition of nitric oxide formation in the nucleus tractus solitarius increases renal sympathetic nerve activity in rabbits. *Circ Res* 1993;72:511-516.

[44] Tseng C.J, Liu H.Y, Lin H.C. et al. Cardiovascular effects of nitric oxide in the brainstem nuclei of rats. *Hypertension* 1996;27:36-42.

[45] Shapoval L.N, Sagach V.F, Pobegailo L.S. Nitric oxide influences ventrolateral medullary mechanism of vasomotor control in the cat. *Neurosci Lett* 1991;137:47-50.

[46] Krukoff T.L, Khalili P. Stress-induced activation of nitric oxide-producing neurons in the rat brain. *J Comp Neurol* 1997;377:509-519.

[47] Hironaga K, Hirooka Y, Matsuo I. et al. Role of endogenous nitric oxide in the brainstem on the rapid adaptation of baroreflex. *Hypertension* 1998;31:27-31.

[48] Di Paola E.D, Vidal M.J, Nistico G. L-Glutamate evokes the release of an endothelium-derived relaxing factor-like substance from the rat nucleus tractus solitarius. *J. Cardiovas. Pharmacol.*1991;17:S269-S272.

[49] Ashley E.A, Sears C.E, Bryant S.M. et al. Cardiac nitric oxide synthase 1 regulates basal and β-adrenergic contractility in murine ventricular myocytes. *Circulation* 2002; 105:3011-3016.

[50] Rabelo F.A.W, Russo E.M, Salgado M.C.O, Coelho E.B. Nonendothelial NO blunts sympathetic response of normotensive rats but not of SHR. *Hypertension* 2001; 38:565-568.

[51] Dobesova Z, Kunes J, Zicha J. The altered balance between sympathetic nervous system and nitric oxide in salt hypertensive Dahl rats: ontogenic and F_2 hybrid studies. *J Hypertens* 2002; 20:945-955.

[52] Dessy C, Saliez J, Ghisdal P, Daneau G. et al. Endothelial β_3-adrenoreceptors mediate nitric oxide-dependent vasorelaxation of coronary microvessels in response to the third-generation β-blocker nebivolol. *Circulation* 2005;112:1198-1205.

[53] Smyth HS, Sleight P, Pickering GW. Reflex regulation of arterial pressure during sleep in man: a quantitative method of assessing cardiac baroreflex sensitivity. *Circ Res.* 1969;24:109-121.

[54] Piccirillo G, V. Di Giuseppe, Nocco M, Lionetti M, Bucca C, Moisè A, Naso C, Tallarico D, Marigliano V, Cacciafesta M. Influence of aging and other cardiovascular risk factors on baroreflex sensitivity. *J Am Ger Soc.* 2001;49:1059-1065.

[55] Piccirillo G, Cacciafesta M, Viola E, Santagada E, Nocco M, Lionetti M, Bucca C, Moisè A, Tarantini S, Marigliano V. Influence of ageing on cardiac baroreflex sensitivity determined noninvasively by power spectral analysis. *Clin Sci.* 2001:100; 267-274.

[56] Task force of the European Society of Cardiology and the North American Society of Pacing and Electrophysiology. Heart rate variability. Standard of Measurements, physiological interpretation and clinical use. *Circulation.* 1996; 93:1043-1065.

[57] Piccirillo G, Nocco M, Moisè A, Lionetti M, Naso C, Di Carlo S, Marigliano V. Influence of vitamin C on baroreflex sensitivity in chronic heart failure. *Hypertension.* 2003;41:1240-1245.

[58] Gribbin B, Pickering GW, Sleight P, Peto R. Effect of age and high blood pressure on baroreflex sensitivity in man. *Circ. Res.* 1971;29:424-431.

[59] Duke PC, Wade JG, Hickey RF, Larson CP. The effects of age on baroreceptor reflex function in man. *Can Anaesth Soc J.* 1976;23:111-124.

[60] Shimada K, Kitazumi T, Ogura H, Sadakane N, Ozawa T. Differences in age-independent effects of pressure on cardiac baroreflex sensitivity between normal and hypertensive subjects. *Clin Sci.* 1986;70:489-494.

[61] James MA, Robinson TG, Panerai RB, Potter JF. Arterial baroreceptor-cardiac reflex sensitivity in the elderly. *Hypertension.* 1996;8:953-960.

[62] Dawson SL, Robinson TG, Youde JH, Martin A, James MA Panerai RB, Potter JF. Older subjects show no age-related decrease in cardiac baroreceptor sensitivity. *Age Aging* 1999;28:347-353.

[63] Spieker LE, Corti R, Binggeli C, Luscher TF, Noll G. Baroreceptor dysfunction induced by nitric oxide synthase inhibition in humans. *J Am Coll Cardiol.* 2000 Jul;36(1):213-8.

[64] Dimmeler S, Zeiher AM.Reactive oxygen species and vascular cell apoptosis in response to angiotensin II and pro-atherosclerotic factors. *Regul Pept.* 2000 Jun 30;90(1-3):19-25.

[65] Mortara A, La Rovere MT, Signorini MG, Pantaleo P, Pinna G, Martinelli L, Ceconi C, Cerutti S, Tavazzi L. Can power spectral analysis of heart rate variability identify a high risk subgroup of congestive heart failure patients with excessive sympathetic activation? A pilot study before and after heart transplantation. *Br Heart J* 1994;71:422-430.

[66] Guzzetti S, Cogliati C, Turiel M, Pantaleo P, Pinna G, Martinelli L, Ceconi C, Cerutti S, Tavazzi L. Sympathetic predominance followed by functional denervation in progression of chronic heart failure. *Eur Heart J* 1995;16:1100-1107.

[67] Van de Borne P, Montano N, Pagani M, Oren R, Somers VK. Absence of low-frequency variability of sympathetic nerve activity in severe heart failure. *Circulation* 1997;95:1449-1454.

In: Frontiers in Antioxidants Research
Editor: Harold V. Panglossi, pp. 103-131
ISBN 1-60021-273-5

Chapter 5

HEMORHEOLOGICAL EFFECTS OF ANTIOXIDANT COMPLEX COMPRISING DIHYDROQUERCETIN AND ASCORBIC ACID (ASCOVERTIN) – A NEW ASPECT OF ANTIOXIDANTS APPLICATION

Mark B. Plotnikov*[1]*, Oleg I. Aliev*[1]*,
***Nonna A. Tyukavkina*[2] *and Tatyana M. Plotnikova*[3]**
[1]Laboratory of Blood Circulation Pharmacology, Institution for Pharmacology, Scientific Center of Russian Academy of Medical Sciences, Tomsk, Russia
[2]Department of Organic Chemistry, I.M. Sechenov Moscow Medical Academy, Moscow, Russia
[3]Department of Pharmacology, Siberian Medical University, Tomsk, Russia

ABSTRACT

Cardiovascular diseases develop on the background of the marked oxidative stress, erythrocytes being an important “target” for reactive oxygen species. The effect of reactive oxygen species on erythrocytes causes a pathological increase in their aggregation and a decrease in deformability. The disturbance of the rheological properties of erythrocytes induced by reactive oxygen species contributes to the formation of the high blood viscosity syndrome developing in cardiovascular diseases.

During in vitro experiments under blood hyperviscosity model conditions there has been established a hemorheological effect of dihydroquercetin (a bioflavonoid isolated from larch wood) and ascorbic acid. This effect has manifested itself by reduction in hyperaggregation of erythrocytes and improvement in their deformability. A synergistic effect of a combination of dehydroquercetin and ascorbic acid has been demonstrated, it being more pronounced than individual effects of the antioxidants studied. Under the same conditions optimal ratio of antioxidant concentrations in the compound have been selected.

In experiments on spontaneously hypertensive rats with high blood viscosity syndrome, the use of the antioxidant complex (AOC) comprising dihydroquercetin and ascorbic acid (20 mg/kg and 50 mg/kg, respectively) during 14 days improved the reduced erythrocytes deformability and decreased their hyperaggregation. It was shown that the mechanism due to which the AOC had a beneficial effect on rheological properties of erythrocytes was mediated by its action on the morphofunctional state of these cells. The AOC decreased a high level of lysophospholipids in erythrocyte membranes in the spontaneously hypertensive rats, promoted preservation of the normal phospholipid spectrum and phospholipid balance in the external and internal layers of erythrocyte membranes. The capacity of the AOC to preserve the lipid composition of erythrocyte membranes provided an increase in the number of discocytes and a decrease in pathological shapes of erythrocytes in their population.

A clinical study of the AOC involved patients suffering essential hypertension grades I–II with manifestation of high blood viscosity syndrome. During 21 days the patients received Ascovertin (20 mg dihydroquercetin and 50 mg ascorbic acid in a tablet) 3 times a day in addition to a standard antihypertensive therapy. A group of clinically healthy people (10 volunteers) was used as normotensive control. By day 21 of treatment Ascovertin application resulted in decreased contents of lipid peroxidation products in erythrocyte membranes and in blood plasma. In this period the patients with arterial hypertension experienced abatement of high blood viscosity syndrome manifestations mainly because of a beneficial effect of the preparation on the cellular rheological indices, i.e. improvement in deformability of erythrocytes and a decrease in their aggregation. A correlation between a decrease in the amount of conjugated dienes in erythrocyte membranes and improvement of erythrocyte deformability was established. An integral effect of the hemorheological therapy with Ascovertin was a reduction in blood viscosity resulting in a moderate decrease of systolic and diastolic arterial blood pressure and of peripheral resistance. In addition, the patients demonstrated a decrease in manifestation of discirculatory encephalopathy clinical signs and improvement in cognitive and neurodynamic functions.

INTRODUCTION

Atherosclerosis, diabetes, cardiovascular diseases occur against the background of the marked oxidative stress [2, 37, 44, 51, 61, 76]. In the same clinical situations hemorheological disorders resulting in the development of high blood viscosity syndrome are observed; moreover, erythrocytes are directly involved in the process: their aggregation increases and deformability decreases [16, 19, 27, 28, 29, 65, 112]. Oxidative modification of erythrocyte membranes in this pathology is not the only damaging mechanism [113], however there is abundant evidence of the association between the disturbance of morphofunctional properties of erythrocytes and activation of lipid peroxidation processes [5, 21, 69, 114, 117].

The data on the ability of antioxidants and antihypoxants to prevent a negative effect of lipid peroxidation processes on rheology functions of erythrocytes [40, 69, 82, 83] spurred us on to the search of promising hemorheological preparations among natural compounds having antioxidative activity. For this purpose extracts and individual substances of Siberian and Far Eastern plants were studied, among which we selected two promising groups: flavonoid-containing and ecdysteroid-containing plants [80, 81]. Of the extracts and individual substances studied the most pronounced activity was shown by dihydroquercetin isolated from Siberian larch wood (*Larix sibirica* Ledeb.) [110], dihydroquercetin being related to a group of flavanones. Dihydroquercetin is known also as taxifolin.

A great deal of reports summarized in a number of substantial reviews [15, 52, 53, 67, 74, 89, 90, 99] was devoted to the study of flavonoid antioxidant activity. Thus, it was demonstrated that dihydroquercetin possesses antioxidant properties in a variety of model systems for oxidation. It slows the oxidation of ethylbenzene initiated by azo-bis-isobutyronitrile [118]. It also slows the free radical oxidation of liposomes from egg phospholipids, induced with the help of the Fe^{2+}/ascorbate system [104], or photosensitization by hematoporphyrin derivatives [56]. Antioxidant properties of dihydroquercetin are demonstrated on other model systems as well [33, 44, 50, 84, 85]. A number of studies are concerned with investigating antioxidant properties of dihydroquercetin using models of oxidative stress *in vivo*. Dihydroquercetin was shown to slow the development of free radical oxidation of lipids in the plasma and in the liver of mice after whole body irradiation [105] and in rats after tetrachloromethane poisoning [106]. In rats receiving dihydroquercetin (130 mg/kg daily for 2 weeks) *ex vivo* resistance of the liver microsomes to induction of lipid peroxidation increased. The basis for antioxidant properties of dihydroquercetin is its ability to function as a free radical scavenger and a chelator of metal with variable valency [8, 84].

I. Evaluation of the Effect of Dihydroquercetin and Ascorbic Acid on Cell Rheology Indices in Vitro

At stage I of the *in vitro* study on a blood hyperviscosity model, an evaluation of dihydroquercetin effect on cell rheology indices – erythrocyte aggregation and deformability – was carried out. For a possible enhancement of hemorheological activity of dihydroquercetin we used ascorbic acid, the property of which to reduce the oxidized forms of flavonoids and to potentiate their pharmacologic effects is well known [8, 67].

The objectives of this stage were (1) to reveal a possible effect of dihydroquercetin and ascorbic acid on rheology properties of erythrocytes, (2) to determine the kind of interaction between dihydroquercetin and ascorbic acid and (3) to choose an optimal concentration of the given antioxidants, which is necessary for achieving a maximum hemorheological effect of the antioxidant complex (AOC).

The model of blood hyperviscosity *in vitro* was reproduced by incubation of the blood at 42.5 °C [39]. The prominence of shifts in some hemorheological indices under these conditions are comparable with changes occurring in a number of pathological conditions, such as diabetes, disturbances of the cerebral and coronary blood circulation, arterial hypertension [22, 28, 31, 36, 102, 108, 112]. This enables to use this model for choosing drugs possessing hemorheological properties. To evaluate the prominence of hemorheological effects of the investigated compounds, at the stage of screening we used the standardized *Ginkgo biloba* extract containing flavone glycosides, ginkgolides, as a reference drug. The choice of the drug of comparison was conditioned by the ability of the extract to improve rheological properties of blood and microcirculation, as well as to protect cell membranes from damage mediated by the processes of lipid peroxidation [59, 75].

For the experiments we used arterial blood collected from anaesthetized rats through catheter in the carotid artery. The blood was stabilized by 3.8% solution of sodium citrate in the ratio 9:1. Erythrocyte aggregation was evaluated by selectrometric technique using a microcolorimeter MKMF-2 (Russia) [79]. To assess erythrocyte aggregation we determined aggregation half-period $T_{1/2}$, the time over which the value of the photometric signal is reduced by half; a decrease in the value of $T_{1/2}$ reflects an increase in erythrocyte aggregation. Erythrocyte deformability was measured by laser ektacytometry; the degree of deformability was evaluated by the index of erythrocyte deformability (IED) [9]. The preparations were added to the blood 10 min before the incubation.

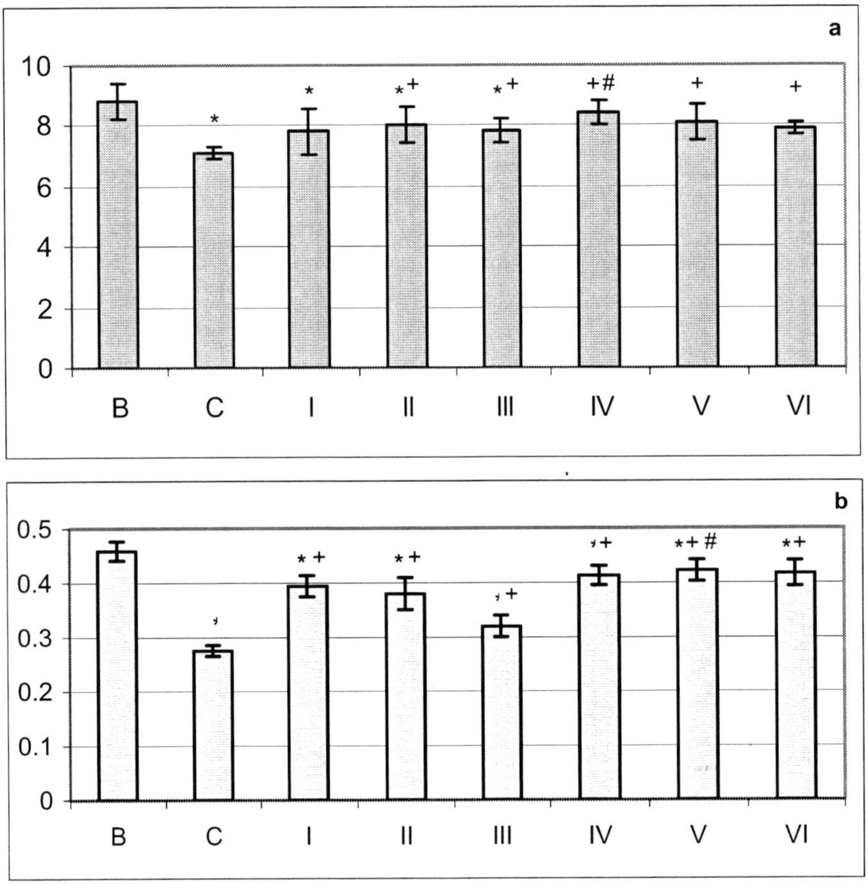

Figure 1. The effect of *Ginkgo biloba* extract, dihydroquercetin, ascorbic acid, and a combination of dihydroquercetin and ascorbic acid in various concentrations on the indices of cell rheology. a – erythrocyte aggregation half-period (s), b – index of erythrocyte deformability at the shear rate 890 s^{-1} (relative units). B – baseline values, C – control values (after 1-hour incubation of the blood at 42.5 °C), I – *Ginkgo biloba* extract, II – dihydroquercetin, III – ascorbic acid, IV, V, and VI – a combination of dihydroquercetin and ascorbic acid in the ratio 1:1, 1:2, and 1:3, respectively. * – $p<0.05$ compared to baseline value; + – $p<0.05$ compared to control; # – $p<0.05$ compared to *Ginkgo biloba* extract.

In control experiments a thermal exposure of the blood for 1 hour resulted in an increase in erythrocyte aggregation (by 20%) and a decrease in the degree of erythrocyte deformability (by 40%) (Figure 1). The *Ginkgo biloba* extract in a concentration $1{\cdot}10^{-5}$ g/ml enhanced the erythrocyte deformability index (by 26%) compared with the control, but an antiaggregant effect of the preparation with regard to erythrocytes did not reach the significant level. Dihydroquercetin of this concentration significantly limited both erythrocyte aggregation (by 12%) and deformability reduction (by 22%). Therefore, under the conditions used for this blood hyperviscosity model, the effects of dihydroquercetin and *Ginkgo biloba* extract were comparable.

Ascorbic acid in the concentration $1 \cdot 10^{-5}$ g/ml rendered a slight but significant effect on the cell rheology indices: it reduced erythrocyte aggregation and increased the deformability of erythrocytes (Figure 1). The AOC (dihydroquercetin and ascorbic acid in the ratio 1:1–1:3 and concentration $1 \cdot 10^{-5}$g/ml, respectively) abated the aggregation of erythrocytes (by 10–16%) and enhanced their deformability (by 27–30%). The AOC hemorheological effect surpassed in intensity the efficacy of separate components.

By its effect on the studied hemorheological parameters, the AOC (dihydroquercetin and ascorbic acid in the ratio 1:1 and 1:2) exceeded the effect of the drug of comparison – *Ginkgo biloba* extract (Figure 1).

Thus we were the first to establish hemorheological activity of dihydroquercetin and to demonstrate synergism between dihydroquercetin and ascorbic acid in their action on the cell rheological parameters – erythrocyte aggregation and deformability. Subsequently, in a depth study of the AOC hemorheological activity using the model of high blood viscosity syndrome *in vivo* and in the investigation of its action mechanism we used dihydroquercetin and ascorbic acid in doses of 20 and 50 mg/kg, respectively, i.e., their ratio (1:2.5) was within the effectiveness range.

II. A Study of Hemorheological Effects of the Antioxidant Complex on the Model of High Blood Viscosity in Rats with Arterial Hypertension

Blood viscosity is an integral, registered *ex vivo*, rheological index, the values of which are the function of shear rate [28, 101]. Blood viscosity is defined by the level of macrorheological indices: volume part concentration of blood cells (hematocrit), plasma viscosity (depends on the type and concentration of proteins) and parameters of cell rheology, i.e. erythrocyte deformability (depends on viscosity of membrane and viscosity of internal contents) and erythrocyte aggregation [19, 101]. Pathologic changes in these factors form a so-called "high blood viscosity syndrome" [28] due to (1) increased hematocrit, (2) increased plasma viscosity (mainly because the plasma contents of fibrinogen and other proteins with a large molecular weight grow), (3) enhanced erythrocyte aggregation, and (4) reduced erythrocyte deformability (at the expense of an increase in viscosity of erythrocyte contents and/or viscosity of cell membranes) [101].

We studied the effect of the AOC including dihydroquercetin and ascorbic acid on the viscosity of whole blood and major hemorheological parameters (plasma viscosity, hematocrit value, total blood plasma fibrinogen and cell rheology indices – erythrocyte aggregation and deformability) in spontaneously hypertensive rats (SHR line). The rats of this line are considered to be the most adequate model of essential hypertension in humans [42]. Wistar rats were used as normotensive control.

For blood sampling the common carotid artery was isolated and catheterized in animals under anesthetic (diethyl either). The blood was stabilized with 3.8%-sodium citrate solution in the ratio 9:1. The whole blood viscosity and the plasma viscosity were determined with the help of rotation viscometer AKR-2 (Russia). The hematocrit was measured by centrifuging of whole blood in glass capillary tubes (650 g, 20 min). The level of total fibrinogen in plasma was measured with a hemocoagulometer Cormey KG–4 (Poland) using a Fibrinogen Kit. The methods of studying cell rheology indices are shown above. The membrane charge of erythrocytes was assessed by means of determination of erythrocyte electrophoretic mobility values [5]. The latter enabled us to judge the amount of the erythrocyte surface charge – zeta potential and therefore their functional properties, particularly the processes of reversible spontaneous aggregate formation [54].

The SHR rats in the experiment AOC group (20 mg/kg dihydroquercetin and 50 mg/kg ascorbic acid) were daily administered intragastrically 1% starch mucilage containing active substances in a suspension form for 14 days. The control SHR rats received the same amount of 1% starch mucilage.

As compared with Wistar rats, in the SHR rats we observed a moderate increase in the hematocrit and in the plasma viscosity (by 5% and 15%, respectively; $0.05<p<0.1$). A marked rise in plasma fibrinogen (1.6 times greater) was noted (Table 1). We also saw an increase (by 44%) in erythrocyte aggregation, which probably may be connected with not only enhancement of fibrinogen content in the SHR rats plasma, but with significantly reduced (by 52%) electrophoretic mobility of erythrocytes. In spontaneously hypertensive rats, viscoelastic properties of erythrocytes were also disturbed, to which testified a decrease in their deformability index (by 24%) in comparison with the index values in Wistar rats.

A correlation analysis of hemorheological indices in spontaneously hypertensive rats showed a significant link between blood viscosity and half-period of erythrocyte aggregation ($r = -0.71$; $p<0.05$), blood viscosity and fibrinogen contents in plasma ($r = 0.72$; $p<0.05$). In its turn, an increase of plasma fibrinogen contents is interrelated with a decrease in half-period of erythrocyte aggregation ($r = -0.85$; $p<0.01$).

Therefore a hemorheological status in SHR rats may be considered to be an adequate model of high blood viscosity syndrome, since in these animals, as compared with Wistar rats, the shifts of all main rheological indices are noted [78]. Moreover these changes in their trend correspond to clinical findings obtained in studying the blood in patients with arterial hypertension [12, 22, 57, 62, 65, 109, 111].

The introduction of the AOC as a course of treatment did not reflect on the macrorheological indices values, namely, plasma viscosity and hematocrit, but manifested itself as moderate but significant reduction of fibrinogen contents in blood plasma (Table 1). Pronounced shifts were seen in cell rheology indices in rats in the experimental group. Under the influence of the AOC a decrease in erythrocyte aggregation occurred, which showed itself as an elevation of $T_{1/2}$ (by 20%). Besides the reduction of the fibrinogen level in the blood, probably, an influence of the AOC on zeta-potential of erythrocytes may also significantly contribute to a decrease in erythrocyte aggregation. So, the value of electrophoretic mobility in the animals receiving the drug was 0.43 ± 0.03 $\mu m \cdot s^{-1} \cdot cm \cdot B^{-1}$, i.e., 1.5 times as much as that in the controls (0.28±0.02 μm·s^{-1}·sm·B^{-1}) but was less than in the Wistar rats (0.59±0.04 μm·s^{-1}·sm·B^{-1}).

Table 1. The effect of AOC on blood viscosity at shear rate 10 s^{-1} (BV_{10}, mPa·s), plasma viscosity (PV, mPa·s), hematocrit (Ht, %), blood plasma fibrinogen (Fbg, mg%), half-period of erythrocyte aggregation ($T_{1/2}$, s), erythrocyte deformability index at shear rate 890 s^{-1} (EDI_{890}, relative units) in rats with arterial hypertension (means±SEM)

Groups of animals		BV_{10}	PV	Ht	Fbg	$T_{1/2}$	EDI_{890}
Wistar		5.8±0.2	1.3±0.1	45±1	180±62	9.7±0.7	0.369±0.012
SHR	Control	8.5±0.3*	1.5±0.1	47±1	327±14*	5.4±0.2*	0.277±0.008*
	AOC	7.6±0.2^{*+}	1.4±0.1	47±1	271±14^{*+}	6.5±0.1^{*+}	0.365±0.014^{*+}

$^{*}p<0.05$ compared to values in Wistar rats; $^{+}p<0.05$ compared to controls.

It is evident that a positive effect of the AOC on erythrocyte aggregation manifested itself in a reduction of blood viscosity at a low shear rate (10 s^{-1}) where the main factor determining viscous properties of blood is erythrocyte aggregation [19]. We should specially point out the marked influence of the AOC on erythrocyte deformability, which was established by us. It made itself evident in a significant increase of erythrocyte deformability index and in the fact that it approached the level of this index in Wistar normotensive rats.

Thus the introduction of the AOC including dihydroquercetin and ascorbic acid as a course of treatment can decrease the manifestation acuty of high blood viscosity syndrome in spontaneously hypertensive rats mainly due to the effect on the factors of cell rheology (aggregation and deformability of erythrocytes), as well as because of the reduction in the concentration of blood plasma fibrinogen, the important macrorheological factor.

The evident positive effect of the AOC on the indices of cell rheology impelled us to undertake an in-depth study of the effect of the AOC on the structural and metabolic state of erythrocytes using arterial hypertension model.

III. The Effect of an Antioxidant Complex on Shape of Erythrocytes and Composition of Erythrocyte Membrane in Spontaneously Hypertensive Rats

According to the results of the *in vitro* and *in vivo* investigations of all hemorheological indices the most stable and pronounced effect was exhibited by the antioxidant complex on deformability of erythrocytes.

Deformability of erythrocytes is a relatively general term that describes the ability of red blood cells to change their shape in response to a deforming force [19]. The ability of erythrocytes to deform is a function of their structural-functional organization: the shape of the cells, viscoelastic properties of membranes, surface area to volume ratio (the higher the ratio, the greater is the degree of deformation which erythrocytes may undergo) and intercellular factors (degree of hemoglobin oxidation and the content of ATP and Ca^{2+} in cytoplasm) [10, 43, 92].

The major function of such highly specialized cell as erythrocyte is oxygen transport. The successful implementation of blood gas transport function is effected by two interrelated properties of the red blood cell: its ability to deform and the optimal biconcave discoid shape (discocyte or normocyte). The discocyte has a high surface area to volume ratio with each hemoglobin molecule being close to the surface of the cell (not farther than 1 μm) which facilitates maximally rapid gas exchange [18]. The erythrocyte has in its discoid shape a maximum "reserve" area for deformation that enables it to travel through capillary blood vessels with a diameter less than the size of the cell [10, 88]. Since erythrocytes are quantitatively predominant cell elements, blood viscosity essentially depends on their properties and, above all, their deformability [28].

Only discocytes can easily change their shape even when acted upon by a slight force. They tend to elongate assuming a "funnel-like" shape which enables them to pass through the capillaries. As erythrocytes age or are exposed to various pathologic factors, the cell shapes become transformed from a disk to a sphere via echinocytosis or stomatocytosis. Subsequently erythrocytes transform to spheroechinocytes, spherostomatocytes and finally to spherocytes, the latter structure being very rigid and nondeformable, and usually preceding destruction of the cell [87]. It has been shown that increased content in the blood of stomatocytes leads to disturbed microcirculation while increased amount of echinocytes can cause impaired blood flow in large vessels due to higher blood viscosity [87].

In experiments on SHR rats an effect of the AOC on an erythrocyte shape in arterial hypertension was studied. The investigation of erythrocyte morphology peculiarities was conducted by means of scanning electron microscopy. Erythrocytes were related to different types in accordance with the classification suggested by G.I. Kozinets and S.A. Simovart [60].

In Wistar rats the bulk of erythrocytes in peripheral blood was represented by discocytes (85%). The content of transitional shapes did not exceed 13 percent while the proportion of prehemolytic and degenerative shapes was minimal (Table 2, Figure 2). The content of discocytes in peripheral blood of SHR rats showed a significant decrease down to 80.60±0.24% versus Wistar rats. The proportion of transitional shapes showed a statistically significant increase (up to 15.21±0.10%) due to an increased number of ellipsoid erythrocytes, flat disk-shaped erythrocytes and discocytes with processes and crests. The content of erythrocytes with other morphological shapes relating to transitional shapes was not significantly increased. The increase in the proportion of erythrocytes of transitional shape is not viewed as a severe pathologic change. These cells retain the common discoid structure and under favorable conditions may revert to discocytes [60]. It may well be that transitional shapes provide a kind of reserve which can be mobilized, pharmacological means included, to yield greater number of discocytes.

Hypertensive rats exhibited a substantially higher proportion of irreversibly altered erythrocytes of both prehemolytic and degenerative shapes (Table 2, Figure 2). The number of prehemolytic shapes increased in comparison with Wistar rats by a factor of 1.8 and reached 2.99±0.14%. Among prehemolytic shapes of cells predominant were dome-shaped erythrocytes while erythrocytes resembling a flat ball were very few in number. The number of degenerative erythrocytes constituted 1.21±0.07% which was 2.1 times higher than in Wistar rats. These are cells of varying shape with clear signs of membrane destruction and their number tends to increase as destructive processes become activated in the body. Considering the fact that shape-altered erythrocytes are less valuable than discocytes in terms of microcirculation, oxygen transport function and capacity to deformation, an increase in their number is an adverse sign [71].

Table 2. Effect of AOC on morphological shapes of erythrocytes (% of total count) in SHR rats

Morphological shapes of erythrocytes		Wistar rats	SHR	
			Control	AOC
Discocytes		85.03±0.15	80.53±0.24*	86.53±1.02^{+}
Transitional shapes	Ellipses	0.33±0.04	0.86±0.04*	0.18±0.08^{+}
	Flat discs	5.18±0.19	6.04±0.13*	4.98±0.34^{+}
	Discocytes with processes	4.97±0.12	5.60±0.18*	4.53±0.12^{+}
	Discocytes with crests	1.81±0.07	2.29±0.12*	1.80±0.15^{+}
	Discocytes with multiple processes	0.42±0.03	0.39±0.04	0.05±0.03^{*+}
	Mulberry-like red cells	0.05±0.02	0.03±0.02	0.08±0.06
	Total	12.76±0.12	15.21±0.10*	11.60±0.51^{+}
Prehemolytic shapes	Dome-shaped erythrocytes	0.55±0.07	1.54±0.10*	0.83±0.37
	Spherical erythrocytes	0.71±0.06	0.95±0.03*	0.53±0.08^{+}
	Erythrocytes in form of flat ball	0.36±0.06	0.50±0.03*	0.28±0.09^{+}
	Total	1.62±0.10	2.99±0.14*	1.63±0.05^{+}
Degenerative shapes		0.56±0.07	1.21±0.07*	0.25±0.05^{+}

* $p<0.05$ compared to values in Wistar rats; $^{+}$ $p<0.05$ compared to controls.

A course treatment of SHR rats with AOC had a positive effect on the quantitative relationship between erythrocyte morphological shapes (Table 2, Figure 2). The discocyte count showed a significant increase (up to 86.52±1.02%) as compared to the control group and did not differ.from the indices of Wistar rats. Among transitional shape erythrocytes the proportion of ellipsoids, flat discs, discocytes with processes and discocytes with crests on their surface was significantly less than in the control group and showed values similar to those in normotensive rats. The SHR rats treated with AOC had a drastic decrease (8.4 times) in the number of discocytes with multiple processes. The drug also had the effect of reducing the fraction of prehemolytic shapes of erythrocytes to the level of Wistar rats. The reduction was due to a decrease in the number of spherical erythrocytes and cells resembling flat ball. Also there was a marked decrease in the number of degeneratively altered erythrocytes (down to 0.25±0.05%), which is statistically significantly less compared to both control and normotensive rats.

The pronounced effect of AOC on the structure of erythrocyte population in spontaneously hypertensive rats correlates with data obtained when investigating its hemorheological effect: in rats of this group the drug was found to improve the deformability of erythrocytes and eliminate their hyperaggregation.

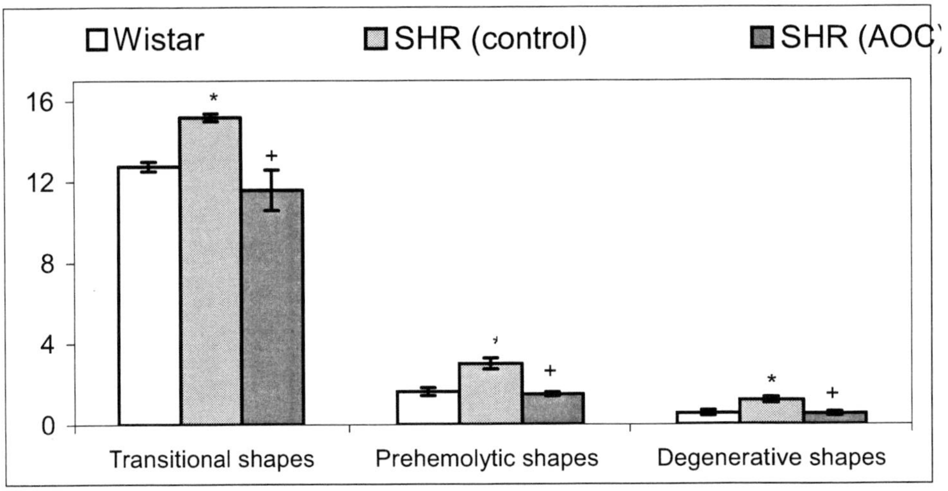

Figure 2. The effect of AOC on the number of abnormal shapes of erythrocytes (%) in spontaneously hypertensive rats. * – $p<0.05$ compared to values in Wistar rats; + – $p<0.05$ compared to controls.

Another important factor that helps secure an optimal for deformation shape of erythrocytes is the viscoelastic properties of their membranes. This is evidenced by the fact that not only erythrocytes can assume a disk shape but also ghosts, that is, erythrocytes devoid of their intercellular content [18]. A balanced lipid and protein composition of membrane components allows the erythrocyte to maintain its biconcave disk shape [41, 64]. The impairment in erythrocyte shape and deformability occurring as a result of various diseases may be precipitated by a variety of factors including changes in composition and structure of membrane components [41]. It has been found that it is lipid components of cell membranes (mainly phospholipids and cholesterol) that determine their fluidity or microviscosity [18].

To study the lipid composition of the membranes using the method developed by J.T. Dodge et al. [32] ghosts of erythrocytes were obtained. In erythrocyte ghost suspension the amount of protein was determined with microbiuret test. The lipid extract was produced by the method given by J. Folch et al. [38]. The total lipid content was estimated in the lipid extract by the reaction with phosphovanillic reagent and phospholipids using the method developed by A.A. Pentiuk et al. [73]. The content of separate phospholipid fractions was evaluated after their separation by thin-layer chromatography [11].

The foregoing changes in erythrocyte surface architectonics in hypertensive rats were accompanied by a pronounced shift in the lipid composition of red cell membranes (Table 3, Figure 3). A significant decrease in the content of lipids in hemoglobin free ghosts of erythrocytes of up to 1.294±0.042 mg/mg protein was observed in SHR rats. The total amount of phospholipids was 0.587±0.09 mg/mg protein, a 39 percent decrease over corresponding indices in normotensive rats. Among the phospholipids the maximum decrease was seen in comparison with normotensive rats in the content of phosphatidylcholine (down to 0.110±0.011 mg/mg protein) and sphingomyelin (down to 0.067±0.004 mg/mg protein). The observed decrease in the amount of phosphatidylethanolamine and phosphatidylserine did not reach the level of statistical significance. The content of the lysophospholipid fraction in red cell membranes of hypertensive rats was 0.049±0.003 mg/mg protein. The varying degrees of change in the contents of individual phospholipid fractions led to a pronounced shift in their ratio. The proportion of phosphatidylethanolamine and phosphatidylserine showed a maximum increase of up to 30±2% and 31±1%, respectively. The percentage of phosphatidylcholine showed a marked decrease (down to 20±1%) whereas that of sphingomyelin despite a reduction in its content remained unchanged (11±1%).

The distribution of phospholipids in the erythrocyte membrane shows an asymmetric pattern [18, 116]. Phosphatidylcholine and sphingomyelin which are the choline-containing lipids are concentrated in the outer layer of erythrocyte membrane while phosphatidylserine and phosphatidylethanolamine which are essentially lipids containing a free amino acid group are concentrated largely in the inner monolayer. Maintaining a definite relationship between phospholipid fractions is an important precondition for normal functioning of erythrocytes. Disruption of membrane lipid bilayer compromises the cell's ability to regulate ionic and antioxidant homeostasis, thereby effecting a change in cell metabolism and irreversible impairment in structural and functional status of erythrocytes [7]. A significant reduction in membranes of the amount of phosphatidylcholine and sphingomyelin which are concentrated in the outer membrane layer and a negligible reduction in the content of inner layer phospholipids – phosphatidylethanolamine and phosphatidylserine – causes a reduction in the surface area of outer lipid monolayer relative to the inner layer which may be important reason for the above change in erythrocyte morphology. Activation of lipid peroxidation provides a mechanism whereby asymmetrical distribution of phospholipids in erythrocyte membrane monolayers can be disrupted [4].

Enhanced lipid peroxidation triggers many processes in the cell which ultimately cause disturbance in erythrocyte structure and function [14, 20 48]. Lipid peroxidation causes a dramatic decrease in the amount of polyunsaturated fatty acids which determine the fluidity of the lipid bilayer. Diffusion of a portion of phospholipids from the interior of the membrane to the surface layer and their reorientation toward the aqueous phase induce the change in erythrocyte surface and shape [14, 96].

Activation of lipid peroxidation in erythrocyte membranes renders them more permeable to penetration of phospholipases into membrane lipid phase which induces the activation of phospholipolysis [68]. Enhanced activity of phospholipases induces hydrolysis of phospholipids while high-polar compounds such as lysophospholipids and free fatty acids may cause shape transformation of discocytes toward echinocytes or stomatocytes [17, 70].

In our studies the absolute quantity of lysophospholipids in spontaneously hypertensive rats did not significantly exceed a similar index for Wistar rats, however, against a background of an overall reduction in the phospholipid fraction their percentage in total number of phospholipids showed a two-fold increase. The accumulation of lysophospholipids in the outer layer of erythrocyte membranes may result in increased erythrocyte aggregation [72].

The course administration of AOC in rats with arterial hypertension was shown to limit disturbances in the composition of the lipid spectrum of erythrocyte membranes (Table 3, Figure 3). There was observed an increase in the quantity of lipids of up to 1.685±0.056 mg/mg protein which statistically significantly exceeds the comparable value in the control group. Total number of phospholipids reliably increased up to 0.769±0.067 mg/mg protein compared to controls. The amount of phosphatidylethanolamine and phosphatidylcholine in hypertensive rats treated with AOC compared to indices of the control animals showed no significant change. The content of phosphatidylserine and sphingomyelin made up

0.241±0.012 mg/mg protein and 0.116±0.010 mg/mg protein, respectively, which was significantly higher than in the control group and did not differ from indices in normotensive rats. During the course administration of AOC a significant decrease was observed in the amount of lysophospholipids (down to 0.029±0.004 mg/mg protein) in hypertensive rats. The animals treated with AOC were found to have a higher sphingomyelin fraction and a twice as low lysophospholipid fraction compared to control rats with percentage of lysophospholipids in treated SHR rats being similar to that of Wistar rats.

Table 3. The effect of AOC on the content in erythrocyte membranes of protein (mg/ml suspension of erythrocyte membranes), total lipids (mg/mg protein), total phospholipids and separate phospholipid fractions (mg/mg protein) in SHR rats

Indices	Wistar	SHR	
		Control	AOC
Protein	4.14±0.49	4.00±0.58	4.86±0.51
Total lipids	1.968±0.104	1.294±0.042*	1.685±0.056+
Total phospholipids	0.960±0.050	0.587±0.029*	0.769±0.067+
Phosphatidylethanolamine	0.226±0.024	0.180±0.018	0.230±0.019
Phosphatidylserine	0.231±0.015	0.181±0.017	0.241±0.012+
Phosphatidylcholine	0.354±0.020	0.110±0.018*	0.152±0.021+
Sphingomyelin	0.110±0.008	0.067±0.004*	0.116±0.010+
Lysophospholipids	0.039±0.002	0.049±0.004*	0.029±0.004+

* – $p<0.05$ compared to values in Wistar rats; + – $p<0.05$ compared to controls.

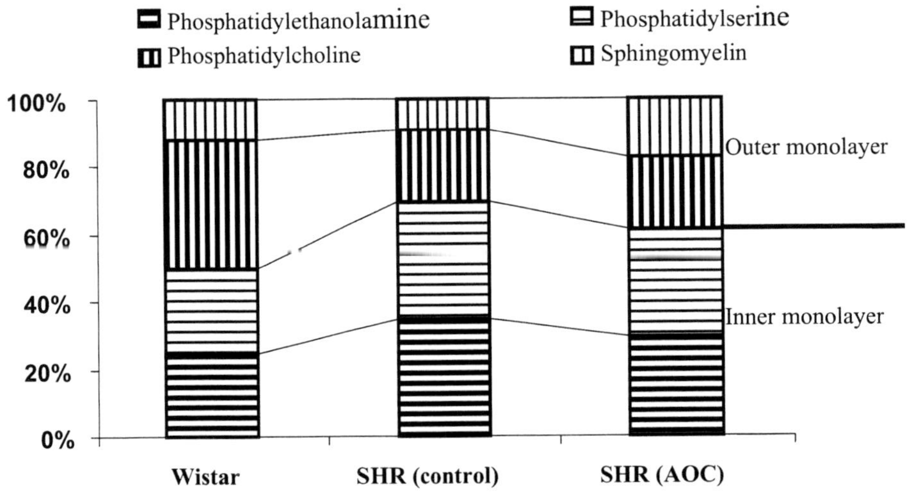

Figure 3. The effect of course administration of AOC on ratio of phospholipids in the inner (phosphatidylethanolamine and phosphatidylserine) and outer (phosphatidylcholine and sphingomyelin) layers of erythrocyte membrane in SHR rats.

IV. A STUDY OF THE EFFICACY OF ASCOVERTIN TREATMENT IN PATIENTS WITH ESSENTIAL ARTERIAL HYPERTENSION

Recent years have seen greater attention being devoted to the study of microcirculatory disorders in arterial hypertension. An increasing research interest in changes in microcirculation associated with this pathology was spurred by the publication of the metaanalytical data showing a reduction in the incidence of cardiovascular complications during long-term treatment with antihypertensive agents [26]. It was found that the actual incidence was far less than the expected value which was calculated with regard to normalizing the blood pressure. The evidence obtained suggests that for preventation of cardiovascular complication due to arterial hypertension to be effective it is essential not only to lower blood pressure but also to correct the disturbed microcirculation.

Being an important component for maintenance of adequate perfusion of bodily organs and tissues, microcirculation undergoes substantial changes in hypertension triggered by at least two pathological processes. First, there is a lack of microcirculatory bed resulting from reduced number or density of capillaries both in patients with borderline blood pressure and in those with a stable form of arterial hypertension [3].

Another pathological process occurring in patients with arterial hypertension at the level of microcirculation are considerable shifts in the rheological properties of blood. In this case the values of blood viscosity are correlated over a wide range of shear rates with arterial pressure value [62], reflecting a close interrelation of these processes. High blood viscosity syndrome in these patients is formed as a result of impaired macrorheological indices (increase in the hematocrit value, plasma viscosity, fibrinogen content) as well as cell rheology parameters (increased rate of erythrocyte aggregation and strength of aggregates, reduced RBC deformability) [12, 22, 30, 57, 62, 65, 93, 109, 112, 119]. Moreover, there is evidence to show that these two pathological processes implicated in microcirculation disorder – rarefaction and blood hyperviscosity – are closely interrelated. Hypertensive patients with lower capillary density and elevated systolic pressure have much higher indices of erythrocyte aggregation and blood viscosity at low shear rates [25].

The disturbances of major hemorheological parameters in patients with arterial hypertension tend to become progressively worse as blood pressure is increased and the disease persists [23, 112], reaching its peak when target organs are damaged [109].

A salient feature of blood rheology in arterial hypertension are elevated hematocrit value [62, 94, 107, 112]. The phenomenon of erythrocytosis in arterial hypertension is attributed both to reduced blood plasma volumes as a result of its redistribution due to high intravascular pressure from the vascular bed into intercellular spaces and to increased erythropoietic activity of bone marrow resulting from tissue hypoxia [97]. At the same time no correlation between the hemoglobin level in blood and blood pressure indices was found [58].

In arterial hypertension it is the erythrocytic link of rheology that undergoes the most substantial changes, yet the contribution of disorders due to erythrocyte aggregation and erythrocyte deformability to enhanced blood viscosity is different [98].

Erythrocyte deformability disorders during arterial hypertension should be considered as crucial since lower erythrocyte deformability leads to an increase in peripheral vascular resistance [47]. Moreover, erythrocyte deformability disorder during arterial hypertension constitutes a specific phenomenon of cell rheology disturbance which tends to progress along with the stage of disease [98]. As the disease advances reduced oxygenation of peripheral tissues correlates with reduced deformability of erythrocytes [24]. The patients exhibit a disk-spherical transformation of erythrocytes with increased content in erythrocyte population of pathological shapes which disturbs the microcirculation [98].

Unlike deformability, disorders associated with erythrocyte aggregation usually evolve when the disease has become complicated and persisted over a long period of time. In patients with hypertension grade I and II a trend is observed toward accelerated rate of spontaneous erythrocyte aggregation which manifests itself in non-significant increase of blood viscosity at low shear rates. And only patients with hypertension grade III with complicated course of the disease show a regular increase both in erythrocyte aggregation and blood viscosity [97]. It is assumed that the occurrence of substantial increase in erythrocyte aggregation in patients with arterial hypertension may serve as a predictor of potential subsequent clinical complications [63, 111].

Alterations in rheological parameters of blood combined with reduced density of microvessels are responsible for decrease in tissue perfusion and transport of oxygen to tissues [101] as well as for increased peripheral resistance [113] and blood pressure [22]. This being so, arterial hypertension is perceived as a progressive ischemic syndrome which affects both macro- and microcirculation [22]. This may be the reason why monitoring of blood pressure falls short of the desirable target of ensuring effective prevention of cardiovascular complications during hypertension and new therapeutic approaches are needed that could improve blood microcirculation. Analysis of blood rheological disorders in hypertensive patients and assessment of their role in pathogenesis and progression of the disease warrant the assumption that blood viscosity reducing medications are an important factor in normalizing microcirculation and reducing the risk of cardiovascular complications. The foregoing also implies that involvement in the pathological process of primarily cell rheology indices requires administration of specific hemorheological remedies.

These notions provide valid reasons for prescribing specific hemorheological drugs for treatment of hypertensive patients in conjunction with antihypertensive drugs. For this purpose Ascovertin tablets were used which contain an antioxidant complex: 20 mg dihydroquercetin and 50 mg ascorbic acid.

Clinical trials of Ascovertin involved 48 patients with essential arterial hypertension grade II or III considered at high or median risk of developing complications [1]. The patients were randomized to the main group (n=38) and a comparison group (n=10). The mean age of the patients was 60±5 years. An ECG revealed signs of left ventricular hypertrophy in all patients while fundus examination revealed hypertensive retinal angiopathy. All patients received a standard antihypertensive therapy (ACE inhibitors, calcium channel blockers, beta-blockers, diuretics). During the course of the investigation no correction was made to baseline therapy. None of the patients in the study received antiaggregants, nootropic drugs or other medications which could directly or indirectly affect the blood parameters under study.

Moreover, the patients in the main and comparison groups had a verified diagnosis of discirculatory encephalopathy stage I or II. The diagnosis of vascular cerebral insufficiency was established on the basis of anamnestic and paraclinical signs, the presence of neurological symptoms, due to vascular cerebral insufficiency and the patients' subjective complaints. The patients with arterial hypertension complained mainly of headache, varying in intensity, localization and character and often associated with fluctuations in blood pressure or weather changes, general weakness and fatigue, dizziness, difficulty in walking and head noise.

The patients' complaints of headache, vertigo, cerebri and tinnitus aurium, easy fatiguability and sleep disturbance were rated according to a 5–point scale, where each symptom scored 0 to 4 (0 – no disorder, 1 – a little, 2 – moderate, 3 –pronounced, 4 – severe with disadaptation disturbances).

The most frequently used neuropsychological tests were performed twice (in the first and final day of the study) on patients of the main and comparable groups to evaluate the brain functional status and to identify the range of cognitive function impairment (short-term memory, concentration and attention stability, psychomotor functions). The tests comprised a memory retention test in which the patients had to memorize and immediately recite 10 double-digit numbers, a serial count (100–7=93, 93–7=86 etc), a Schulte table test and reciprocal coordination test (alternately clenching and unclenching the hands within 30 s with tallying the number of clenches of each hand).

In assessing the clinical efficacy of Ascovertin the focus was on investigating the effects of the drug on the hemorheological status of patients. Hemorheological parameters were defined prior to commencement of the treatment course and on the 21st day of the study. A 3.8 % solution of sodium citrate to whole blood ratio of 1: 9 was used as anticoagulant. Fasting blood samples were collected from the ulnar vein into a plastic tube in the morning. The whole blood viscosity (at shear rates of 3, 10, 50, 100, 300 s^{-1}) and plasma viscosity (at shear rate of 300 s^{-1}) were defined with the help of rotational viscometer AKP-2 (Russia). Erythrocyte aggregation, erythrocyte deformability, hematocrit and total fibrinogen levels in blood plasma were measured using the above methods. In addition, for comparison of hemorheological indices, blood of 10 clinically healthy people (control group) was examined, who were quite similar in age to patients in the main groups (mean age 55±6 years) and had never been diagnosed with cardiovascular diseases.

The blood samples of the main group patients collected to determine their hemorheological status were also checked for the content of initial and end products of lipid peroxidation. Once lipids had been extracted from the erythrocyte mass [38] the content of conjugated dienes and thrienes was determined on spectrophotometer Model 557 Hitachi [77] and fluorescent products were measured using a fluorescent spectrophotometer Model 850 Hitachi [103]. The content of malondialdehyde (MDA) was assessed in blood plasma [95].

The main group patients have undergone a 3-week Ascovertin treatment course. In the first week the patients were given two tablets three times a day after meals and in the second and third week one tablet three times a day.

Early in the study the main group patients and those the comparison group presented on examination with cardiovascular condition specific syndrome of high blood viscosity which was manifested with primary shifts of cell rheology, namely, increased erythrocyte aggregation ($T_{1/2}$ was less by 25%) and a manifest reduction in erythrocyte deformability (IED dropped by 28–54%) (Table 4, Figure 4, 5). Also patients in these groups demonstrated changes in other indices as well: they tended to have elevated levels of blood fibrinogen and the main group patients showed a slight but significant increase in hematocrit. Plasma viscosity indices were normal which supports the view that this is a stable "conservative" link of hemorheology which prevents pathological changes in blood viscosity [27]. The shifts in rheological properties in hypertensive patients were manifested as enhanced viscosity of whole blood (by 21–28%) over the entire investigated range of shear rates as compared to corresponding indices for control group patients (Figure 4). An analysis of changes in individual hemorheological parameters unequivocally suggests that increase in blood viscosity is due to primary impairment of cell rheology indices.

Table 4. Changes in hemorheological profile indices in hypertensive patients (mean ±SEM)

Indices	Controls	Main group		Comparison group	
		Before treatment	21st day	1st day	21st day
Plasma viscosity, mPa·s	1.5±0.1	1.5±0.1	1,5±0.1	1,5±0.1	1,5±0.1
Hematocrit, %	42±1	44±1*	42±1	43±2	42±2
Plasma fibrinogen, g/l	2.11±0.3	2.52±0.11	2.36±0.08	2.58±0.05	2.58±0.03
Half-period of erythrocyte aggregation, s	10.1±0.5	7.5±0.5*	9.5±0.7+	6.1±0.9*	7.1±0.9*

+ – $p<0.05$ compared to baseline; * – $p<0.05$ compared to normal controls.

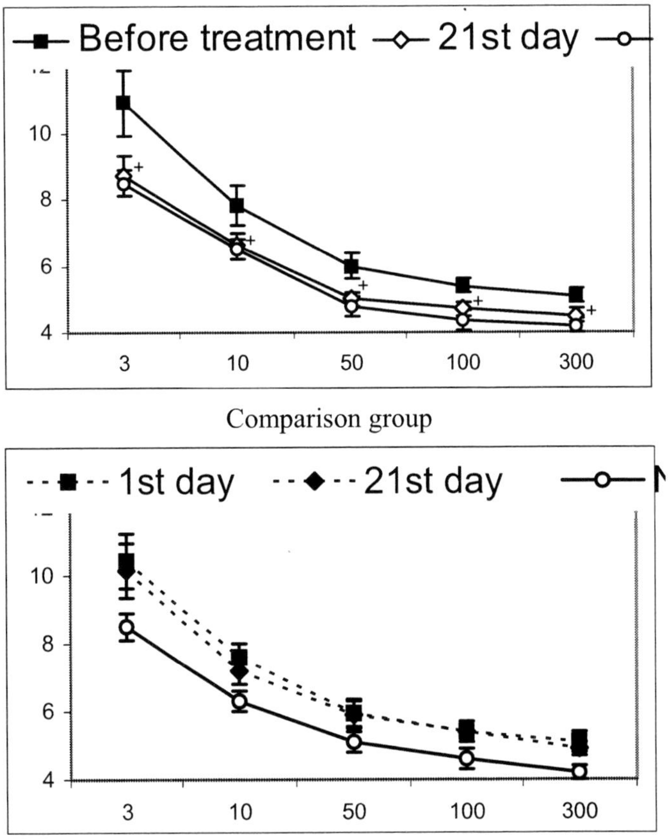

Figure 4. Changes in blood viscosity in hypertensive patients. Along the abscissa axis – shear rate, s^{-1}; along the ordinate axis – blood viscosity, mPa·s. + – $p<0.05$ compared to baseline. Black marks – $p<0.05$ compared to normal controls.

Evaluation of hemorheological profile of the main group patients after completion of Ascovertin administration course reflects positive dynamics of rheological indices (Table 4, Figure 4, 5). Whole blood viscosity tended to significant decrease compared with baseline level over the entire shear rate range. By the end of the third week the erythrocyte deformability index had shown a regular increase of 88, 27 and 20 percent at low, medium and high shear rates respectively while the half-period of erythrocyte aggregation had risen by 27 percent against the baseline value. The plasma viscosity remained unchanged and there was a tendency to reduced fibrinogen content. In the comparison group no significant changes in the investigated hemorheological parameters have been ascertained.

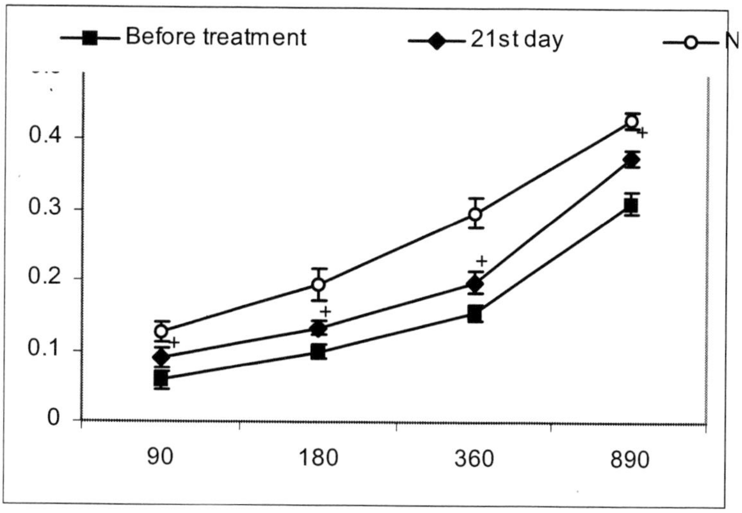

Comparison group

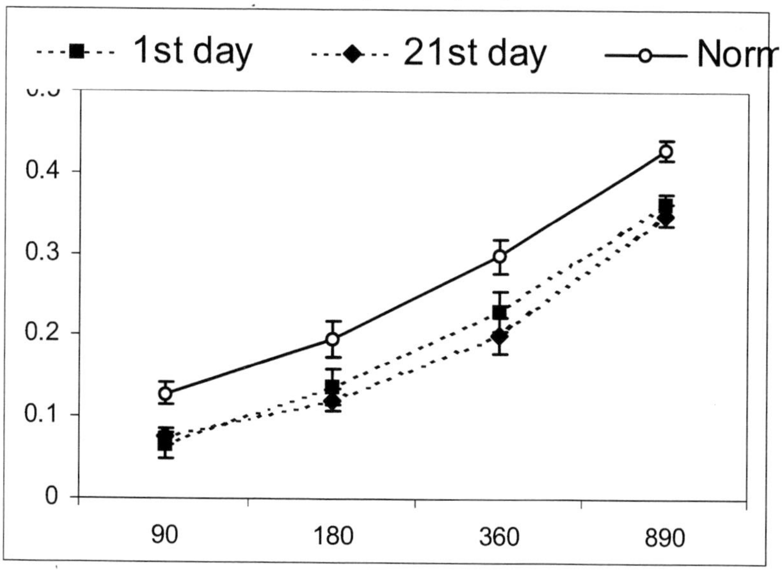

Figure 5. Change in the index of erythrocyte deformability (IED) in hypertensive patients. Along the abscissa axis – shear rate, s^{-1}; along the ordinate axis – IED, rel. units. + – $p<0.05$ compared to baseline. Black marks – $p<0.05$ compared to normal controls.

Arterial hypertension like other cardiovascular disorders is classified among the so-called oxidative stress mediated diseases. The blood of affected people shows increased production of active forms of oxygen, activation of lipid peroxidation processes and lower levels of antioxidants, notably of ascorbic acid in blood plasma and alpha-tocopherol in erythrocyte membranes [61, 91, 115]. In the blood of hypertensives there was detected significant decrease of the activity of enzymes which utilize superoxide radical and lipoperoxides (superoxide oxidase and glutathione peroxidase), especially when the disease reaches a critical stage [49].

Free radical processes occurring in erythrocytes have the effect of modifying the viscoelastic properties of their membranes with a resultant impairment of cell deformability [5, 13, 21, 100, 114] and hence an impairment in the oxygen transport function of blood. This study explored the effect of Ascovertin on lipid peroxidation processes in erythrocytes and in blood plasma because of all hemorheological indices it was the erythrocyte capacity for deformation that showed a significant change under the action of the drug.

A significant decrease of the content of conjugated dienes (56%), conjugated thrienes (51%) and fluorescent products (72%) in erythrocyres and malondialdehyde (16%) in blood plasma was manifested in the main group patients following a 21-day course of Ascovertin (Table 5). Therefore, it is valid to say that this administration of Ascovertin had a limiting effect on the processes of lipid peroxidation both in erythrocyte membranes and in blood plasma. Correlation between reduced content of conjugated dienes in erythrocyte membranes and improved cell deformability ($r=0.527$; $p=0.05$) provides further evidence in support of the hypothesis that there is a link between the antioxidant effect of the drug and its ability to improve the rheological properties of erythrocytes.

Table 5. The effect of Ascovertin on the content of conjugated dienes (CD, OD /mg lipids), conjugated thrienes (CT, OD/mg lipids), fluorescent products (FP, OE/mg lipids) in erythrocytes and malondialdehyde (MDA, nmol/ml) in blood plasma of hypertensive patients (mean ±SEM)

Period	CD	CT	FP	MDA
Before treatment	0.382±0.078	0.732±0.149	1.551±0.545	17.31±1.06
After treatment	0.106±0.010*	0.363±0.008*	0.445±0.219*	14.53±1.28*

* – $p < 0.05$ compared to values before treatment.

The formation of high blood viscosity syndrome in hypertensive patients tends to aggravate the impairment of basic hemodynamic parameters. Since total peripheral resistance is determined not only by the vessel lumen (primarily resistive) but also by the viscous resistance of blood [19] the high blood viscosity in hypertensive patients manifests itself in increased peripheral resistance and may lead to complications of the disease [55, 57, 98]. Moreover, it is well known that these hypertensive cases have a reduced dilator reserve of arterioles and therefore an increase in blood viscosity can cause a greater increase in total peripheral resistance and arterial blood pressure in these patients than is the case with normotensive subjects [86]. The results of the study of correlation dependence between hemodynamic indices (peripheral resistance, cardiac index) and rheological indices show evidence that in hypertensive patients there exists a relationship between changes of microrheological characteristics (erythrocyte deformability and aggregation) and indices of systemic hemodynamics (notably in stage II and III arterial hypertension) but no significant correlations are detected between hemodynamic indices and hematocrit [97]. These findings lend support to the belief that disturbances in blood rheological properties are a major factor in hypertension pathogenesis. In this connection, modifying the blood's viscous properties appears to be an important but as yet not actively pursued complementary strategy of arterial hypertension therapy.

Table 6. The effect of Ascovertin on the dynamics of systolic arterial pressure (SAP, mmHg), diastolic arterial pressure (DAP, mmHg), heart rate (HR, beats/min) and total peripheral resistance (TPR, dyne·cm^{-5}·s) in hypertensive patients (mean ±SEM)

Indices	Groups	Period	
		1st day	21st day
SAP	Main	153±5	132±4*
	Comparison	150±10	148±9
DAP	Main	103±4	90±3*
	Comparison	99±7	95±6
HR	Main	78±5	74±5
	Comparison	76±7	73±7
TPR	Main	1910±27	1507±28*
	Comparison	1989±22	2013±14

* – $p < 0.05$ compared to values before treatment.

In our investigations the treatment of main group patients with Ascovertin apart from the hemorheological shifts also caused favourable hemodynamic changes: a moderate but reliable reduction of systolic (14%) and diastolic (13%) arterial pressure (Table 6). Studies by J.A. Dormandy [34] also prove the possibility of reducing arterial pressure by diminishing the viscosity of blood in hypertensive patients.

It may also be assumed that one of the mechanisms for reducing arterial blood pressure and total peripheral resistance is the antiaggregant effect of Ascovertin on erythrocytes. This effect has been demonstrated by our studies *in vitro*, in spontaneously hypertensive rats and in patients with arterial hypertension. Our assumption is also based indirectly on the results of fundamental investigations by G. Mchedlishvili et al. [66] which using an array of methodological approaches demonstrated a relationship between erythrocyte aggregation and systemic arterial pressure / total peripheral resistance.

High blood viscosity syndrome in hypertensive patients contributes dramatically to progression of the disease (elevation of blood pressure) due to increased viscodynamic resistance to blood flow while the impairment of erythrocyte rheological properties makes for inadequate tissue and organs perfusion and thus fosters development of chronic cerebral ischaemia. In our studies hypertensive patients have initially demonstrated characteristic for chronic cerebral ischaemia disorders such as deterioration in short-term memory, slowing of mental function, reduced attention span with concomitant easy fatiguability, sleep disturbances and practically all patients were suffering from vertigo, headache, and head noise. The course treatment with Ascovertin was instrumental in reducing manifestations of the main subjective complaints, especially headache, sleep problems, and fatigue. No significant changes were observed in the comparison group (Figure 6).

Neuropsychological tests have revealed a significant improvement in immediate memory and attention and brain psychomotor functions in patients of the main group (Table 7). The short-term memory improvement was demonstrated by the increase in the number of figures recited by the patients in the "10 double-digits" test: from 4.4±1.0 prior to commencement of Ascovertin therapy to 5.1±1.2 following completion of the course, a 14 percent increase ($p<0.05$). In serial count test the time it took the patients to perform the test decreased by 14 percent ($p<0.05$).

No noticeable change occurred in performance time in Shulte attention test. In reciprocal coordination test the number of clenches of each hand within 30 sec significantly increased by 23 percent. In the comparison group no substantial changes in the investigated parameters were recorded (Table 7).

Table 7. Dynamics of the results of neuropsychological tests in hypertensive patients (mean±SEM)

Period	Groups	Shulte test, s	Serial cont, s	«10 double-digits»	Kinetic test
1st day	Main	75.4±3.9	64.3±4.7	4.5±0.3	34.3±2.8
	Comparison	80.9±9.0	69.5±12.9	4.8±0.7	32.9±5.1
21st day	Main	76.7±5.7	55.4±4.3*	5.2±0.3*	42.1±2.6*
	Comparison	77.5±7.4	63.8±11.1	5.0±0.6	33.9±3.9

* – $p< 0.05$ compared to values before treatment.

The results of neuropsychological tests in hypertensive patients clearly demonstrate the effectiveness of hemorheological treatment with Ascovertin targeted at improving the cell rheology indices, namely, aggregation and deformability of erythrocytes. The validity of the chosen therapeutic approach is indirectly corroborated by findings showing that other blood viscosity reducing modalities were found to be inadequate in terms of their effect on cognitive function. Reduction in hematocrit (hemodilution) is by far the simplest method for lowering blood viscosity [36]. However, the relationship between cognitive function and hematocrit shows a U shaped pattern in the elderly, that is to say, the elderly perform at their best when their average hematocrit level equals 0.46. Changes in hematocrit value in the direction of both increasing and decreasing value were accompanied by a similar weakening of cognitive functions [35].

To sum it up, the three-week course of Ascovertin therapy applied to patients suffering from discirculatory encephalopathy with attendant hypertension resulted in improved physical health of patients, reduction of systolic and diastolic arterial pressure and total peripheral resistance. There was observed a reduction in the expression of the syndrome of high blood viscosity which was largely due to the positive effect of Ascovertin on cell rheology indices, in particular, on erythrocyte deformability and to a lesser extent on erythrocyte aggregation. The content of products of lipid peroxidation in cell membranes and blood plasma tended to diminish. The patients also showed positive dynamics in the condition of cognitive and neurodynamic functions. Neurological symptoms in this patient group remained at baseline level.

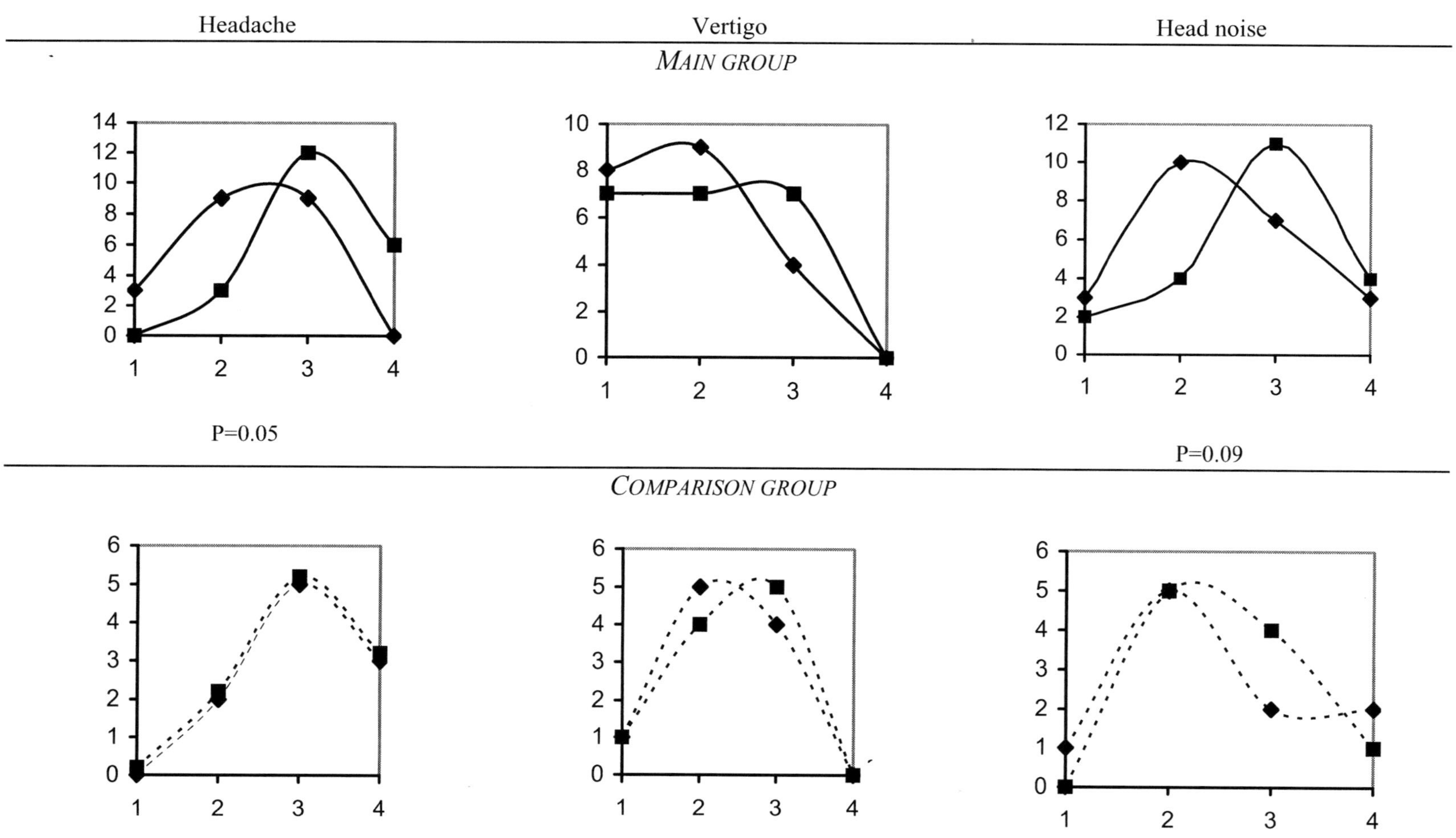

Figure 6. Continued on next page.

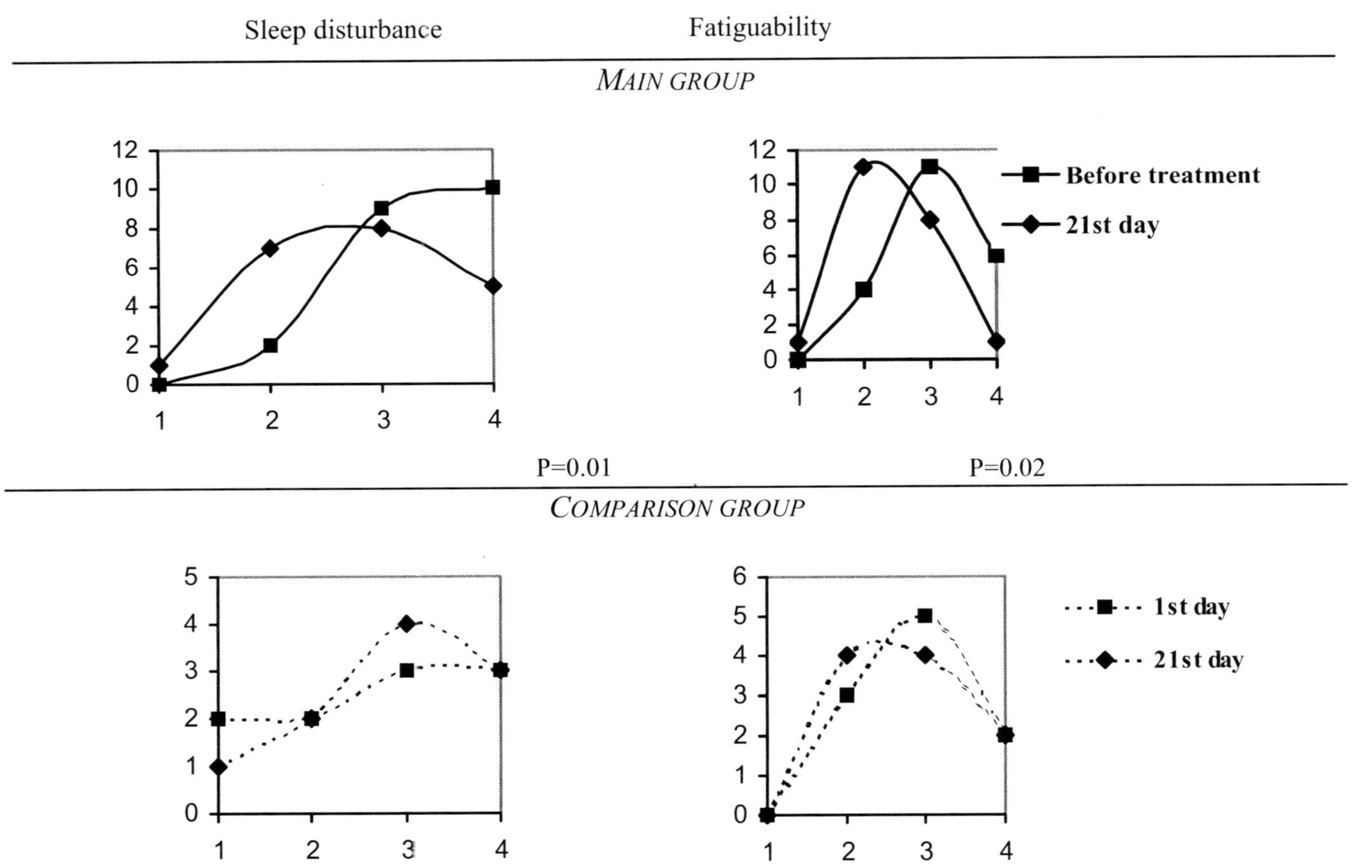

Figure 6. The effect of Ascovertin on the expression of clinical signs in hypertensive patients. Along the abscissa axis – points; along the ordinate axis – number of patients with varying degree of clinical expression of a given sign.

CONCLUSION

Essential hypertension is characterized by enhanced blood viscosity, increased aggregation ability of erythrocytes, impairment of their plasticity, elevated plasma fibrinogen and increased hematocrit [22, 30, 94, 109]. The use of antihypertensive drugs cannot have a beneficial effect on some hemorheological indices forming high blood viscosity syndrome. Furthermore, a negative effect of antihypertensive therapy, especially a combination of beta-adrenergic blockers and diuretics, on rheological properties of blood in patients is known [98].

These findings, as well as a high degree of correlation between pathologic changes of hemorheological parameters and risk of acute cardiovascular disorders [57, 98], between the arterial pressure and blood viscosity [12] justify the necessity of a purposeful correction of hemorheological shifts in hypertensive patients.

One of the promising approaches to the treatment of microcirculaton disturbances in arterial hypertension may be an application of antioxidants. Despite a considerable number of reports testifying to the fact that during intensification of free radical reactions there occurs an impairment of blood rheological properties, mainly at the expense of disturbances in erythrocyte functioning [5, 13, 21, 100, 114], investigations devoted to the efficacy evaluation of antioxidants as specific rheological agents are of single occurrence [83, 69].

The main objective of our research was to obtain experimental and clinical evidence on the possibility to use antioxidants as hemorheological therapeutic agents. It was shown that under *in vitro* conditions and under *in vivo* conditions with an adequate model of high blood viscosity syndrome (spontaneously hypertensive rats), the AOC, dihydroquercetin and ascorbic acid included, can make the syndrome not so pronounced. This is achieved through an action on aggregation and deformability of erythrocytes. It has been established that the mechanisms of the AOC effect are based on its ability to protect erythrocyte membranes in spontaneously hypertensive rats. It was manifested by the restoration of a normal ratio between phospholipids of the outer and inner layers of erythrocyte membranes, as well as the reduction of lysophospholipids content in them. This is presumed to lead to a better erythrocyte population composition, specifically, to a decreased number of their pathologically changed shapes and accordingly to an increased proportion of discocytes, which eventually resulted in an improvement of red blood cells rheological properties.

The AOC efficacy is supported by clinical trials during which patients with arterial hypertension grades I–II received tablets of Ascovertin, a drug form of the AOC. First and foremost it should be noted that in the patients receiving Ascovertin, in addition to a specific antihypertensive therapy a decrease in blood viscosity was observed in contrast to the controls. This effect, also seen in the experimental studies, is mainly governed by a positive influence of Ascovertin on the indices of blood cell rheology. Taking into account the pathogenesis of microcirculatory disturbances in arterial hypertension [22, 24], this trend in the hemorheological effect of Ascovertin is of fundamental importance. The decreased blood viscosity in patients receiving Ascovertin resulted in moderate lowering systolic and diastolic arterial pressure, reducing total peripheral resistance compared to patients who did not take the preparation. In addition, an improvement of short-term memory and attention in patients using Ascovertin was registered by means of relevant tests.

Thus Ascovertin can enhance the effect of specific antihypertensive therapy as it makes high blood viscosity syndrome not so marked in patients suffering from arterial hypertension. The positive results due to Ascovertin therapy enabled us to consider a new approach to using antioxidants for treatment of hemorheological disorders in arterial hypertension.

REFERENCES

[1] 2003 World Health Organization (WHO) – International Society of Hypertension (ISH) statement on management of hypertension. *J. Hypertens,* 2003, 21, 1983–1992.

[2] Abrescia, P; Golino, P. Free radicals and antioxidants in cardiovascular diseases. *Expert Rev. Cardiovasc. Ther.,* 2005, 3, 159–171.

[3] Antonios, TF; Singer, DR; Markandu, ND; et al. Rarefaction of skin capillaries in borderline essential hypertension suggests an early structural abnormality. *J. Hypertens.,* 1999, 34, 655–658.

[4] Arduini, A; Stern, A; Storto, S; et al Effect of oxidative stress on membrane phospholipids and protein organization in human erythrocytes. *Artch. Biochem. Biophys.,* 1989, 273, 112–120.

[5] Baskurt, OK; Meiselman, HJ. Susceptibility of equine erythrocytes to oxidant-induced rheologic alteration. *Am. J. Vet. Res.,* 1999, 60, 1301–1306.

[6] Bascurt, OK; Tugral, E; Neu, B; et al. Particle electrophoresis behavior of red blood cells. *Electrophoresis,* 2002, 23, 2103–2109.

[7] Backman, L; Jonasson, JB; Horstedt, P. Phosphoinositide metabolism and shape control in sheep red blood cells. *Mol. Membr. Biol.,* 1998, 15, 27–32.

[8] Beloborodov, VL; Ilyasov, IR; Tyukavkina, NA; et al. Antiradical activity of diquertin and combinations on its basis. Actual Problems of Creation of New medical preparations of natural Origin: Proc. 8th Int. Congr., *Mikkeli, Finland,* 2004, 60–61.

[9] Bessis, M; Mohandas, N. A defractometric method for the measurement of cellular deformability. *Blood Cells,* 1975, 1, 307–313.

[10] Bessis, M; Mohandas, N. Deformability of normal, sharp-altered and pathological red cells. *Blood Cells,* 1975, 1, 315–329.

[11] Biological membranes: A practical approach. Ed. Findley, JBC; Evans, WH. Oxford, Washington DC: IRL Press; 1987.

[12] Bogar, L. Hemorheology and hypertension: not "chicken or egg" but two chickens from similar eggs. *Clin. Hemorheol. Microcirc.,* 2002, 81–83.

[13] Bolokadze, N; Varazashvili, M; Salia, N; et al. Lipid peroxidation in the erythrocytes under condition of increased erythrocyte aggregation. In: 12th Eur. Conf. Clin. Hemorheol.: Program and Book of Abstracts. Sofia, 2003, 90.

[14] Brunauer, LS; Moxness, MS; Huestis, WH. Hydrogen peroxide oxidation induces the transfer of phospholipids from the membrane into the cytosol of human erythrocytes. *Biochemistry,* 1994, 33, 4527–4532.

[15] Cao, G; Sofic, E; Prior, RL. Antioxidant behavior of flavonoids: structure – activity relationships. *Free Radical Biol. Med.,* 1997, 22, 749–760.

[16] Chang, TW; Chen-Po, H. Changes in viscosity of low share rates and viscoelastic properties of oxidative erythrocytes suspension. *Clin. Hemorheol. Microcirc.*, 1999, 21, 99–103.

[17] Chasis, JA; Schrier, S. Membrane deformability and capacity for shape change in the erythrocyte. *Blood,* 1989, 74, 2562–2568.

[18] Chernetsky, EA; Vorobey, AV. Structure and function of erythrocyte membrane. Minsk: Nauka I Tekhnika; 1981 (in Russian).

[19] Chien, S. Clinical rheology in cardiovascular disease. *Bibl. Anat.,* 1977, 16, 472–474.

[20] Choudhuty, TD; Das, N; Chattopadhyay, A;, Datta, AG. Effect of oxidative stress and erythropoietin on cytoskeletal proteins and lipid organization in human erythrocytes. *Pol. J. Pharmacol., 1999*, 51, 341–350.

[21] Chung, TW; Ho, CP. Changes in viscosity of low shear rates and viscoelastic properties of oxidative erythrocytes suspensions. *Clin. Hemorheol. Microcirc.,* 1999, 21, 99–103.

[22] Cicco, G; Pirelli, A. Red blood cell (RBC) deformability, RBC aggregability and tissue oxygenation in hypertension. *Clin. Hemorheol. Microcirc.,* 1999, 21, 169–177.

[23] Cicco, G; Carbonara, MC; Stingi, GD; Pirrelli A. Cytosolic calcium and hemorheological patterns during arterial hypertension. *Clin. Hemorheol. Microcirc.,* 2001, 24, 25–31.

[24] Cicco, G; Vicenti, P; Stingi, G; et al. Hemorheology in complicated hypertension. *Clin. Hemorheol. Microcirc.,* 1999, 21, 315–319.

[25] Ciuffetti, G; Pascualini, L; Pirro, M; et al. Blood rheology in men with essential hypertension and capillary rarefaction. *J. Hum. Hypertens.,* 2002, 16, 529–531.

[26] Collins, R; Peto, R; MacMahon, S; et al. Blood pressure, stroke, and coronary heart disease. Part 2, Short-term reductions in blood pressure: overview of randomised drug trials in their epidemiological context. *Lancet*, 1990, 335, 827–838.

[27] Crepaldi, G; Calabro, A; Belloni, M. Blood hyperviscosity syndrome. *Ric. Clin. Lab.,* 1983, 13, Suppl. 134, 89–104.

[28] Dintenfass, L. *Rheology of blood in diagnostic and preventative medicine.* London; 1976.

[29] Dintenfass, L. The clinical impact of the newer research in blood rheology: an overview. *Angiology*, 1981, 32, 217–229.

[30] Dintenfass, L; Giromali, A. Rigidity of red blood cells in essential hypertension. *Haemostasis*, 1978, 7, 298–302.

[31] Ditzel, J. The nature of the intravascular erythrocyte aggregation in diseases with particular references to diabetes mellitus. *Acta med. scand.,* 1955, 52, 372–378.

[32] Dodge, JT; Mitchell, C; Hanahan, DJ. The preparation and chemical characteristics of hemoglobin-free ghost of human erythrocytes. *Arch. Biochem. Biophys.,* 1963, 100, 119–130.

[33] Dok-Go, H; Lee, KH; Kim, HJ; et al. Neuroprotective effects of antioxidative flavonoids, quercetin, (+)-dihydroquercetin and quercetin 3-methyl ether, isolated from Opuntia ficus-indica var. saboten. *Brain. Res.,* 2003, 965, 130–136.

[34] Dormandy, JA. Influence of blood viscosity on blood flow and the effect of low molecular weight dextran. *Br. Med. J.,* 1971, 4, 716–719.

[35] Elwood, PC; Pichering, J; Gallacher, JC. Cognitive function and blood rheology: results from the Caerphilly cohor of older men. *Age Aging,* 2001, 30, 135–139.

[36] Ernst, E. Haemorheology, cardiovascular risk factors and disease. *J. Intern. Angiol.*, 1996, 15, Suppl. 1, 36–45.

[37] Flaherty, JT. Myocardial injury mediated by oxygen free radicals. *Amer. J. Med.*, 1991, 91, 79–85.

[38] Folch, J; Lees, M; Sloane-Stanley, G. A simple method for the isolation and purification of total lipids from animal tissues. *J. Biol. Chem.*, 1957, 226, 497–509.

[39] Francis, DA; Francis, JL; Roath, OS. The effect of nifedipine on the deformability of heat-treated red cells. *Clin. Hemorheology,* 1985, 5, 149–153.

[40] Giakoumaki, A; Haritou, M; Galaris, D; Koutsouris, D. A study on the effects of antioxidants on the deformability of human erythrocytes subjected to oxidative stress. Proc. Int. Conf. Hemorheology. Yaroslavl, Russia; 2001, 5–6.

[41] Gimsa, J. A possible molecular mechanism governing human erythrocyte shape. *Biophys. J.* 1998, 75, 568–569.

[42] Gurevich, MI. Experimental models of arterial hypertension and current concepts of the pathogenesis of hypertension. *Fiziol. Zh.*, 1981, 27, 595–602 (in Russian).

[43] Hansen, JC; Skalak, R; Chien, S; Hogen, A. An elastic network model based on the structure of red blood cell membrane skeleton. *Biophys. J.*, 1996, 70, 146–166.

[44] Haraguchi, H; Mochida, Y; Sakai, S; et al. Protection against oxidative damage by dihydroflavonoids in Engelhardtia chrisolepis. *Biosci. Biotechnol. Biochem.*, 1996, 60, 945–948.

[45] Hiramatsu, K; Arimori, S. Increased superoxide production by mononuclear cells of patients with hypertriglyceridemia and diabetes. *Diabetes,* 1988, 37, 832–837.

[46] Hemodilution in Stroke Group. Hypervolemic hemodilution treatment of acute stroke: results of a randomized multicenter trail using pentastarch. *Stroke,* 1989, 20, 317–323.

[47] Hossmann, V; Bonner, G; Wambach, G; et al. Blood viscosity: a pathogenetic factor in the development of essential hypertension. *Clin. Exp. Hypertens.*, 1986, 8, 673–680.

[48] Huang, Y; Liu, D; Sun, S. Mechanism of free radicals on the molecular fluidity and chemical structure of the red cell membrane damage. *Clin. Hemorheol. Microcirc.*, 2000, 23, 287–290.

[49] Iarema, NI; Konovalova, GG; Lankin, VZ. Changes in the activity of antioxidant enzymes in patients with hypertension. *Kardiologiia,* 1992, 32, 46–48 (in Russian).

[50] Igarashi, K; Uchida, Y; Murakami, N; et al. Effect of astilbin in tea processed from leaves of Engelhardtia chrysolepis on the serum and liver lipid concentrations and on erythrocyte and liver antioxidative enzyme activities of rat. *Biosci. Biotechnol. Biochem.*, 1996, 60, 513–515.

[51] Jai, SK; McVie, R; Duett, J; Herbst, JJ. Erythrocyte membrane lipid peroxidation and glycosylated haemoglobin in diabetes. *Diabetes*, 1989, 38, 1539–1543.

[52] Jovanovic, SV; Steenken, S; Tosic, M; et al. Flavonoids as antioxidants. *J. Am. Chem. Soc.,* 1994, 116, 4846–4851.

[53] Kandaswami, C; Middleton, E. Flavonoids as antioxidants. In: Shahidi F, editor. Natural antioxidants: chemistry, health effects, and applications. Illinois: Champaign; 1997; 174–203.

[54] Kharamonenko, SS; Rakitjanskaja, AA. Electrophoresis of blood cells in norm and pathology. Minsk: Belarus'; 1984 (in Russian).

[55] Kitaeva, ND; Shabanov, VA; Levin, GIa; Kostrov, VA. *Microrheological disorders of erythrocytes in patients with hypertension.* Kardiologiia, 1991, 31, 51–54 (in Russian).

[56] Klebanov, GI; Teselkin, you; Babenkova, IV; et al. Effect of lipophilic antioxidants on peroxidation of liposome membranes photosensitized by hematoporphyrin derivatives upon He–Ne laser irradiation. Membr. *Cell Biol.,* 1996, 10, 139–143.

[57] Klein, W; Eber, B; Dusleag, J; et al. Hypertension and hemorheology. *Wien. Med. Wochenschr.,* 1995, 145, 355–357.

[58] Koenig, W; Sund, M; Ernst, E; et al. Association between plasma viscosity and blood pressure: Results from the MONICA-project Augsburg. *Am. J. Hypertens.,* 1991, 4, 529–536.

[59] Koltringer, P; Eber, O; Lind, P; et al. *Microzirkulation und Viskoelastizitat des Vollblutes unter Gingo biloba extract. Eine plazebokontrollierte randomizierte Doppelblind-Stidie.* Perfusion, 1989, 1, 28–30 (in German).

[60] Kozinets, GI; Simovart, YuA. *Surface architectonics of cells of peripheral blood in norm and blood system diseases.* Tallin: Vargus; 1984 (in Russian).

[61] Kumar, KW; Das, UM. Are free radical involved in the pathology of human essential hypertension? *Biochem. J.,* 1993, 19, 59–66.

[62] Letcher, RL; Chien, S; Pichering, TG; et al. Direct relationship between blood pressure and blood viscosity in normal and hypertensive subjects: Role of fibrinogen and concentration. *Am. J. Med.,* 1981, 70, 1195–1202.

[63] Linde, T; Sandhagen, B; Hagg, A; et al. Blood viscosity and peripheral vascular resistance in patients with untreated essential hypertension. *Hypertension,* 1993, 11, 731–736.

[64] McGough, AM; Josephs, R. On the structure of erythrocyte spectrin in partially expanded membrane skeletons. *Proc. Nat. Acad. Sci.* USA, 1990, 87, 5208–5212.

[65] Mchedlishvili, G; Gobejishvili, L; Beritashvili, N. Effect of intensified red blood cell aggregability on arterial pressure and mesenteric microcirculation. *Microvasc. Res.,* 1993, 45, 233–242.

[66] Mchedlichvili, G; Tsinamdzvrishvili, B; Beritashvili, N; et al. New evidence for involvement of blood rheologycal disorders in rise of peripheral resistance in essential hypertension. *Clin. Hemorheol. Microcirc.,* 1997, 17, 31–39.

[67] Middleton, E; Kandaswami, C; Theoharides, TC. The effect of plant flavonoids on mammalian cells: implication for inflammation, heart disease and cancer. *Pharmacol. Rev.,* 2000, 52, 673–751.

[68] Mikaelian, EM; Karagezian, KG; Ovakimian, SS. Dynamics of quantitative changes in total and individual phospholipids from erythrocyte membranes of albino rats during different stages of the stress reaction. *Vopr. Med. Khim.,* 1988, 34, 64–68 (in Russian).

[69] Mo, J; Fan, J; Guo, Z; et al. A new hypothesis about the relationship between free radical reactions and hemorheological properties in vivo. *Med. Hypotheses.,* 1993, 41, 516–620.

[70] Moor, DJ; Sills, RH; Mendelsohn, R. Conformation order of specific phospholipids in human erythrocytes: correlation with changes in cell shape. *Biochemistry,* 1977, 36, 660–664.

[71] Novitsky, VV; Rjazantseva, NV; Stepovaia, EA. Physiology and pathophysiology of erythrocyte. Tomsk: Izd. Tom. Univ.; 2004 (in Russian).

[72] Othmane, A; Bitbol, M; Snabre, P; Mills, P. Influence of altered phospholipid composition of the membrane outer layer on red blood cell aggregation: relation to shape changes and glycocalyx structure. *Eur. Biophys. J.*, 1990, Suppl. 2, 93–99.

[73] Pentiuk, AA; Gutsol, VI; Iakovleva, OA; et al. Determination of phospholipids based on the formation of a hydrophobic complex with ammonium ferrothiocyanate. *Lab. Delo,* 1987, 6, 457–459 (in Russian).

[74] Pietta, PJ. Flavonoids as antioxidants. *J. Nat. Prod.,* 2000, 63, 1035–1042.

[75] Pincemail, J; Dupius, M; Nasr, C; et al. Superoxide action scavenging effect and superoxide dismutase activity of Gingko biloba extract. *Experim.,* 1989, 45, 708–712.

[76] Plachta, H; Bartnikowska, E; Obara, A. Lipid peroxides in blood from patients with atherosclerosis of coronary and peripheral arteries. *Clin. Chem. Acta,* 1992, 211, 101–112.

[77] Plazer, Z; Kusella, L. In vivo Lipoperoxidation in der Leben nach partieller Hepatotectimie. *Acta Biol. Med. Germ.,* 1968, 21, 121–124 (in German).

[78] Plotnikov, MB; Aliev, OI; Koltunov, AA; Maslov, MYu. Increased blood viscosity syndrome in SHR rats: analysis of the model adequacy. *Biull. Eksp. Biol. Med.*, 1998, 126, 150–151 (in Russian).

[79] Plotnikov, MB; Aliev, OI; Popel', FV. Modified microcolorimeter MKMF-1 for recording of erythrocyte aggregation. *Klin. Lab. Diagn.,* 1995, 3, 57–58 (in Russian).

[80] Plotnikov, MB; Koltunov, AA; Aliev, OI. The hemorheological properties of extracts from some flavonoid-containing plants. *Rast. Resursy,* 1998, 1, 87–91 (in Russian).

[81] Plotnikov, MB; Zibareva, LN; Koltunov, AA. The hemorheological properties of extracts from some ecdysteroid-containing plants. *Rast. Resursy*, 1998, 1, 91–97 (in Russian).

[82] Plotnikova, TM; Bazhenova, TG; Plotnikov, MB; Saratikov, AS. The effect of cerebrocrast on microcirculation in acute transient cerebral ischemia. *Russian J. Exper.* Clin. Pharm., 1997, 1, 58–60.

[83] Plotnikova, TM; Firsov, NN; Vaizova, OE. Mechanism of preservation from erythrocyte deformability disturbances after cerebral ischemia and recirculation with means of ethomerzol. *Eksp. Klin. Farmakol.,* 1992, 55, 29–31 (in Russian).

[84] Potapovich, AI; Kostyuk, VA. Comparative study of antioxidant properties and cytoprotective activity of flavonoids. *Biochemistry* (Mosc), 2003, 68, 514–519 (in Russian).

[85] Ratty, AK; Sunamoto, J; Das, NP. Interaction of flavonoids with 1,1-diphenyl-2-picrylhydrazyl free radical, liposomal membranes and soybean lipoxygenase-1. *Biochem. Pharmacol.,* 1988, 37, 989–995.

[86] Redchits, EG; Parfenov, AS; Abshilava, DO; Pronevich, IK. Interrelation of the rheological properties of the blood and the state of central hemodynamics in patients with a stable form of hypertension. *Kardiologiia*, 1988, 28, 77–80 (in Russian).

[87] Reinhart, WH; Chien, S. Red blood cell rheology in stomatocyte-echinocyte transformation. *Blood*, 1986, 67, 1110–1118.

[88] Reinhart, WH; Singh, A. Erythrocyte aggregation: the role of cell deformability and geometry. *Eur. J. Clin. Invest.,* 1990, 20, 458–462.

[89] Rice-Evans, C. Flavonoid antioxidants. *Current Med. Chem.,* 2001, 8, 797–807.

[90] Rice-Evans, CA; Miller, NJ; Paganga, G. Structure–antioxidant activity relationships of flavonoids and phenolic acids. *Free Radical Biol. Med.,* 1996, 20, 933–956.

[91] Russo, C; Olivieri, O; Girelli, D; et al. Anti-oxidant status and lipid peroxidation in patients with essential hypertension. *J. Hypertens., 1998,* 16, 1267–1271.

[92] Sakutá, S; Takamatsu, S. Determination of deformability index. *Microvasc. Res.,* 1982, 24, 215–218.

[93] Sandhagen, B. Red blood cell fluidity in hypertension. *Clin. Hemorheol. Microcirc.,* 1999, 21, 179–181.

[94] Sandhagen, B; Frithz, G; Waern, U; Ronquist, G. Increased whole blood viscosity combined with decreased erythrocyte fluidity in untreated patients with essential hypertension. *J. Intern. Med.,* 1990, 228, 623–626.

[95] Santos, MT; Valles, J; Aznar, J; Vilches, J. Determination of plasma malondialdehyde-like material and its clinical application in stroke patients. *J. Clin. Pathol.,* 1980, 33, 973–976.

[96] Smith, JE. Erythrocyte membrane: structure, function and pathophysiology. *Vet. Pathol.,* 1987, 24, 471–476.

[97] Shabanov, VA; Kitaeva, ND; Levin, GIa; et al. The clinical importance of studying disorders in the rheological properties of the blood in hypertension patients. *Ter. Arkh.,* 1990, 62, 89–94 (in Russian).

[98] Shabanov, VA; Terekhina, EV; Kostrov, VA. Changes in blood rheological properties in patients with hypertension. *Ter. Arkh.,* 2001, 73, 70–73 (in Russian).

[99] Shahidi, F. Natural antioxidants: an overview. In: Shahidi F, editor. *Natural antioxidants: chemistry, health effects, and applications.* Illinois: Champaign; 1997; 1–11.

[100] Srour; Bilto, YY; Juma, M; Irhimeh, MR. Exposure of human erythrocytes to oxygen radicals causes loss of deformability, increased osmotic fragility, lipid peroxidation and protein degradation. *Clin. Hemorheol. Microcirc.,* 2000, 23, 13–21.

[101] Stoltz, JE; Donner, M. New trends in clinical hemorheology: an introduction to the concept of the hemorheological profile. Schweiz. *Med. Wochenschr.,* 1991, 43, Suppl., 41–49.

[102] Sund, M; Filipiak, B; Doring, A; et al. Plasma viscosity and the risk of coronary heart disease: results from the MONICA-Augsburg Cohort Study, 1984 to 1992. Arterioscler. *Thromb. Vasc. Biol.,* 1998, 5, 768–772.

[103] Tappel, AL. Protection against free radical lipid peroxidation reaction. Pharm. Intervent. *Aging Process,* 1978, 9, 111–113.

[104] Teselkin, IuO; Zhambalova, BA; Babenkova, IV; Tyukavkina, NA. Antioxidant properties of dihydroquercetin. *Biofizika,* 1996, 41, 620–624 (in Russian).

[105] Teselkin, YO; Babenkova, IV; Kolhir, VK; et al. Dihydroquercetin as a means of antioxidative defence in rats with tetrachloromethane hepatitis. *Phytother. Res.,* 2000, 14, 160–162.

[106] Teselkin, YO; Babenkova, IV; Tjukavkina NA. Influence of dihydroquercetin on the lipid peroxidation of mice during post-radiation period. *Phytother. Res.,* 1998, 12, 517–519.

[107] Tibblin, G; Bergentz, SE; Bjure, J; et al. Hematocrit, plasma protein, plasma volume, and viscosity in early hypertensive disease. *Am. Heart J.,* 1966, 72, 165–176.

[108] Tozzi-Ciancarelli, MG; Di-Massino, C; Masciou, A; et al. Rheological features of erythrocytes in acute myocardial infarction. *Cardioscience*, 1993, 4, 231–234.

[109] Turchetti, V; Bellini, MA; Guerrini, M; Forconi, S. Evaluation of hemorheological parameters and red cell morphology in hypertension. *Clin. Hemorheol. Microcirc.*, 1999, 21, 285–289.

[110] Tyukavkina, NA; Lapteva, KI; Pentegova, VA. Flavonoids of Larix dahurica. *Khim. Prirod. Soedin.*, 1967, 4, 278–279 (in Russian).

[111] Vaya, A; Martinez, M; Garcia, J; et al. Hemorheological alterations in mild essential hypertension. *Thromb. Res.*, 1992, 66, 223–229.

[112] Vekasi, J; Marton, Z; Kesmarky, G; et al. Hemorheologic factors in hypertensive and diabetic retinopathy. *Orv. Hetil.*, 2001, 142, 1045–1048.

[113] Vicaut, E. Hypertension and the microcirculation: a brief overview of experimental studies. *J. Hypertens.*, 1992, 10, Suppl. 5, S59–S68.

[114] Watanabe, H; Kobayashi, A; Yamamoto, T; et al. Alteration of human erythrocytes membrane fluidity by oxygen derived free radicals and calcium. *Free Radical Biol.* Med., 1990, 8, 507–514.

[115] Wen, Y; Killania, S; McGettingan, P; Feely, J. Lipid peroxidation and antioxidant vitamin C and E in hypertensive patients Ir. *J. Med. Sci.,* 1996, 165, 210–212.

[116] Wustner, D; Pomorski, T; Herrmann, A; Muller, P. Release of phospholipids from erythrocyte membranes by taurocholate is determined by their transbilayer orientation and hydrophobic backlone. *Biochemistry,* 1998, 37, 17093–17104.

[117] Yerer, MB; Aydogan, S. The antioxidant effectiveness of alpha-tocopherol in oxidative stress induced by SNP in red blood cells. In: 12th Europ. Conf. Clin. Hemorheol.: Program and Book of Abstract. Sofia; 2003; 47.

[118] Zakharova, NA; Bogdanov, GN; Zaprometov, MN; et al. Antiradical activity of natural phenolic compounds. Zh. Ob. Khimii, 1972, 42, 1414–1420 (in Russian).

[119] Zannad, F; Voisin, P; Brunotte, F; et al. Haemorheological abnormalities in arterial hypertension and their relation to cardiac hypertrophy. *J. Hyperten.,* 1988, 6, 293–297.

In: Frontiers in Antioxidants Research
Editor: Harold V. Panglossi, pp. 133-200
ISBN 1-60021-273-5

Chapter 6

IMPACT OF OXIDATIVE STRESS ON DIABETES MELLITUS AND INFLAMMATORY BOWEL DISEASES

Jana Varvařovská,[1] Rudolf Štětina,[2] Josef Sýkora,[2] Zdeněk Rušavý,[3] Jaroslav Racek,[4] Silva Lacigová [3] and Konrad Siala [2]

[1]Department of Paediatrics, Faculty of Medicine Plzen, Charles University Prague, and University Hospital Plzen, Plzen, Czech Republic

[2]Department of Toxicology, Faculty of Military Health Sciences Hradec Králové, University of Defence Brno, Czech Republic

[3]Diabetology Center, Ist Clinic of Internal Diseases, Faculty of Medicine Plzen, Charles University Prague, and University Hospital Plzen, Czech Republic

[4]Institute of Clinical Biochemistry and Haematology, Faculty of Medicine Plzen, Charles University Prague, and University Hospital Plzen, Czech Republic

ABSTRACT

Formation of reactive oxygen species (ROS) is a natural process during oxidative metabolism. ROS play an important role not only in pathological processes of human organism as usually presented but less attention is paid to their proper important role in cell signaling, biosynthesis or non-specific antiinfectious defence. Overproduction of ROS during numerous pathological situations in presence of insufficient antioxidant protection leads to substantial oxidative changes of lipids, proteins, sugars, and also DNA. Protection against ROS is assured by different extracellular or intracellular antioxidant mechanisms as studied during last decades. Antioxidant enzymes rectifying the oxidative damage are studied with regard to their different activities and usefulness in body protection. Their genetic polymorphisms are certainly involved in different response to oxidative stress.

Special attention should be devoted to the topic of oxidative nuclear and mitochondrial DNA damage and its restoring via DNA repair process, especially base excision repair (BER). A large scale of antioxidant enzymes is involved in correction of

DNA oxidative damage. Natural trend of worsened DNA repair is usually associated with aging. Other pathologies related with deficient DNA repair are susceptibility to carcinogenesis (lack of apoptosis control) or degenerative diseases.

Oxidative stress is involved in the pathophysiology of diabetes mellitus (DM – oxidative stress of mainly metabolic origin) and inflammatory bowel diseases (IBD – oxidative stress of mainly inflammatory origin). In spite of confirmed OS in DM or IBD, the substantial information about the intensity of DNA repair and its possible relationship to the disease course and development of chronic complications is missing.

Our pilot studies completed both in adult and pediatric patients with DM or IBD confirmed an increased oxidative stress as well as oxidative DNA damage examined with comet assay. The surprising findings were ascertained in intensity of DNA repair (analysed with modified comet assay). DNA repair process was stimulated in Type 1 diabetes adults without diabetic microvascular complications and still more in diabetic children with short disease duration. On the other hand adults with Type 2 diabetes had substantially increased oxidative DNA damage and extremely low DNA repair. This finding could be the link to increased susceptibility of Type 2 DM patients to cancerogenesis. Patients with IBD (Crohn´s disease - both children and adults) had similar tendencies in OS intensity and oxidative DNA damage and repair but less intensive.

Large population studies in DM or IBD studying intensity of OS and expression of DNA repair enzymes are needed in order to get the correlation between individual repair enzymes expression and the long-term course and occurence of complications in DM or IBD.

Key words: oxidative stress, reactive oxygen species, antioxidant defense, oxidative DNA damage, DNA repair, Type 1 diabetes mellitus, diabetic microvascular complications, Crohn´s disease

2. Introduction

2.1 ROS under Physiological Conditions

Formation of reactive oxygen species (superoxide, hydrogen peroxide, hydroxyl radical, *ROS*) is a natural process during oxidative metabolism. ROS play an important role not only in pathological processes of human organism as usually presented but less attention is paid to their proper important role in cell signalling, biosynthesis or non-specific antiinfectious defence.

Triplet-state molecular oxygen *undergoes* process of univalent reduction and formation of superoxide anion ($O_2^{\cdot-}$) nonenzymatically by redox-reactive compounds in the mitochondrial electron transport chain and enzymatically via enzymes such as NAD(P)H oxidases and xanthine oxidase. Further conversion of labile superoxide is into hydrogen peroxide (H_20_2) by superoxide dismutase. In the presence of reduced transition metals (e.g. ferrous or cuprous ions), hydrogen peroxide can be converted (via Fenton reaction) into the highly reactive hydroxyl radical ($^{\cdot}OH$). Alternative conversion of hydrogen peroxide into water is mediated by the enzymes catalase or glutathione peroxidase. In the glutathione peroxidase reaction, glutathione is oxidized to glutathione disulfide, which can be converted back to glutathione by glutathione reductase in an NAD(P)H-consuming process [1](Figure 1). Superoxide and related ROS formed via NAD(P)H oxidase have important physiological functions such as signal transduction from various membrane receptors, control of ventilation, smooth muscle relaxation, and enhancement of immunological functions, control of erythropoietin production and other hypoxia-inducible functions, cell apoptosis.

Under physiological conditions, ROS formation and concentration in biological cells and tissues is determined by the balance between their rates of production and their rates of clearance by various antioxidant compounds and enzymes. Main nonenzymatic compounds are such as α-tocopherol, ascorbate, β-carotene, glutathione, amino acids, albumin, and the most important enzymes involved in antioxidant defence are superoxide dismutase SOD, glutathione peroxidase GPx, glutathione reductase, glutathione transferase, and catalase [1].

Oxidant-antioxidant balance is very important for cells and tissues life and metabolism. A short-term increase in ROS concentrations or a decrease in the activity of one or more antioxidant systems stimulate cell signal cascades and lead to stimulated gene expression and higher production of proteins or antioxidant enzymes (oxidative stress response) [2]. The original balance between ROS production and ROS scavenging capacity is restored and a so-called redox homeostasis is re-established.

ROS play important role in receptor-mediated signalling pathways. Growth factors, cytokines or other ligands trigger ROS production in non-phagocytic cells through NADPH oxidase stimulation. Such ROS production mediates further signal transduction including stimulation of protein tyrosine kinases, mitogen activated protein kinases (MAPK) cascade, oxidative activation of protein kinase C as well as activation of transcription factor AP-1 important for differentiation processes and also transcription factor NF-κB, implicated in inflammatory reactions, growth control and apoptosis.

ROS are involved in the defence against environmental pathogens and immunological response. In phagocytic cells (macrophages, neutrophils), NADPH oxidase produces ROS after stimulation with microbial products, lipoproteins or by cytokines such as interferon-γ, interleukin-1β, or interleukin-8. The stimulated massive production of ROS is called oxidative burst and plays an important role as a first line of defence against environmental pathogens. The following product created by combination activities of NADPH oxidase and myeloperoxidase is hypochlorous acid (HClO), a potent antimicrobial and oxidant agent. ROS production in lymphocytes is mediated by the enzyme 5-lipoxygenase (5-LO) and may influence their response to cytokines. Exposure of T lymphocytes to relevant concentrations of environmental ROS amplify signalling cascades even after mild stimulation and in case of massive ROS production substantially enhances the lymphocyte reactivity and stimulation.

ROS produced during oxidative phosphorylation in mitochondria serve as sensor in carotid body for changes in oxygen concentration and also for expression of erythropoietin. ROS also induce the adherence of leukocytes to endothelial cells in post-capillary venules. ROS are crucial for normal functions of cardiac and vascular cells including vascular tone.

Though the physiological and favourable effect of ROS on a normally functioning cell, there is a propensity for ROS to evade antioxidant defences and to modify cell components – lipids, proteins, sugars, and finally DNA. If ROS impact is short, there is no serious damage to the cell. On the other hand, prolonged ROS effect leads to cell apoptosis, cellular dysfunction, or neoplastic shift.

2.2 ROS under Pathological Conditions

If ROS overproduction during numerous pathological situations in human medicine remains stable and long-lasting, it could be taken as *basic pathological mechanism for many different diseases and complex processes* as aging, neoplasias, infectious diseases, autoimmune disorders, ischaemia-reperfusion syndromes (myocardial infarct, brain stroke, injuries, organ transplantation), atherosclerosis, diabetes mellitus, toxic factors of different origin, irradiation, extreme physical activity and *systemic and organ specific diseases* as pancreatitis, glomerulonephritis or interstitial nephritis, inflammatory bowel diseases, hepatitis, different dermatological diseases (atopic dermatitis, psoriasis, infections, pulmonary affections (asthma, dust diseases, ARDS), rheumatoid arthritis, demyelinating diseases [3].

When considering the origin of non-regulated ROS production, it is necessary to refer to *the most important situations:*

a) Mitochondrial electron transport chain (ETC), b) inflammatory processes with excessive stimulation of NDAPH oxidases and lipoxygenases, c) ischaemia and reperfusion with xanthine oxidase stimulation, d) endogenous or exogenous toxic factors including radiation.

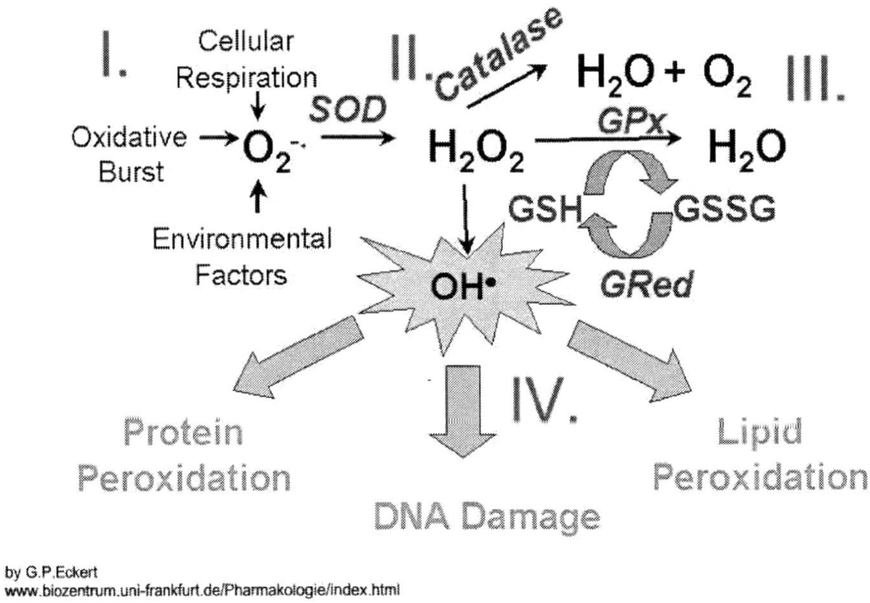

Figure 1. Scheme of oxidative stress in human cell. I. Generation of superoxide, II. Formation of hydrogen peroxide, III. Detoxification of hydrogen peroxide by antioxidant enzymes, IV. Protein, lipid and DNA damage by ROS (hydroxyl radical) (by G.P. Eckert)

Oxidative stress (OS) is then defined as the imbalance between high ROS production and insufficient antioxidant (AO) defence. Once formed, ROS deplete antioxidant defences, rendering the affected cells and tissues more susceptible to oxidative damage. Lipids, proteins and DNA are the cellular targets for oxidation, leading to changes in cellular structure and function. The order of preference for modification depends upon a number of factors, such as location of ROS production, relative ability for the biomolecule to be oxidised, and availability of metal ions. Oxidative changes of lipids and proteins may be removed via normal turnover of the molecules; damage to DNA is required to be repaired. Prolonged oxidative stress leads to serious injuries of cell structures and may be finished by cell apoptosis, dysfunction or uncontrolled cell division and neoplasia. *Diabetes mellitus and inflammatory bowel diseases represent 2 model diseases with important oxidative stress in their pathogenesis and they will be discussed later.*

2.3 Antioxidant Defence of Human Organism

There are several approaches how to distinguish components of defence against oxidative stress. The schedule underlines the process of ROS formation or degradation and hence the defence against them [3, 4].

a) *Substances preventing the formation of ROS* are mainly the compounds binding reduced transition metals (e.g. ferrous or cuprous ions) such as acute-phase proteins (transferrin, ferritin, lactoferrin, haptoglobin, hemopexin, ceruloplasmin), or chelating agents, also inhibitors of enzymes catalysing the formation of ROS (allopurinol blocking xanthine oxidase).
b) *Substances removing previously formed ROS or restoring reducing agents* are either intracellular and extracellular enzymes such as superoxide dismutase, catalase, glutathione peroxidase, glutathione reductase and transferase, or non-enzymatic endogenous and exogenous substances such as glutathione, α-tocopherol, ascorbate, β-carotene, amino acids, uric acid, bilirubin, albumin, and polyphenols.
c) *Repair systems removing molecules damaged by ROS* are principally enzymes degrading modified proteins, or oxidized lipids (phospholipases, glutathione peroxidases), and finally the complex of enzymes repairing DNA damaged by ROS.

2.4 Some Remarks to Antioxidant Enzymes and Substances from the Recent Literature

Antioxidant enzymes are directly implicated in human protection against oxidative stress. Their properties, their known polymorphisms and their corresponding phenotype are target of many studies.

Superoxide dismutase SOD transforms superoxide into hydrogen peroxide. Three isoforms (cytoplasmic CuZn SOD or SOD1, mitochondrial Mn SOD or SOD2, tetrameric CuZn extracellular EC-SOD or SOD3) exist and have been studied for many years *in vitro* and *in vivo*. Relationships among different SOD isoforms and human diseases were found. Down regulated or mutant SOD1 has been associated with stroke, ischaemia/reperfusion syndrome, neurodegenerative disorders (Parkinson's disease) and familial amyotrophic lateral sclerosis with 58 known mutations in the CuZn SOD gene (chromosome 21q22.1). Loss or reduction of the SOD2 activity has been associated with neurodegeneration, heart failure and also death during neonatal period. SOD3 has been detected in several compartments such as the plasma, lymph, ascites, cerebrospinal fluid and lung and is related to inflammation, hyperoxic pulmonary disorders, and focal cerebral ischaemia [5]. The present efforts are done to introduce into clinical practice SOD mimetic drugs [6], either selective (macrocyclics) or non-selective such as manganese metalloporphyrins, manganese salen complexes [7, 8]. Another possibility seems to be dietary delivery system using wheat gliadin biopolymers carrying plant SOD extracts [9].

Glutathione peroxidases GPx scavenge peroxides generated in cells. There are four isoforms with different tissue localisation. Cytosolic GPx1 is ubiquitously expressed in human organism, particularly in erythrocytes, kidney, and liver. Cytosolic GPx2 is expressed primarily in gastrointestinal tissues and plays an important role in protection against ingested lipid peroxides. GPx3 is an extracellular enzyme reducing hydroperoxides of more complex lipids. It is mainly present in plasma, but also in lung, heart, kidney and placenta. GPx4 is detected both in the cytosol and associated with membranes. This enzyme reduces peroxidised phospholipids and cholesterol in membranes [5] (Figure 2).

Glutathione reductase GSR has two isoenzymes (cytosolic and mitochondrial) and its function is to restore glutathione into reduced form [5].

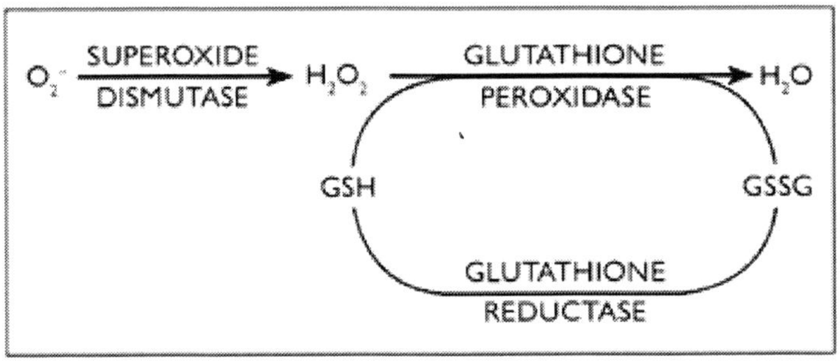

Figure 2. Glutathione peroxidase and glutathione reductase action in antioxidant defence and glutathione metabolism

Catalase decomposes hydrogen peroxide into water and oxygen. This enzyme is particularly abundant in erythrocytes, hepatocytes and the kidney. There are several mutations/polymorphisms in the catalase gene (chromosome 11p13) associated with acatalasemia in erythrocytes, but phenotypes associated with acatalasemia are not prominent [5].

Glutathione transferases GST exist in six cytosolic isoforms and one microsomal GST, the latter now designated membrane associated proteins involved in eicosanoid and glutathione metabolism (MAPEG). GSTs play an important role in detoxification of xenobiotics (chemical carcinogens, environmental pollutants, antitumor agents) and in inactivation of endogenous hydroperoxides and unsaturated aldehydes. GSTs catalyse the conjugation of 4-hydroxynonenal, the degradation product of lipid peroxidation, with glutathione [5, 10, 11]. GST expression is regulated by the cellular redox status and represents a sensor able to transmit the redox variation to the apoptosis machinery. Cytosolic GST isoenzymes are broadly cytoprotective, but their genetic polymorphisms can increase susceptibility to carcinogenesis [12, 13] and inflammatory disease such as chronic obstructive pulmonary disease, asthma, pancreatitis, autoimmune hepatitis, rheumatoid arthritis [5, 14, 15, 16, 17, 18].

It is obvious that cells exposed to oxidative stress express stress-induced genes or genes encoding antioxidant defences [19], and their polymorphisms are certainly involved in various responses to oxidative stress [5].

2.5 Non-enzymatic Substances of Endogenous or Exogenous Origin

Non-enzymatic substances of endogenous or exogenous origin are of great importance for antioxidant defence. Some of them are newly synthesized and classified as antioxidant enzymes mimetics and were mentioned concurrently with antioxidant enzymes. Further new antioxidants are analogues of naturally existing substances.

Glutathione (GSH - γ-glutamylcysteinylglycine) draw attention in context with different diseases. GSH is the major intracellular non-protein antioxidant and is present in all mammalian tissues, where it plays a crucial role in the detoxification of free radicals. Its synthesis serves to maintain a reduced cellular environment. The liver is the main site of inter-organ glutathione synthesis and supplies GSH into circulation and systemic distribution, but the GSH production occurs also in other body cells such as erythrocytes, GIT epithelium, and bronchiolar epithelium. GSH pool is drawn on for three major applications: for direct free radical scavenging and as an antioxidant enzyme cofactor (glutathione peroxidases GPx, glutathione transhydrogenases reconverting dehydroascorbate to ascorbate), and as cofactor for the glutathione transferases GST. Total glutathione has two forms – the free form which is mainly in its reduced form (GSH) and the form bound to proteins (gluthathionylated proteins) [11, 20, 21]. Conversion of GSH reduced form into oxidised glutathione (GSSG) occurs during oxidative stress and can be reverted to the reduced form by the action of glutathione reductase GSR mentioned above (Figure 3). This enzyme uses as its source of electrons the coenzyme NADPH coming mainly from the pentose phosphate shunt. Low GSH, high GSSG, and a higher GSSG/GSH ratio indicates the presence of oxidative stress and consumption of GSH [11].

Glutathione has also profound importance for cellular homeostasis and for diverse cellular functions such as protein synthesis, enzyme catalysis, transmembrane transport, receptor action, intermediary metabolism, cell maturation, and apoptosis [11, 20].

The importance of glutathione and its disturbances has been highlighted in numerous articles [11, 22, 23]. GSH deficiency certainly plays the role in liver diseases such as cirrhosis, hepatitis and non-alcoholic steatohepatitis [20, 21]. Depletion of glutathione was also found in severe acute pancreatitis [16]. Alterations in alveolar and lung GSH metabolism is widely recognized as a central feature of many inflammatory lung diseases such as idiopathic pulmonary fibrosis, acute respiratory distress syndrome, chronic obstructive pulmonary disease (COPD), and asthma [24, 25, 26]. In patients with cystic fibrosis (CF), CFTR channel is no more taken for a primarily „chloride channel" but recognized as a channel that also controls the efflux of other physiologically important anions, such as glutathione and bicarbonate. CF mutations in fact cause a primary dysfunction in the reduced GSH system, e.g. CF mutations significantly decrease GSH efflux from cells and this leads to deficiency of GSH in the epithelial lining fluid of the lung, as well as in other compartments, including immune system cells and the gastrointestinal tract. Following this, other antioxidants are depleted and this may play a role in initiating the over-inflammation characteristic of cystic fibrosis [26, 27]. The role of glutathione is also alleged in neurodegenerative diseases (Parkinson's disease, Alzheimer's disease), in atherosclerosis, and in diabetes whose topic will be discussed later [20, 22].

Strategies for cellular glutathione repletion include mainly dietary interventions. Natural dietary glutathione undergoes hydrolysis by intestinal and hepatic gamma-glutamyltransferase [28], and so food sources or supplements that increase glutathione must either provide the precursors of glutathione, or enhance its production by some other means. Natural foods that boost glutathione levels are fresh and frozen fruits and vegetables (asparagus, broccoli, avocado, spinach, walnuts), fish, and meat [29]. N-acetyl cysteine takes on significance as a dietary GSH source. N-acetylcysteine has been used in several indications, such as the treatment of paracetamol (acetaminophen) intoxication [30], prevention of contrast-induced nephropathy after intravascular angiography [31], treatment of chronic obstructive pulmonary disease [32]. Its application in the treatment of severe sepsis and septic shock remains controversial [33, 34, 35]. N-acetylcysteine amide is currently studied as another possible substance for treatment of neurodegeneration and other oxidation-mediated disorders [36].

Thioredoxin (Trx)

Thioredoxin (Trx)is a small multifunctional protein involved in cellular thiol-redox processes. It contains two redox-active cysteine residues in its active sites. The protein is stress-inducible and enhanced by various types of stresses including ROS. The thioredoxin is kept in the reduced state by the flavoenzyme thioredoxin reductase, in a NADPH-dependent reaction. It acts as an electron donor to peroxidases and ribonucleotide reductase and the administration of recombinant Trx protein, induction of endogenous Trx, or gene therapy can be a therapeutic modality for oxidative stress-associated disorders [37,38, 39, 40].

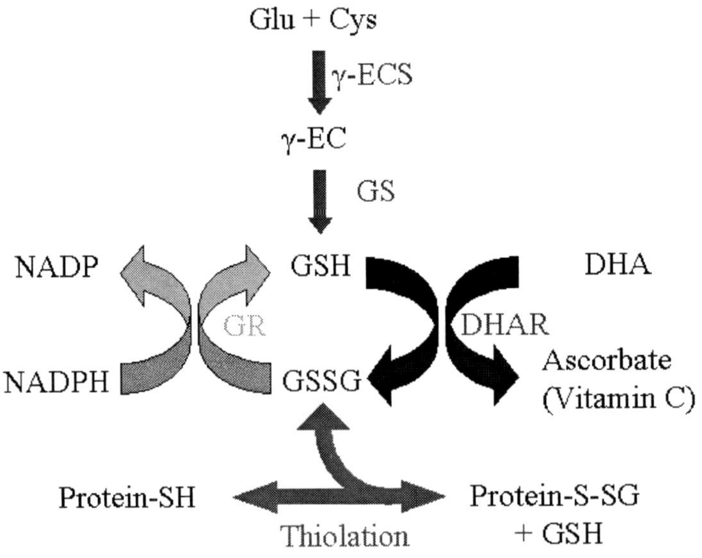

Figure 3. Metabolism of glutathione in the cell. GR-glutathione reductase (NADPH-dependent), GS-glutathione synthase, γ-ECS- gamma-glutamylcysteine synthase, DHA-dehydroascorbate, DHAR-dehydroascorbate reductase, GSSG- oxidized glutathione, GSH-reduced glutathione

Coenzyme Q10 (CoQ)

Coenzyme Q10 (CoQ)known as ubiquinone, CoQ, and vitamin Q10 is a fat-soluble vitamin-like quinone present in every cell of the body. It is naturally present in different amounts in foods (mostly high in beef meat, soy oil, sardines, mackerel, and peanuts), but it is also synthesized from its precursors Q1-9 or *de novo* synthesized from acetyl coenzyme A in liver. CoQ-10 is found throughout the body in cell membranes, especially in the mitochondrial membranes and is particularly abundant in the heart, lungs, liver, kidneys, spleen, pancreas and adrenal glands.Q10 is a mobile electron carrier from NADH dehydrogenase complex to cytochrome b-c_1 complex within the mitochondrial electron transport chain enabling the H^+ flow out of the mitochondrial matrix. Thus electrochemical proton gradient across the inner membrane is formed and finally drives the H^+ flow through the ATP synthase, that uses the energy of the H^+ flow to synthesize ATP as a carrier of free energy [39]. Q10 is also a powerful antioxidant both on its own and in combination with vitamin E. CoQ is present not only in mitochondria, where bound to mitochondrial membranes serves also as an antioxidant. It is also present in cell membranes where in its reduced form ubiquinol can neutralize a lipid peroxyl radical. The CoQ radical ubisemiquinone is stable and its formation is a normal intermediate between ubiquinone (CoQ) and ubiquinol ($CoQH_2$), and is restored to a non-free-radical state by the respiratory chain Q cycle. Ubisemiquinone and ubiquinol can also regenerate the vitamin E tocopheroxyl radical by electron donation and this is very important as vitamin E neutralizes lipid peroxyl radicals far more readily and is less hydrophobic, allowing it to more freely move throughout the mitochondrial membrane. CoQ is more confined to the centre of the phospholipids layer. Its importance as an endogenously produced lipid-phase antioxidant is indicated with its high concentration not only in cell membranes, but also in Golgi vesicles and microsomes [4, 41, 42]. Supplementation of CoQ is recommended in patients with Parkinson's disease, mitochondrial encephalomyopathies, with chronic heart failure [41], as CoQ is needed for energy production and antioxidant protection. The problem in question is the supplementation of CoQ in patients treated with statins as HMG-CoA reductase is also the first committed rate-limiting step for the synthesis of a range of other compounds including steroid hormones and ubiquinone. Currently, there is insufficient evidence from human studies to link statin therapy unequivocally to pathologically significantly decreased tissue CoQ levels [43]. Cosupplementation with vitamin E and CoQ reduces circulating markers of inflammation as proved on animal models and this example can be used for further studies dealing with vascular diseases [44].

Vitamin C

Vitamin C is essential for human organism. Under physiological conditions, vitamin C predominantly exists in its reduced form, ascorbic acid (AA), it also exists in trace quantities in the oxidized form – dehydroascorbic acid (DHA). AA functions as a cofactor for enzymes involved in the biosynthesis of collagen, carnitine, norepinephrine, and in the amidation of hormones. In plasma and cells, AA is a powerful antioxidant, quenching ROS. During the process of quenching free radicals, ascorbate donates an electron, becoming the unstable intermediated ascorbyl radical that can be reversibly reduced back to ascorbate via glutathione oxidation. Ascorbyl radical can also donate a second electron and be converted to DHA that can efflux from the cells via the glucose transporters and functions as a readily transportable form of vitamin C. As mentioned above, ROS activate transcription factors, such as NF-κB, that are important in host defence, inflammation, and apoptosis. AA directly quenches ROS intermediates involved in the activation of NF-κB, and is oxidized to DHA, which directly inhibits IκBα kinase (IKKβ) and thus NF-κB cannot be activated [45].

Vitamin E

Vitamin E is a fat-soluble vitamin present in many foods, especially certain fats and oils. There are α, β, γ, and δ forms, among them α-tocopherol (α-TOH) is the most abundant and active form with the referring term vitamin E. It is a natural, lipophilic radical-scavenging antioxidant and is described as the most important lipophilic antioxidant in vivo, which has been the subject of many extensive studies [46]. Vitamin E localization in the lipophilic domain of the membranes and lipoproteins inhibits lipid peroxidation, i.e. α-TOH reacts with peroxyl radicals much faster than lipids do and thus it may scavenge the majority of peroxyl radicals before they attack lipids. The efficacy of α-TOH is better when a radical scavenging occurs near the membrane surface. If the radical went deeper into the interior of the membranes, scavenging activity of α-TOH decreased significantly [47]. α-TOH is converted to α-TO· radical which may undergo several reactions. Preferentially, it is reduced by ascorbate in order to regenerate α-TOH provided that α-TO· radical is localized in the membranes and LDL. If the radical goes deeper into the interior of cell or is localized in the LDL core, ascorbate is unable to reduce the radicals. The α-TO· radical can be reduced by other reductants, such as ubiquinol and polyphenolic compounds. Vitamin E may exert its effect by acting as a radical-scavenging antioxidant whose activity depends on many factors (localization, mobility, presence of other collaborating antioxidants). These factors influencing vitamin E efficiency and impact on oxidative stress can explain certain controversies in the antioxidant studies with vitamin E. Nevertheless, vitamin E remains a perspective antioxidant in combination with synergistic antioxidant compounds [46, 47].

Phytochemicals

Phytochemicals are a wide range of different naturally plant compounds, such as carotenoids, polyphenols including flavonoids. Their antioxidant effects depend on their chemical structure and lipophilic or hydrophilic character. *Carotenoids* are plant pigments and animals do not synthesize them. They are responsible for the red, yellows, and orange colour of fruits and vegetables, their number in nature exceeds 600 and can be grouped into carotenes, xanthophylls and lycopene. Carotenoids have been intensively studied in the last decade and as proved by several epidemiological studies, they showed certain preventive or inhibitory effect on atherosclerosis, degenerative diseases, cancer and other diseases [48, 49, 50]. The antioxidant activity of carotenoids arises as a result of the ability to delocalise any unpaired electrons. β-carotene has an excellent ability to quench singlet oxygen without degradation and reacts with free radicals such as peroxyl radical, hydroxyl radical. This is the way that assures lipid protection from peroxidative damage. *Polyphenols, among them flavonoids* existing for example in green tea, black currant, blackberries, form stable phenolic radicals with ROS, regenerate vitamin C and E and bind transition metals [4]. *Resveratrol* is a naturally occurring polyphenol (phytoalexin) produced by some higher plants in response to injury of fungal infection. Resveratrol is found in grapevines, also in peanuts and mulberries. It has several activities which include inhibition of the oxidation of low-density lipoproteins, blockade of superoxide anion and hydrogen peroxide in macrophages stimulated by lipopolysacharides (LPS), decrease of arachidonic acid release induced by LPS or by exposure to superoxide or hydrogen peroxide, glutathione-sparing activity thanks to hydroxyl-radical scavenging activity, suppression of lipid peroxidation both by chelation of copper and by scavenging of the free radicals. Resveratrol action is explained by its influence on NADPH-dependent oxidases, xanthine oxidase, 5-lipoxygenase and 15-lipoxygenase, myeloperoxidase. It seems to be a good candidate protecting the vascular walls from oxidation, inflammation, platelet aggregation, and thrombus formation, i.e. atherosclerotic process [51]. The French paradox (low incidence of coronary heart in France) is attributed to the complex antiatherosclerotic role of grape polyphenols regularly consumed in red wine. Isorhapontigenin (ISO), a new resveratrol analogue, has been isolated from Belamcanda chinensis (blackberry lily). Its chemical structure is very similar to that of resveratrol. ISO significantly inhibits malondialdehyde formation induced by hydrogen peroxide and the increase in lipid peroxidation, ISO also inhibits oxidative DNA damage [48, 52].

Figure 4 shows the cellular distribution of some enzymatic and non-enzymatic antioxidants.

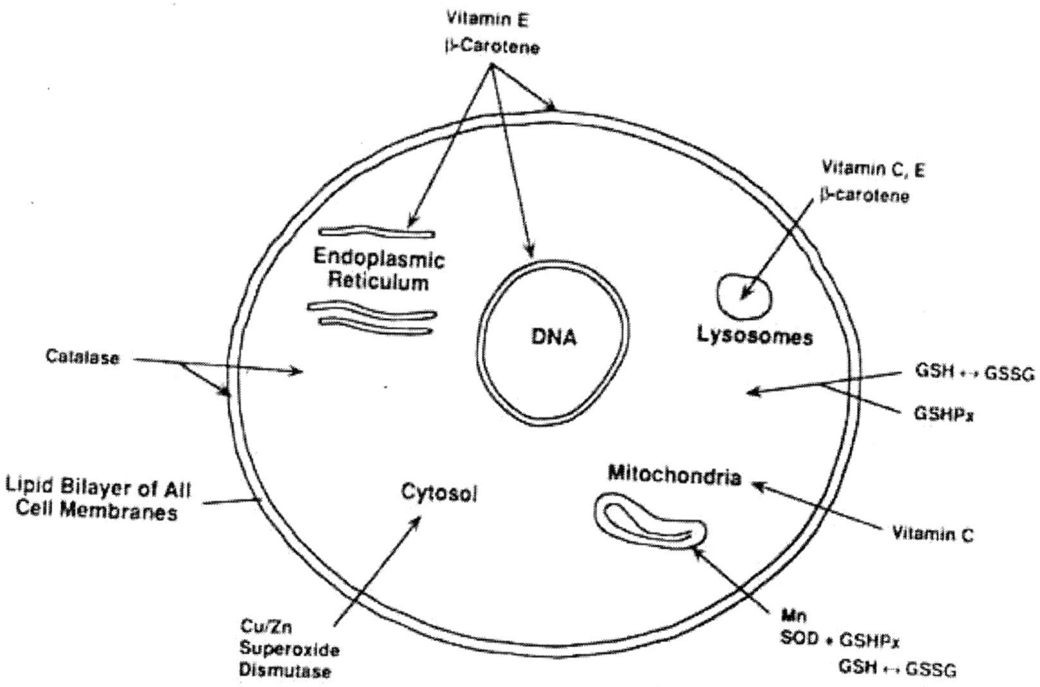

Figure 4. Cell structure and location of different endogenous and exogenous antioxidants. Available from: www.involuntaryweightloss.org, by RH Demling and L De Santi

2.6 Catalytic Antioxidants – New Therapeutic Possibilities

As mentioned above, superoxide $O_2^{\cdot-}$ and hydrogen peroxide H_2O_2 participate in the formation of several reactive species that have been directly implicated in tissue damage. Cellular antioxidant enzymes as SODs and catalase detoxify ROS. Unfortunately, their large size, short circulating half-life, and antigenicity are not suitable for therapeutic use in free radical diseases. To overcome many of these limitations, an increasing number of low molecular-weight catalytic antioxidants have been developed. They are designed with redox-active metal centres that catalyse the dismutation reaction of $O_2^{-\cdot}$ and/or H_2O_2 by a mechanism that is similar to the mode of action of the active-site metals of SOD and catalase. An ideal mimetic is stable and non-toxic and its size and charge of a mimetic can be exploited to target crucial cellular sites of oxidative stress. Three classes of metal-containing catalytic antioxidants, i.e. macrocyclic (M40403), salen (EUK series), and metalloporphyrin mimetics (AEOL series) seem to be important for future clinical use as shown on *in vitro* and *in vivo* models. Their potential includes lung fibrosis, chronic obstructive lung diseases, asthma, acute respiratory distress syndrome, bronchopulmonary dysplasia, shock, myocardial infarction, liver failure, colitis, diabetes, ischaemia-reperfusion, transplantation, arthritis, amyotrophic lateral sclerosis, neurodegenerative diseases, stroke [7, 8].

3. DNA Oxidative Damage and DNA Repair

Nuclear DNA Damage and Repair

DNA is constantly exposed to damaging agents from both endogenous and exogenous sources. If these lesions are not repaired, they can lead to mutations and result in cellular dysfunction with either further uncontrolled cell proliferation, or apoptosis. In order to maintain the integrity of the genome, a complicated network of DNA repair pathways remove the majority of deleterious lesions. There are six major repair pathways of DNA repair [53, 54, 55]. The number of human DNA repair genes exceeds 140 and keeps growing [56, 57]. Direct reversal (DR) consists of repair proteins acting directly on a damaged base and re-establishing the correct structure in situ without removing the damaged nucleotide. Exogenous agents such as ionising radiation, tobacco smoke, cytostatics generate larger DNA lesions with abnormal structure or abnormal chemistry (24-29 nucleotides) which are repaired via nucleotide excision repair (NER). NER steps involves a) damage recognition, b) binding of a multi-protein complex at the damaged site, c) double incision of the damaged strand several nucleotides away from the damaged site, on both the 5′and 3′sides, d) removal of the damage-containing oligonucleotide from between the two nicks, e) filling in of the resulting gap by a DNA polymerase and f) final ligation. The genes encoding many of the human NER proteins were first identified in genetic complementation studies of the human DNA repair disease – xeroderma pigmentosum (XP) with mutations in any of 7 genes. In addition to XP, Cockayne′s syndrome (CS) and trichothiodystrophy (TTD) are two other human genetic disease with defects in NER [58, 59].

The *mismatch repair (MMR)* is a post-replicative DNA repair system contributing to the fidelity of replication and the maintenance of the genome. Recombinational repair (RER) restores deleterious double-strand breaks via *homologous recombinational repair (HRR) or non-homologous end-joining (NHEJ)*. Genes and proteins related to HRR are implicated in chromosomal stability and are critical in maintaining cellular resistance to ionising radiation [60]. Ataxia teleangiectasia (AT) and Nijmegen breakage syndrome (NBS) are chromosome instability syndrome with mutated genes, such as ataxia teleangiectasia mutated (ATM - chromosome 11q23) or NBS respectively. AT is an autosomal recessive disease and affected patients develop cerebellar ataxia, teleangiectasia, combined cellular and antibody immunodeficiency, sinopulmonary infections, and malignancies. The Nijmegen breakage syndrome (NBS – chromosome 8q21) is also an autosomal recessive disease characterized by microcephaly, growth retardation, immunodeficiency and cancer predisposition [61, 62]. Germline and somatic mutations of certain HRR genes contribute inevitably to carcinogenesis (e.g. BRCA1, BRCA2 proteins)[63].

Finally, *base excision repair (BER)* is the most important pathway for oxidative DNA damage. Free radicals, most notably ·OH, react with DNA compounds and form radicals of DNA bases and the sugar moiety. Further reactions of these radicals result in a variety of final products. Major products of oxidative damage to the DNA bases are numerous, among them thymine glycol, 5-formyluracil, 5-hydroxyuracil, 5-hydroxycytosine, 8-hydroxyadenine, 8-hydroxyguanine, 2,6-diamino-4-hyroxy-5-formamidopyrimidine. In addition to sugars modified by oxidative stress (e.g. 2-deoxyribonolactone), unaltered sugar moieties within DNA, called base-free sites (or apurinic/apyrimidinic site – AP site) are formed from the elimination of modified DNA bases due to the weakening of the glycosidic bond. These lesions can result in single strand breaks.

ROS-reactive oxygen species, 4-HNE- 4-hydroxy-2-nonenal, MDA-malondialdehyde, M_1G pyrimidopurinone, edG ethenodeoxyguanosine, edA etheno-deoxyadenosine, hOgg1 human 8-oxoguanine DNA glycosylase 1, MPG N-methylpurine DNA glycosylase, FapyG 2,6-diamino-4-hydroxy-5-formamidopyrimidine, 8-oxo-G 8-oxo-7,8-dihydro-2′-guanosine

As ROS are continuously generated in all organisms, the oxidized bases, single-strand breaks and AP sites in DNA are repaired primarily via the DNA base excision repair pathway (BER) (Figures 5, 6). NER is implicated as a back-up system for BER, so oxidative DNA lesions containing oligonucleotide are removed via NER and is taken as a back-up system for BER.

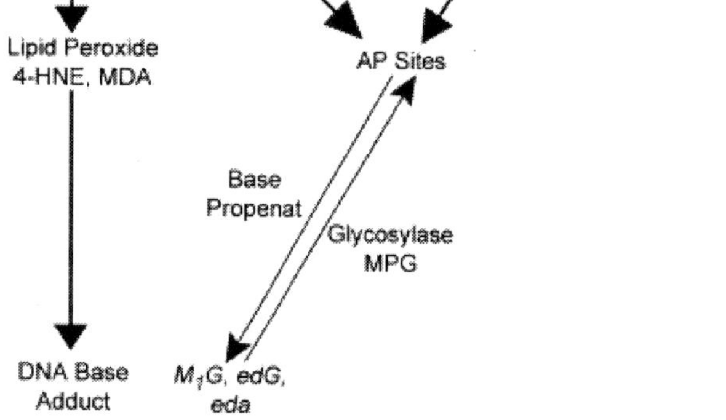

Figure 5. Schematic diagram of types of DNA damage induced by ROS (published by Powell, CL, Swenberg, JA and Rusyn, I. in Cancer Letters, 2005, 229, 1-11)

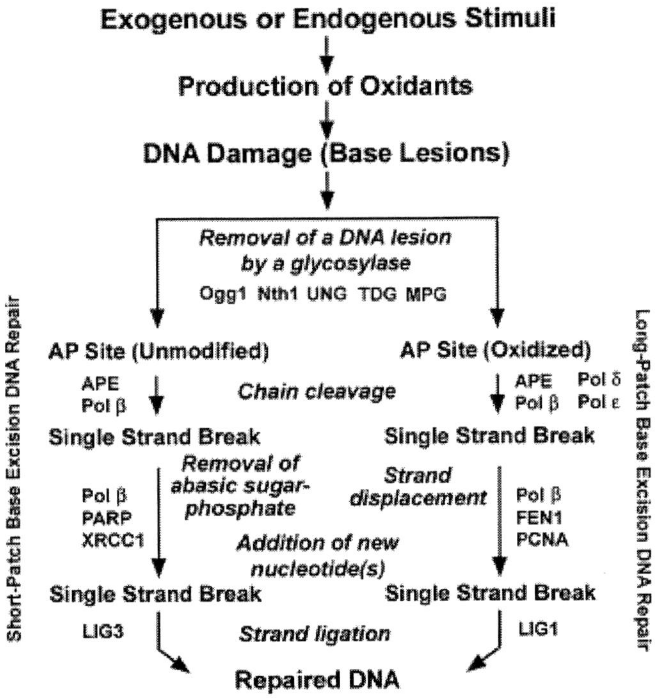

Figure 6. Base excision repair pathway (published by Powell, CL, Swenberg, JA and Rusyn, I. in Cancer Letters, 2005, 229, 1-11)

The developing knowledge about DNA repair processes is bringing the detailed information about *purine- and pyrimidine-derived lesions and their removal from DNA*. 8-OH-guanine glycosylase OGG1 has 2 major forms hOGG1-1a being targeted to the nucleus and hOGG1-2a being targeted to the mitochondrial inner membrane and protecting mitochondrial DNA. OGG1 is a constitutively expressed gene and its expression can vary with tissue source and between individuals. MutY homologue (hMYH) glycosylase repairs mismatches 8-OH-Gua:A and 8-OH-Gua:G. Human MutT homologue (hMTH1) degrades 8-OH-dGTP to 8-OH-dGMP and pyrophosphate. N-methylpurine-DNA glycosylase (MPG protein or 3-methyladenine-DNA glycosylase) has a relatively broad range of substrates including 8-OH-Gua and 3-methyladenine by BER mechanism. Endonuclease III homologue (hNTH1) is involved in the repair of oxidized pyrimidines. Another guanine-derived 2,6-diamino-4-hydroxy-5-formamidopyrimidine (FapyGua) is removed via hOGG1 or NEIL1 (glycosylase excising FapyGua). Adenine-derived lesions such as 8-hydroxyadenine (8-OH-Ade) are removed also via hOGG1 when 8-OH-Ade pairs opposite cytosine. 2-OH-adenine is the substrate for hMTH1. 4,6-diamino-5-formamidopyrimidine (FapyAde) is released by the activity of hNTH1 and also NEIL1 glycosylase. The same enzyme is targeted at 5-hydroxycytosine (5-OH-Cyt), 5-OH-uracil lesions and thymine glycol. Thymine glycol could be removed also by thymine glycol glycosylases (primarily mitochondrial TGG1 and nuclear TGG2) [2, 64].

Removal of a damaged nucleotide by a glycosylase forms an AP site. *Repair of AP sites* inhibits both the mutational and cytotoxic effects of nucleic acid loss. AP endonucleases (APEX1, APEX 2) recognize abasic site and cleave the phosphodiester DNA backbone. Subsequent step is up to the *DNA polymerase β* which removes the deoxyribose phosphate and adds a nucleotide. Finally, *DNA ligase III in partnership with the XRCC1 protein (ligase accessory factor)* seals the nick. Cells deficient in polymerase β showed hypersensitivity to monofunctional alkylating agents. The described pathway is called *short patch-BER* (Figure 6) [54, 59].

The second BER pathway - *long patch-BER* is a little bit complicated and involves the activities of glycosylase, AP-endonuclease I, replication factor C, proliferating cell nuclear antigen (PCNA), DNA polymerase δ or ε, flap-endonuclease 1 (FEN1 – 5′nuclease) and DNA ligase I. This involves removal and re-synthesis of a 2-6 nucleotide patch (Figure 6)[54, 59, 64].

Whichever pathway is used, the product secreted from the cell will be the modified base, because they both pathways involve a glycosylase activity. These *excreted oxidized bases* could be measured as a marker of endogenous oxidative DNA damage i.e. oxidative stress [2]. There is a large scale of methods for measuring oxidative DNA damage: chromatographic assessment of oxidized purines and pyrimidines, comet assay (or single cell gel electrophoresis SCGE) for determination of single-strand breaks [65], when lesion-specific endonucleases are included, allows detection of oxidized purines and pyrimidines. Slot-blot assays enables the measurement of abasic (AP) sites and with addition of lesion-specific endonucleases allows detection of oxidized purines and pyrimidines [66]. For example, an intensively studied 8-OH-guanine was measured in blood and especially in urine as a marker of oxidative stress in different diseases. Parkinson's and Alzheimer's disease, multiple sclerosis, amyotrophic lateral sclerosis, breast cancer, colorectal cancer, haematological disorders, chronic hepatitis, haemochromatosis, Wilson's disease, cystic fibrosis, lung and gastric cancer, rheumatoid arthritis, systemic lupus erythematosus, Down's syndrome, diabetes mellitus [2].

Repair enzymes are constitutively expressed, their expression and/or activity may be modulated in response to various potential genotoxic stress or in concert with the cell cycle. Levels of oxidative bases in DNA are the consequence of a balance between lesion induction from radical processes and repair. Reduced repair will result in elevated lesion and an increased risk of disease. Genetic polymorphisms in repair proteins could also affect the relative propensity of individuals to develop various pathologies including even human inherited disease. Biallelic mutations in the BER DNA glycosylase MYH were found in an autosomal recessive syndrome of adenomatous colorectal polyposis with very high risk of colorectal cancer [67]. Several studies focusing the tissue expression of BER enzymes, and their relationship to diseases have been accomplished or are in motion using animal models or human samples [66, 68, 69]. Variable population distribution of polymorphisms in DNA repair genes and inter-individual differences in the DNA-repair efficiency are referred to the different occurrence of oxidative stress related diseases in the world [69, 70].

MItochondrial DNA Damage and Repair

BER repair pathway comes about not only in nucleus, but also in mitochondria. Mitochondria (originated from maternal egg) are present in many copies in mammalian cells, except for mature erythrocytes (Figure 7). Each mitochondrion has a few identical copies of its own circular DNA, which codes for 13 mitochondrial enzymes involved in cellular respiration (using a slightly different genetic code than does nuclear DNA). Nuclear genes code for several other mitochondrial proteins. In somatic cells, mitochondrial DNA mutates about 10 to 20 times faster than nuclear DNA, because mitochondria are a major source of reactive oxygen species. These mutations accumulate with age in postmitotic tissues such as neurons, and in cardiac and skeletal muscle. As studied in multiple reports [71] and brilliantly summarized in one of the latest reports [72], there is an evidence that multiple DNA repair pathways exist also in mitochondrion (DR, BER, MMR, RER). BER pathway in mitochondrion shares similar steps like in nuclear BER but taking into account that the responsible enzymes have nuclear and mitochondrial isoforms (OGG1, TGG, APE, MYH). The presence of the only strand could also contribute to the observed increased mutation frequencies of mtDNA compared to nDNA. Though this fact, other non-mutated copies of mtDNA are present and thus mitochondrial function does not necessarily be compromised. Repair of mtDNA and nDNA in principle could be very similar with the difference being that nDNA repair pathways involve a larger number of proteins.

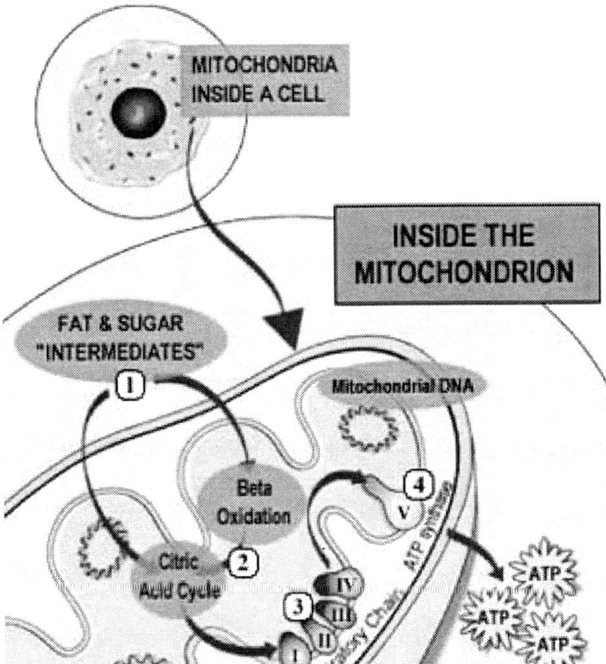

Figure 7. Metabolic pathways in mitochondrion. available from http://www.mitoresearch.org/images/q64bigmito.jpg

If oxidative *DNA damage is not repaired completely*, several situations can come about. Many oxidative base lesions are mutagenic, other can induce conformational changes in DNA. Lesions as thymidine glycol can block replication one nucleotide before and after the lesion. The length of repetitive sequences of DNA (microsatellites) is constant in normal cells, but microsatellite instability (i.e. variable number of repeats) derives from oxidative DNA damage. If the DNA oxidative lesions are present in the transcribed regions of genes they can lead to mutation. But if they are localized in promoter, elements they can affect transcription factor binding [4, 64].

3.3 Poly(ADP-ribose) Polymerase

Poly(ADP-ribose) polymerase 1 (PARP) plays an important role in oxidative DNA damage repair. Poly(ADP-ribose) polymerase 1 (PARP-1) is the 113-kDa enzyme, mostly found in nucleus, member of the PARP enzyme family consisting of PARP-1 and several recently identified poly(ADP-ribosylating) enzymes. PARP-1 represents the best studied PARP enzyme and is responsible for more than 90% of the cellular poly(ADP-ribosyl) capacity. The process of poly(ADP-ribosyl)ation plays the role in a variety of physiological and pathophysiological phenomena, such as signalling of DNA damage induced by ionising radiation, alkylating agents and oxidants, DNA-base excision repair, regulation of genomic stability in cells under genotoxic stress, transcriptional regulation, stimulation of nuclear proteasomal function, ageing and longevity, further in pathophysiology of acute and chronic inflammatory disorders (e.g. Crohn´s disease), diabetes mellitus, ischaemia-reperfusion damage in tissue, septic and haemorrhagic shock [73]. The primary signal that cause PARP-1 activation is the recognition of single or double strand DNA breaks caused by various genotoxic agents inclusive oxidative stress in the course of different pathological situation as described above. Activated PARP-1 dimerizes at recessed DNA ends and cleaves NAD+ into nicotinamide and ADP-ribose which forms long branching $(ADP\text{-}ribose)_n$ polymers. The latter product is then attached to glutamate or aspartate residues of nuclear acceptor proteins, including PARP itself (PARP automodification) (Figure 8). As described by Virag [74], by conferring negative charges to acceptors, this covalent protein modification alters the physico-chemical properties of the modified target proteins and thus regulates their function. The set of polymer acceptor proteins includes various DNA repair proteins, transcription factors, histones, other proteins, and PARP-1 itself. This PARP-1 automodification represents a negative feedback mechanism causing the down regulation of PARP-1 enzyme activity, the poly(ADP-ribosyl)ation is reversible and the enzyme poly(ADP-ribose)glycohydrolase (PARG) degrades the polymer (Figure 8)

Free radicals and other agents as UV light, ionising radiation or alkylating agents may cause DNA strand breakage. PARP-1 binds to recessed DNA ends resulting in the activation of the enzyme. Active PARP-1 cleaves NAD+ into ADP-ribose (ADPR) and nicotinamide (NA). Then PARP-1 polymerises ADPR covalently linked to itself and histones leading to recruitment of various DNA repair adapter and effector proteins. Poly(ADP-ribosyl)ation of histones causes relaxation of chromatin structure rendering the site of DNA damage accessible to the repair machinery. Automodified PARP-1 detaches from DNA and the repair machinery seals broken DNA ends. PARG (poly(ADP-ribose) glycohydrolase) decomposes the polymer and the chromatin regains its original structure.

As described, nuclear *ADP-ribosylation induced by the presence of DNA strand breaks stimulates DNA r*epair, and finally leads to the cell recovery from moderate DNA damage (Figure 8). If DNA damage is excessive and unrepairable, PARP is overactivated and mediates a futile energy-consuming cycle inactivating the stress response of the cells [73, 74].PARP-1 depletes the cellular stores of its substrate NAD+ , and in turn NAD+ resynthesis also consumes ATP. Hence, NAD+ and ATP depletion as two key energy metabolites leads to cell death, apoptosis or necrosis (Figure 9). The switching from apoptosis to necrosis by PARP-1 overactivation may aggravate tissue damage, as leakage of cellular content from necrotic cells is pro-inflammatory. It is necessary to stress that the intensity of cellular poly(ADP-ribosyl)ation decreases with age either in humans or in animals [73].

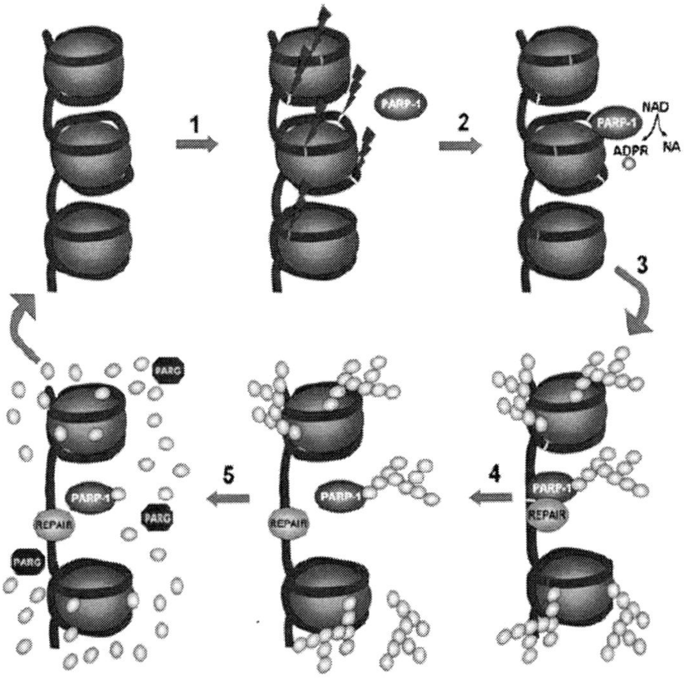

Figure 8. DNA damage-induced activation of PARP-1 (published by Virag L. Current Vascular Pharmacology, 2005, 3, 209-214, with the kind permission of the author)

The central role of PARP-1 in oxidative stress-related pathology. Oxidative-stress-induced DNA strand breakage triggers the activation of PARP-1, leading to apoptosis inducing factor (AIF) release from the mitochondria and AIF-mediated, caspase independent apoptotic cell death NAD/ATP consumption and consequent necrotic cell death. Oxidative stress also stimulates activation of redox-sensitive transcription factors such as NfκB and activator protein 1 AP-1, key regulators of inflammatory cytokines and chemokines.

Except for the role of PARP-1 in regulation of genomic stability and cell survival, it has also an impact on gene expression. Gene interaction with PARP-1 had either positive or negative effects on the specific transactivation process. An important example is the involvement of PARP-1 in the regulation of NFκB, the specific transcription factor involved in the control of numerous genes, including those of many cellular genes involved in immune responses and inflammation. PARP- has also been implicated in the regulation of activator protein (AP-1)-driven transcriptional activity (Figure 9). The activites of PARP shows certainly the role in many pathological processes, such as acute ischaemia-reperfusion damage, allergen-induced asthma, septic or haemorrhagic shock, and chronic including cancer, cardiac disorders, Parkinson´s diesease, inflammatory bowel disease and diabetes mellitus. It is necessary to emphasize the fact that the function of PARP-1 and poly(ADP-ribosyl)ation as a regulator of inflammatory signal transduction and transactivation shows marked cell-type and stimulus dependency [75]. This finding might certainly play the role in possible usage of envisaged PARP inhibitor therapy as will be mentioned later.

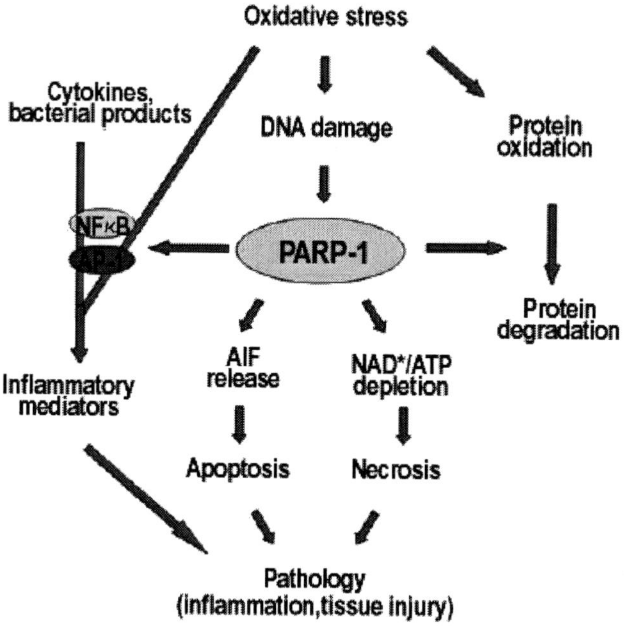

Figure 9. The role of PARP-1 in oxidative stress-related pathology (published by Virag L. Current Vascular Pharmacology, 2005, 3, 209-214, with the kind permission of the author)

A close association was described between PARP-1 and *p53 protein* in DNA damage-induced apoptosis [74, 76]. p53 protein is a nuclear protein that plays an essential role in the regulation of cell cycle, specifically in the transition from G0 to G1, the cell cycle arrest at the G1/S transition (which prevents the manifestation of unrepaired chomosome alterations), and also on cell cycle arrest at the G2/M transition, which inhibits the distribution of defective genomes. P53 also initiate apoptosis after the introduction of irrepairable DNA damage. At this point, both PARP-1 activation and p53 activation occur rapidly following DNA damage. The activation of these two mediators is likely to be linked to each other, as PARP-1 has been shown to interact with and poly(ADP-ribosyl)ate p53 [74, 76].

The described activities of PARP-1 in DNA base excision repair, in apoptosis or cell necrosis induction, stimulation of inflammatory mediators via NFκB and AP-1 transcription factors, and protein degradation have been taken into consideration in several studies with *PARP inhibitors* on animal models or cell cultures [77](Figure 10) and recently also in clinical trials on oncological or diabetic patients [78, 79, 80]. Most PARP inhibitors developed to date have structural similarity to the substrate NAD+, thus competing for the active centre of the enzyme. The compounds are non cytotoxic on their own at concentrations necessary to achieve PARP inhibition. PARP inhibitors are used for cancer treatment with regard to the effect of PARP inhibition and potentiation of cell necrosis [77]. Another indication is to turn down the stimulation of pro-inflammatory mediators like in chronic obstructive lung disease, diabetes mellitus, or congestive heart failure, and Parkinson´s disease [80]. The question remains what side effects might be observed after a long PARP inhibitor application with regard to the blockage of DNA repair in non-cancerous diseases.

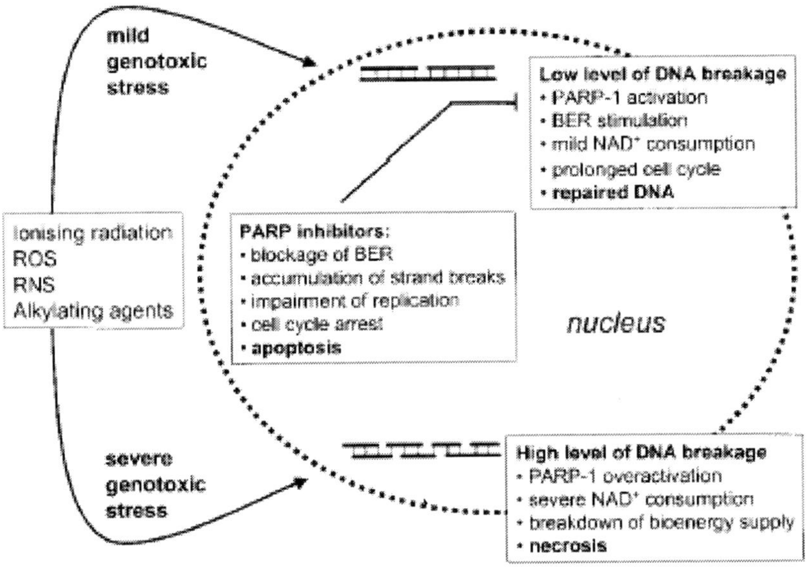

Figure 10. DNA breakage and the activity of PARP inhibitors (published by Beneke, S; Diefenbach, J; Bűrkle, A. Poly(ADP-ribosyl)ation inhibitors: promising drug candidates for a wide variety of pathophysiologic conditions. Int J Cancer, 2004, 111, 813-818, with the kind permission of the author A. Bűrkle)

Oxidative-stress-induced DNA strand breakage triggers the activation of PARP-1. If the DNA breakage is low, BER is stimulated, cell cycle is prolonged (in cooperation with p53 protein activation) and DNA is finally repaired. If DNA breakage is high, PARP-1 is over activated, severe NAD+ consumption is in progress and apoptosis or even necrosis is started. PARP inhibitors may block the inflammatory pathways but also BER.

3.4 Diseases Related with Oxidative Stress and DNA Damage

Natural trend of worsened DNA repair is usually associated with aging. *Aging* as a constant and inevitable process has been related to oxidative stress for many years. Telomere shortening related to a finite number of replication (*Hayflick´s model*) is observed in normal human somatic cells and is considered as one of the mechanisms of the senescence (in this case – replicative senescence) [81].

Aged cells show age-dependent accumulation of 8-oxoguanine in the nucleus and age-dependent decrease in the activity of OGG1 imported into the nuclei and into mitochondria

[82, 83]. Also AP endonuclease showed age-associated decreased activity, i.e. less intensive BER corresponds with the *theory of aging associated with oxidative stress* [83, 84].

Another cause of aging is related to mutation of human WRN gene. The role of normal Werner protein (or *RECQ3 helicase*) *is to interact with many proteins involved in BER,* and in this way to facilitate BER by unwinding BER intermediates. Mutated WRN gene give rise to a rare autosomal recessive genetic disorder Werner syndrome with premature aging, predisposition to cancer and early onset of aging symptoms such as osteoporosis, ocular cataracts, greying, loss of hair, diabetes mellitus, atherosclerosis [85, 86, 87].

Facts related to aging and *polymorphisms of antioxidant enzymes* have not yet been fully established. Reports on mutations of SOD causing amyotrophic lateral sclerosis are known [5].

The *mitochondrial theory of aging* states that senescent cellular changes are related to the balance between inherited healthy mitochondrial DNA and repaired mtDNA and the load of age-related unrepaired mutations in this DNA [84]. Eventually, damage or loss of mitochondrial DNA prevents postmitotic cells from regenerating new mitochondria, thereby reducing the production of ATP and leading to cell death. Oxidative damage of mtDNA, accumulating with age, should affect mitochondrially encoded proteins, but the high number of mitochondrial genomes allows a certain degree of heteroplasmy (different genomes within a mitochondrion) without effects on phenotype. Clonal accumulations of damaged/mutated mtDNA within individual cells up to homoplasmy of mutant mtDNA, which could be either neutral with regard to phenotype or which could cause substantial phenotype alterations. The degree of age-induced mutations in mitochondrial DNA varies in people and may be under genetic control. Some mitochondrial DNA haplotypes are more common in centenarians than in the general population [88, 89, 90]. *Mitochondrial oxidative stress should be considered a hallmark of cellular aging.* Mitochondrial ROS production mediates signal transduction pathways sensitive to oxidative stress and this would be involved in the onset and development of age-related degenerative diseases and that limit the mean life span. The second pathway is related to oxidative damage to mitochondrial DNA, proteins, and lipids and would determine the maximum life span [91].

Other pathologies related with oxidative stress and DNA damage are susceptibility to carcinogenesis (lack of apoptosis control), and other non-cancerous pathological conditions, such as degenerative diseases (Alzheimer's disease, Parkinson's disease), metabolic diseases (haemochromatosis, Wilson disease, diabetes mellitus), inflammatory diseases of infectious and non-infectious origin (atherosclerosis, autoimmune, and allergic diseases), ischaemia-reperfusion injury. *The intensity and quality of DNA repair are studied particularly in tissue sections, or tissue cultures, human leucocytes, or on animal models in some pathological conditions,* such as malignant tumours [2, 64, 92, 93, 94], neurodegenerative diseases [68, 95], atherosclerosis [88, 96, 97], inflammatory bowel diseases [98], diabetes [99, 100], and in workers exposed to genotoxic effects of different chemicals [101].

The foregoing condensed summary dealing with oxidative stress and oxidative DNA damage and particularly BER serves for further elucidation of specific changes in two models of free radical diseases – diabetes mellitus and inflammatory bowel diseases.

4. Oxidative Stress and Pathophysiology of Diabetes Mellitus and Inflammatory Bowel Diseases

Among human diseases mentioned above, diabetes mellitus (DM) and inflammatory bowel diseases (IBD) represent 2 chronic lifelong diseases that could be present as 2 model free radical diseases. ROS in DM are produced via different pathways, among them the most important is the ROS overproduction by the mitochondrial ETC and glucose autoxidation, i.e. *oxidative stress of predominantly metabolic origin with consequent inflammatory processes.* In IBD, mainly Crohn's disease, excessive stimulation of otherwise tightly regulated NADPH oxidases during inflammatory process contributes to the ROS formation and the presence of *oxidative stress of predominantly inflammatory origin.*

4.1 Diabetes Mellitus

Diabetes mellitus is defined as a group of chronic, metabolic heterogeneous disease marked by high levels of sugar in the blood. It results from insufficient action of insulin in consequence of its absolute or relative deficiency or both. Diabetes as a life-long disease is accompanied with complex disturbances of sugar, lipid and protein metabolism. The clinical features of diabetes are well-known, such as polyuria and polydipsia, nycturia, loss of weight, fatigue, loss of consciousness even coma, acetone in breath, recurrent infection of skin and urogenital system, later occurs the development of microvascular complications (retinopathy even blindness, nephropathy even renal failure, peripheral and autonomic neuropathy) and atherosclerosis with accompanied hypertension, heart attack, brain stroke, claudication [102] (Figure 11).

Type 1 diabetes (T1DM) develops as a result of autoimmune insulitis in genetically predisposed individuals, typically is diagnosed in childhood, adolescence, or early adulthood. Autoimmune destruction of the ß-cells of the pancreas is reflected with markers of the immune destruction of the ß-cell include islet cell autoantibodies (ICAs), autoantibodies to insulin (IAAs), autoantibodies to glutamic acid decarboxylase (GAD_{65}), and autoantibodies to the tyrosine phosphatases IA-2 and IA-2ß. Also, the disease has strong HLA associations, with linkage to the DQA and B genes, and it is influenced by the DRB genes, these genes being either predisposing or protective. These patients are also prone to other autoimmune disorders such as Graves' disease, Hashimoto's thyroiditis, Addison's disease, vitiligo, and pernicious anaemia. Incidence of the disease is variable with regions, and in Europe an increasing tendency from the South to the North is reported with the highest number of 50/100000 children up to 15 years/year in Finland. The age-related incidence has its peak at the age of 13-15 years. T1DM dominates in childhood and adolescence. The disease onset in adulthood is no more rare (LADA - latent autoimmune diabetes of adults) and has been intensively studied. As T1DM is insulin dependent, different insulin intensified therapies are applied. Besides insulin, also diet, and regular physical activity are necessary for T1DM successful treatment.

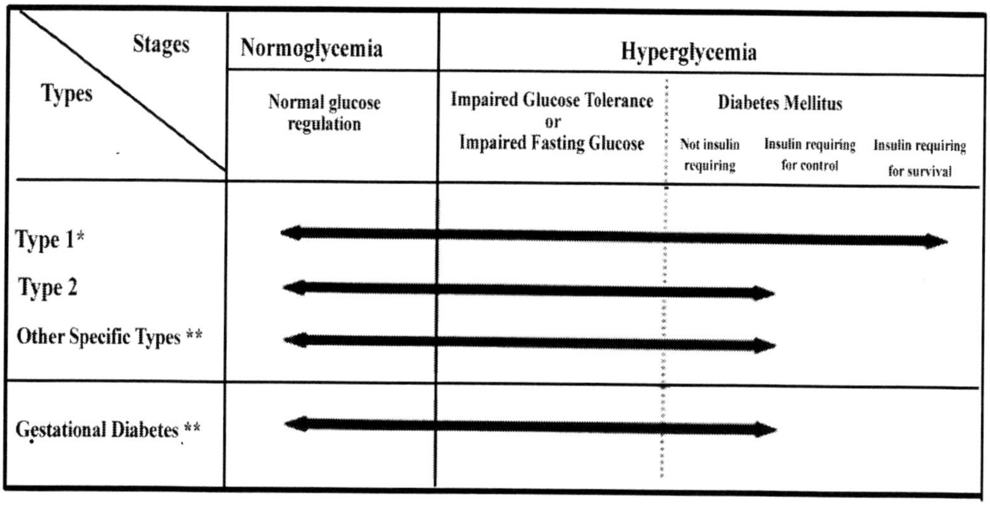

Figure 11. The Expert Committee on the Diagnosis and Classification of Diabetes Mellitus ADA (Diabetes Care 26: S5-20, 2003)

Type 2 diabetes (T2DM) is characterized by peripheral insulin resistance with an insulin-secretory defect that varies in severity. For type 2 diabetes to develop, both defects must exist: all overweight individuals have insulin resistance, but only those with an inability to increase beta-cell production of insulin develop diabetes. 90% of patients who develop type 2 diabetes are obese. Patients with type 2 diabetes often do not need treatment with oral antidiabetic medication or insulin if they lose weight. There are probably many different causes of this form of diabetes, and it is likely that the proportion of patients in this category will decrease in the future as identification of specific pathogenic processes and genetic defects permits better differentiation among them and a more definitive subclassification. Autoimmune destruction of ß-cells does not occur, and patients do not have any of the other specific causes of diabetes. Both genetic and environmental factors (above mentioned obesity) contribute to insulin resistance. Adipose tissue plays a central role in the pathogenesis of insulin resistance that induces a compensatory increase in β cell mass, which results in normal glucose levels. In other people, β cell response is not adequate and leads to impaired glucose tolerance or even type 2 diabetes. The presence of chronic hyperglycaemia i.e. glucotoxicity induces multiple defects in β cells, including early decreases in glucose-stimulated insulin secretion, and late irreversible changes in insulin-gene transcription and β cell mass with consequent low insulin production. The world epidemic of obesity and thus the related increased incidence of T2DM threatens developed countries and represents a serious problem to public health. Worldwide prevalence of T2DM is estimated as 150 million cases in 2002 (Report of a WHO Meeting).

Other specific types of diabetes includes genetic defects of the ß-cell (monogenetic defects in ß-cell function - MODY), *point mutations in mitochondrial DNA, genetic defects in insulin action* (mutations of the insulin receptor), *diseases of the exocrine pancreas* (acquired processes include pancreatitis, trauma, infection, pancreatectomy, cystic fibrosis and haemochromatosis), *endocrinopathies* (e.g. acromegaly, Cushing's syndrome, glucagonoma, pheochromocytoma), *drug- or chemical-induced diabetes, infections* (rubella, coxsackievirus B, cytomegalovirus, adenovirus, and mumps), *uncommon forms of immune-mediated diabetes* (systemic lupus erythematosus and other autoimmune diseases), *other genetic syndromes sometimes associated with diabetes* (Down's syndrome, Klinefelter's syndrome, and Turner's syndrome. Wolfram's syndrome).

Gestational diabetes mellitus (GDM) is defined as any degree of glucose intolerance with onset or first recognition during pregnancy.

The increasing number of diabetic patients all over the world is an important problem of public health. Quality of life of diabetic patients, chronic diabetic complications, treatment of all types of diabetes and its complications at vast expenses represent important challenges not only for medical science, but also for human society.

4.1.1 ROS and Diabetes

Hyperglycaemia is common for all types of diabetes. This metabolic finding is the key for all important consequences related to oxidative stress. High constant influx of glucose under hyperglycaemia via GLUT 1 transporters leads to ROS overproduction at the mitochondrial level (Figure 12). In diabetic cells with high glucose inside, there is more glucose being oxidized in the citrate cycle (TCA cycle), which in effect pushes more electron donors (NADH and $FADH_2$) into the electron transport chain. As a result of this, the voltage gradient across the mitochondrial membrane increases until a critical threshold is reached. At this point, electron transfer inside complex III is blocked, causing the electrons to back up to coenzyme Q, which donates the electrons one at a time to molecular oxygen, thereby generating superoxide (Figure 13). *Overproduction of superoxide is the first and key event in the activation of all other pathways of hyperglycemic damage involved in the pathogenesis of diabetic complications* [103, 104, 105, 106, 107], such as *formation of advanced glycation end-products AGEs, stimulation of protein kinase C and transcription factor NFκB, polyol pathway and hexosamine pathway* (Figure 12, 14, 15, 16, 17). The cited work of Brownlee presents an integrated approach to the oxidative stress in diabetes.

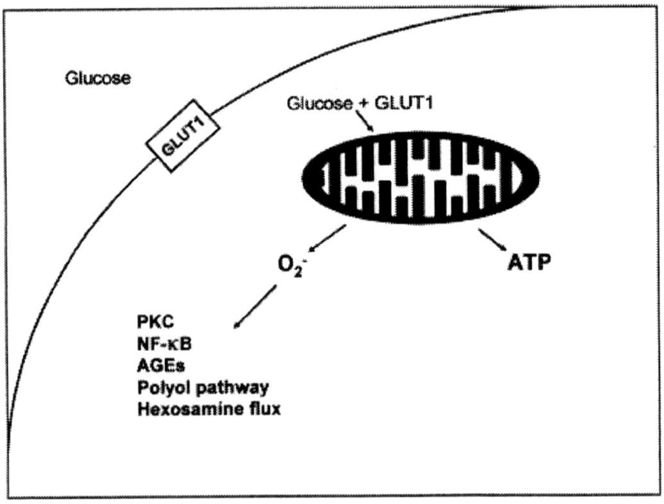

Figure 12. The role of increased flux of glucose into the cell and mainly to the mitochondrion (published by Ceriello, A. New insights on Oxidative Stress and Diabetic Complications May Lead to a "Causal" Antioxidant Therapy. Diabetes Care, 2003, 26, 1589-1596, with the kind permission of the author)

In endothelial cells, glucose can pass freely through the cell membrane in an insulin-independent manner via GLUT1. Intracellular hyperglycaemia induces overproduction of superoxide at the mitochondrial level. Overproduction of superoxide is the first and key event in the activation of all other pathways involved in the pathogenesis of diabetic complications, such as polyol pathway flux, increased advanced glycosylation end product (AGE) formation, activation of protein kinase C (PKC) and NF-B, and increased hexosamine pathway flux.

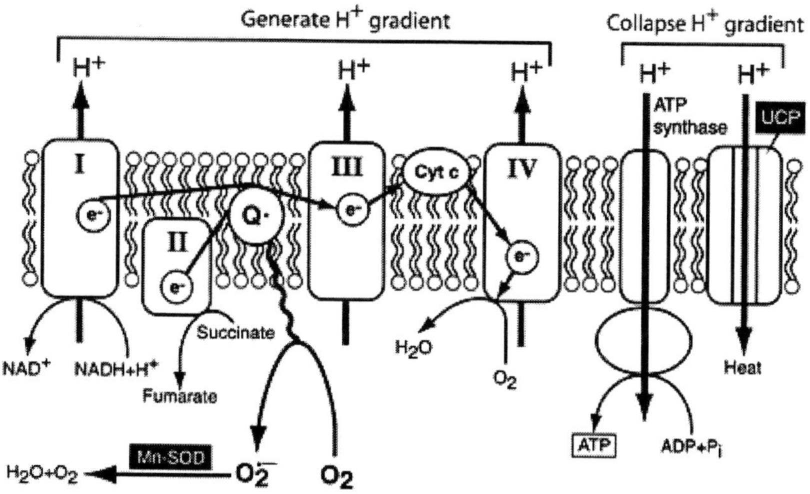

Figure 13. Hyperglycaemia-induced production of superoxide by the mitochondrial electron transport chain (published by Brownlee, M. The Pathobiology of Diabetic Complications. Diabetes, 2005, 54, 1615-1625, with the kind permission of the author)

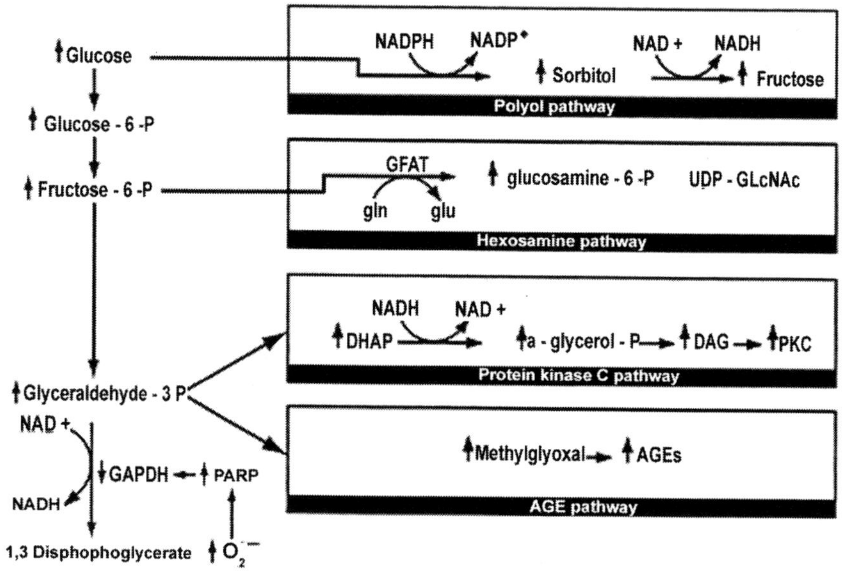

Figure 14. Mitochondrial overproduction of superoxide activates four major pathways of hyperglycaemic damage by inhibiting GAPDH (published by Brownlee, M. The Pathobiology of Diabetic Complications. Diabetes, 2005, 54, 1615-1625, with the kind permission of the author). GAPDH - glyceraldehyde-3-phosphate dehydrogenase, GFAT – glutamine:fructose-6-phospate

amidotransferase, GLN-glucosamine, glu-glutamine, UDP-uridine diphosphate, GlcNAc- N-acetylglucosamine, DHAP –dihydroxyacetone phosphate, DAG-diacylglycerol (activator of protein kinase C)

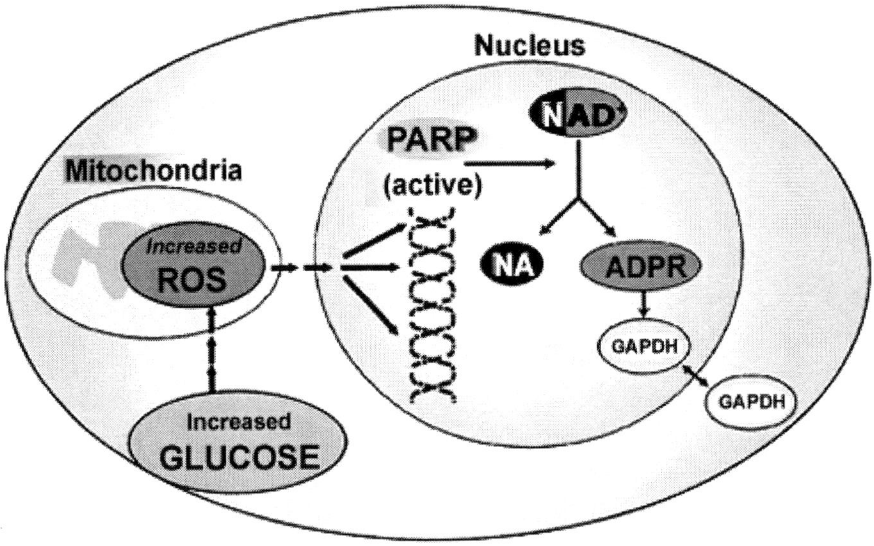

Figure 15. ROS-induced DNA damage activates PARP and modifies GAPDH (published by Brownlee, M. The Pathobiology of Diabetic Complications. Diabetes, 2005, 54, 1615-1625, with the kind permission of the author). ADPR – ADP-ribose, NA- nicotinic acid, GAPDH- glyceraldehyde-3-phosphate dehydrogenase, PARP- poly(ADP-ribose)polymerase

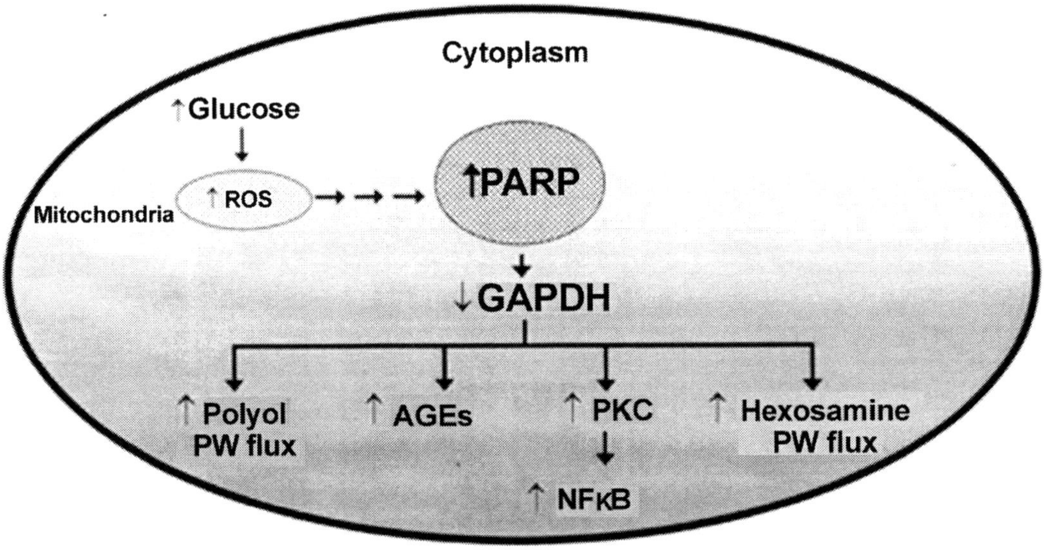

Figure 16. The unifying mechanism of hyperglycaemia-induced cellular damage (published by Brownlee, M. The Pathobiology of Diabetic Complications. Diabetes, 2005, 54, 1615-1625, with the kind permission of the author). AGEs- advanced glycation endproducts, PKC – protein kinase C, NFκB- nuclear factor κB proinflammatory transcription factor, PW - pathway

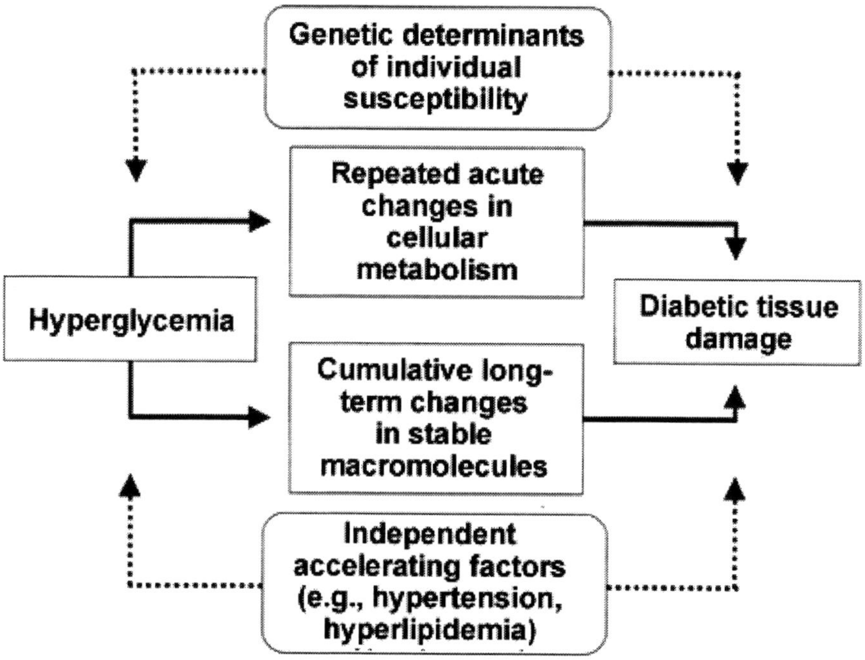

Figure 17. General features of hyperglycaemia-induced tissue damage. (published by Brownlee, M. The Pathobiology of Diabetic Complications. Diabetes, 2005, 54, 1615-1625, with the kind permission of the author)

Many previous studies analysed the influence of glucose on protein glycation and formation of advanced glycation end-products [108, 109, 110, 111, 112, 113, 114]. As shown for example by Kalousova and Skrha [115], accumulated glycation products (AGEs, but also advanced oxidation protein products – AOPP and advanced lipoperoxidation end products ALEs) exert not only direct effect on the extracellular matrix, but they are also bound to RAGE specific receptors. Beside other AGE-binding receptors, RAGE receptors are the best known and characterized as a 35kDa protein classified as a member of the immunoglobulin superfamily. RAGE can be expressed on the surface of various cell (e.g. monocytes, macrophages, mesangial cells, neurons, endothelial cells, smooth muscle cells and fibroblasts). It is a multiligand receptor and recognizes also β-amyloid, amphoterins and calgranulins involved in inflammatory processes. RAGE has also physiological function for the development of the central nervous system but during maturation, its presence decreases and is minimally expressed in adults. Under pathological conditions, such as diabetes melllitus, immune-inflammatory processes, Alzheimer´s disease, and cancer, RAGE expression is increased and binds AGE. AGE-RAGE interaction results in the activation of intracellular signal transduction pathways, such as MAPK and JNK kinases, activator protein 1 (AP-1) and nuclear factor NFκB. Subsequently, this activation is followed by overexpression of genes for cytokines (TNF-α, IL-1, IL-2, interferon γ, IL-8), growth factors (platelet-derived growth factor PDGF, insulin-like growth factor IGF-1), adhesion molecules (ICAM-1, VCAM-1). Other processes are also stimulated, among them stimulation of cell proliferation, increased vascular, migration of macrophages, formation of endothelin-1, increased synthesis of collagen IV, fibronectin and proteoglycans, increased procoagulant state [116, 117]. Little is known about the formation and accumulation of AGEs in young patients with T1DM. Tsukuhara [118] described increased urinary concentrations of pentosidine as AGE, and 8-hydroxy-2′-deoxyguanosine and acrolein-lysine as markers of OS in children with type 1 diabetes when compared with age-matched healthy control subjects. The mean age of 38 diabetic children was 12.8±4.5 years and their disease duration 5.7±4.3 years and HbA_{1c} 8.0±1.6%, 11 subjects had microalbuminuria >15 mg/g creatinine. The study indicated that the accumulation of AGEs is closely linked to oxidative stress and the subsequent endothelial dysfunction may start early in the course of type 1 diabetes. This means that the risk of vascular complications may be present at an early age and that the best possible glycemic control should be emphasized from the diagnosis of diabetes. Regarding these results, it is important to take into consideration also high and low haemoglobin glycation phenotypes in type 1 diabetes as presented by Hempe [119]. Different glycation phenotype are also associated with susceptibility to the glycation of other proteins, increased AGE synthesis, and greater risk of diabetes complications. Though there are analogies in hyperglycemia, oxidative stress and stimulation of consequent metabolic and inflammatory processes in different types of diabetes, T1DM and T2DM as the most frequent types of diabetes differ in their character. T1DM as autoimmune disease develops towards other autoimmunities and microvascular complications. T2DM (besides microvascular complications) inclines to atherosclerotic (macrovascular) complications, and to carcinogenesis [120, 121]. With regard to a variety of AGEs, there is also a large scale of AGE-inhibitors and AGE-breakers. These substances, either natural or synthetic, could display different reactions. They react with free amino groups of protein to modify them in order to prevent sugar attachment to protein, or they inactivate aldose and ketose sugars before reacting with amino groups of proteins. They could also be metal chelators, and antioxidants themselves like vitamin C or E. Another group are inhibitors trapping reacative dicarbonyl intermediates to form substituted triazines. There are Amadori adducts inhibitors, compounds inducing for enzymatic deglycation at the Amadori level. Finally, inhibitors called cross-link breakers are able to selectively cleave and break the established AGE-protein cross-links *in vitro* and *in vivo.* AGE-inhibitors and breakers for clinical use should be non-toxic, well absorbed across the gastrointestinal tract and achieve a broad distribution throughout various tissues. Their therapeutic impact can include not only diabetes, but also other diseases with AGE-formation and accumulation [114, 122].

Also the antioxidant defence is the focus of an intensive research in diabetes. The polymorphisms in the *Mn-SOD* and *EC-SOD* (CuZn-SOD) genes play certainly the role in the intensity of detoxifying superoxide. Chistyakov [123] found the relationship between Ala(-9)Val substitution in the *Mn-SOD* gene and diabetic neuropathy in a Russian population. The antioxidant gene enzyme expression and protein activity was studied on skin fibroblast cultures in type 1 diabetic patients with and without nephropathy, and nondiabetic control subjects. Skin fibroblasts of T1DM patients with diabetic nephropathy exposed to long-term hyperglycemia displayed unchanged expression and activity of Mn-SOD, catalase and GPx, whereas T1DM patients without complications, non-diabetic nephropathic patients, and control subjects had an intact stimulated antioxidant response to glucose-induced oxidative stress [124]. The present oxidative stress and low antioxidant defence was found not only in diabetic children, but similar tendency was observed also in their non-diabetic siblings, but not in their non-diabetic parents [125].

ROS, DNA Damage and DM

As mentioned at the beginning of this chapter, oxidative stress injures also DNA. It is impossible to enumerate all articles studying the intensity of oxidative stress and DNA damage in diabetic patients. Krapfenbauer [126] examined in 1998 type 1 and type 2 adult patients and compared them with age-matched non-diabetic controls. He confirmed the increased pentosidine and 8-hydroxy-2′-deoxyguanosine in urine in both diabetic groups and made conclusion that increased glycoxidation was approved but 8-OHdG could be taken either as consequence of increased DNA oxidation or reflection of DNA repair. Collins [127] used comet assay with endonuclease III to detect oxidized pyrimidines, and formamidopyrimidine glycosylase to detect damaged purines including 8-oxo-guanine. The increased formamidopyrimidine glycosylase-sensitive (FPG) sites were found in diabetic patients and the strong correlation was displayed between those sites and serum glucose concentrations. Another studies [128] summarized the importance of detection of 8-hydroxy-2′-deoxyguanosine (8-OHdG) in urine in different diseases. The methods for 8-OHdG detection and normal reference range for women and men were also discussed. Special attention was paid to 8-OHdG levels in patients with cancer , chronic inflammation, atherogenesis, and diabetes. An outline was made with regard to the levels of urinary 8-OHdG as oxidative stress marker and the presence of accelerated vascular dysfunction, and development of microvascular complications. The level of 8-OHdG could be also used as a marker of the effectiveness of dietary supplements with regard to whether they will reduce the oxidative damage. The review published by Samcova [129] described free radical different diseases and levels of 8OhdG. DNA damage and antioxidant defence were examined in peripheral leukocytes of T1DM patients by Dincer [130]. Comet assay was used in this study that confirmed increased DNA strand breakage and FPG-sensitive sites in diabetic patients. SOD and GPx activities in leukocytes were decreased. The presented findings showed increased oxidative DNA damage and impaired antioxidant defence in leukocytes of adult patients with T1DM. Similar findings of increased DNA damage in diabetic patients were confirmed in another study using comet assay [131].

ROS, DNA Repair and DM

The information about DNA repair process in relation to diabetes and oxidative DNA damage is scarce in humans. Attention is mostly paid to PARP and its inhibitors than to DNA repair process itself. PARP activates three major pathways of hyperglycemic damage in endothelial cells via inhibition of GAPDH activity (Figure 16)[132].

Activity of PARP was found to be increased in whole retina and in endothelial cell and pericytes of diabetic rats. Long-term administration of PARP inhibitor (PJ-34) led to significantly inhibited death of retinal microvascular cell and prohibited from the development of early lesions of diabetic retinopathy in those animal models. In another experiment, PARP interaction directly with both subunits of NFκB (p50 and p65), mainly under hyperglycemic condition. The usage of PJ-34 blocked the PARP mediated activation of NFκB [133].

Japanese study published in 2004 [134] showed in a large group of T1DM patients that human *MTH1* gene Val83Met was associated with type 1 diabetes, particularly in females. The product of *MTH1* gene human mutT homologue 1 hydrolyzes 8-hydroxy-deoxyguanosine triphosphate (8-OHdGTP) to 8-hydroxy-deoxyguanosine monophosphate in order to prevent transversion mutation. MTH1 is localized not only in nucleus but also in the mitochondrial matrix assuring here the integrity of mitochondrial DNA. Val83Met polymorphism of *MTH1* gene leads to labile type of MTH1 and its decreased activity, both in nuclear and also in mitochondrial DNA. 8-OHdGTP can pair in DNA with cytosine or adenine and induce transversion mutations in mitochondrial DNA (mtDNA) as well as in nuclear DNA (nDNA). Such accumulated mutations would cause mitochondrial dysfunction, consequently more ROS production, leading to DNA strand breaks and the resultant recruitment of poly(ADP-ribose) polymerase for the repair.

Free-radical mediated ß-cell damage has been intensively studied in type 1 diabetes, but not in human type 2 diabetes. Oxidative DNA damage and intensity of DNA repair in pancreatic islets was assessed on pancreatic specimens (post mortem or post surgery) from patients with diabetes for 2-23 years and healthy controls. 8-OH-hydroxyguanine glycosylase (OGG1) DNA repair enzyme expression was examined using immunofluorescent staining of OGG1. The intensity and islet area stained for OGG1 displayed a significant increase in islets from T2DM subjects compared to the healthy controls. A correlation between increased OGG1 fluorescent staining intensity and duration of diabetes was also found. Most of the observed staining was cytoplasmic, suggesting that mitochondrial OGG1 accounts primarily for the increased OGG1 expression. The authors [135] concluded that oxidative stress related DNA damage may be a novel important factor in the pathogenesis of human type 2 diabetes and stimulates OGG1 islet expression. Blasiak [99] published in 2004 the results of study aimed at the intensity of DNA repair in patients with T2DM. Comet assay was used for the assessment of the level of endogenous basal DNA damage (DNA strand breaks and alkali labile sites), as well as endogenous oxidative and alkylative DNA damage (using DNA repair enzymes endonuclease III, formamidopyrimidine-DNA glycosylase and 3-methyladenine-DNA glycosylase II) in peripheral lymphocytes. Finally, the measurement of the sensitivity to DNA-damaging agents (hydrogen peroxide and doxorubicin) and the efficacy of removing this induced DNA damage in peripheral blood lymphocytes was performed. The levels of basal endogenous and oxidative DNA damage in diabetic patients were higher than in control subjects. There was no difference between the level of alkylative DNA in the patients and the controls. Diabetic patients displayed higher susceptibility to hydrogen peroxide and doxorubicin and decreased efficacy of repairing DNA damage induced by these agents than healthy control. The conclusion was made that patients with T2DM had the elevated level of oxidative DNA damage and the decreased efficacy of DNA repair and this may be the link between diabetes and cancer. At the same time, Varvarovska [136] published the study comparing the degree of DNA damage and the intensity of DNA repair in T1DM adults and children. Also in this case, comet assay was used for the evaluation of DNA damage and repair. Diabetic adults displayed higher DNA strand breaks and lower DNA repair capacity (measured in peripheral blood lymphocytes) than diabetic children. When adult patients were divided into 2 groups according the presence or absence of diabetic microvascular complications (DMC), the differences were more expressed, i.e. adults with DMC had higher DNA strand breaks and lower DNA repair capacity. The ratio between those two parameters was expressed as DNRI index that displayed large variations in adults without DMC and mainly in children.

Some Contributions to Antioxidant Therapy in Diabetes Mellitus

Advance in research of oxidative stress and developing knowledge of its impact on human metabolism has brought new therapeutic possibilities into experiments, clinical trials or clinical practice. In a review published by Schultz Johansen [137] there is a instructive summary of current antioxidant interventions. Several experiments on animal models were mentioned, among them usage of α-lipoic as antioxidant or SOD mimetic experiments in diabetic animals. Recently performed clinical trials with different antioxidants were enumerated. The HOPE trial was the largest trial conducted thus far for the use of antioxidants in diabetes, unfortunately no beneficial effect of vitamin E was approved on cardiovascular outcome or diabetic nephropathy. The Steno-2 trial compared the effect of a multifactorial intensive therapy with that of conventional treatment on modifiable risk factors for cardiovascular disease in T2DM patients. In the intensive treatment group, patients received combined pharmacotherapy (vitamin C, E, folic acid, chromium piconlinate and drugs lowering hyperglycemia, dyslipidemia and hypertension) plus behavior modification including low-fat diet, exercise and smoking cessation. Patients in intensive groups had a 50% decrease in the risk of cardiovascular events than a control group. Evidence is that a multifactorial approach is superior to conventional therapy for the prevention of oxidative stress-induced vascular complications in diabetes. Application of α-lipoic acid in the treatment of diabetic neuropathy had promising results and significantly improved patient symptoms were reached. A number of commonly used drugs have shown promising anitoxidant activity in addition to their primary pharmacological activity, such as thiazolidinediones, 3-hydroxy-3-methyl-glutaryl-Coenzyme A reductase (HMG-CoA) inhibitors (statins), and inhibitors of the renin-angiotensin system (inhibitors of angiotensin II activity, such as angiotensin converting enzyme inhibitors ACEIs and angiotensin II receptor blockers ARBs). In vitro and animal studies confirmed antioxidant effect of those drugs. These antioxidant properties may be a contributing factor to the therapeutic efficacy of these agents. Based on the new developments in the understanding of the pathophysiology of oxidative stress, new agents emerge and seems to be beneficial for the treatment of OS associated clinical problems (SOD and catalase mimetics, L-propionyl carnitine, PKC-β inhibitor). Another review published by Ceriello [106] summarized the choice of different antioxidant drugs and emphasized the importance of thiazolidinediones, statins, ACE inhibitors and AT1 inhibitors (Figure 18). Da Ros summarized similarly causal antioxidant therapy with new promising tools influencing mitochondrial function and reducing DNA damage, blocking PKC, PARP and peroxynitrite [138, 139]. Reusch [140] reviewed the recent knowledge about diabetic complications and mechanism of glucotoxicity. It is emphasized that conventional antioxidants scavenge free radicals in an inefficient stoichiometric manner so that one molecule of the antioxidant would be neede to neutralize each free radical generated. Novel small mollecular weight compounds functioning as superoxide dismutase mimetics have more reliable benefits due to the catalytic properties that could permit enzymatic detoxification. Suggestion of PARP inhibitors is another therapeutic possibility for diabetic complication prevention. Li [141] pointed to the risk of long-term inhibition of PARP, e.g. premature aging, loss of genome stability. In animal experiment, low-dose PARP inhibitor-containing combination therapies (PARP inhibitor+vasodilators) showed beneficial effect on early peripheral diabetic neuropathy. Another approach how to face diabetic microvascular complications could be the application of aldose reductase inhibitors that block sorbitol formation [142].

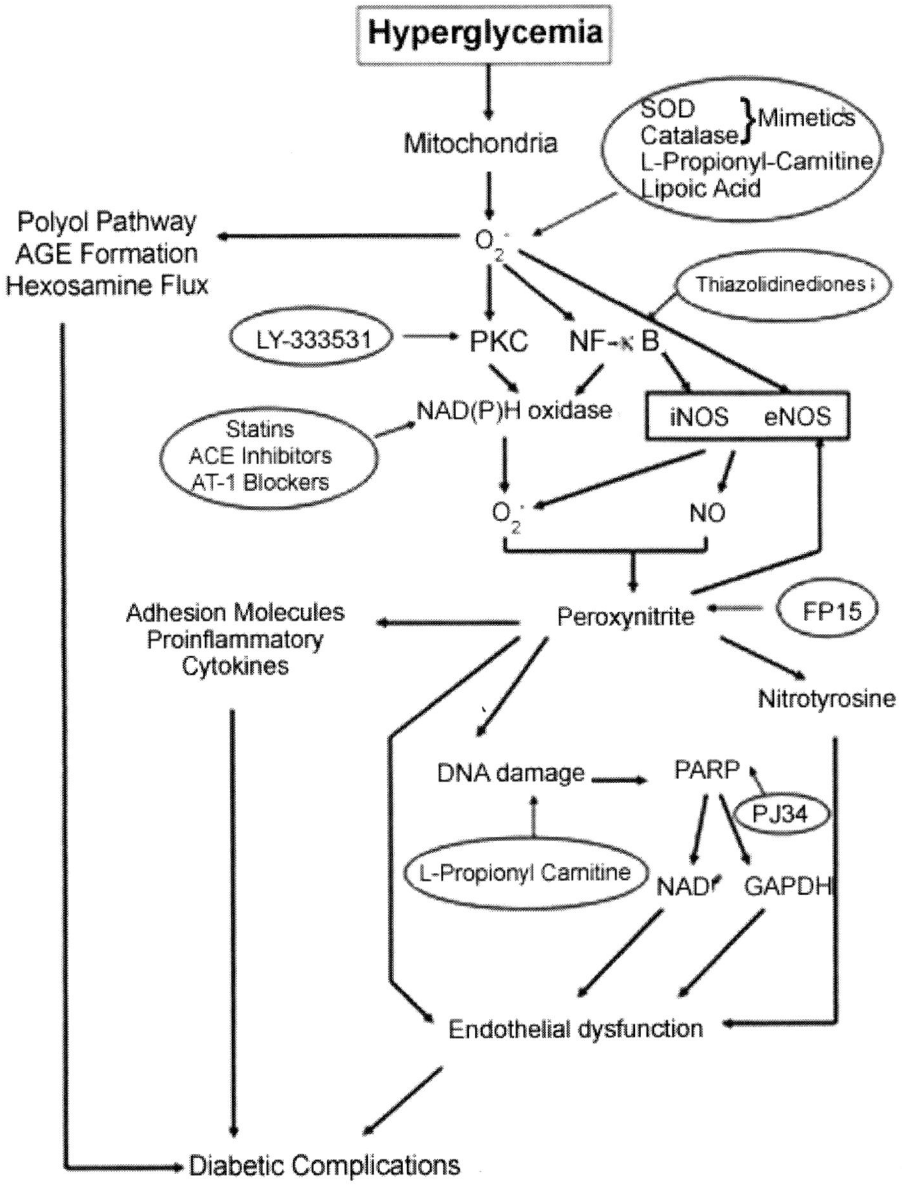

Figure 18. Location of action of different types of antioxidants in the treatment of diabetes mellitus (published by Ceriello, A. New insights on Oxidative Stress and Diabetic Complications May Lead to a “Causal” Antioxidant Therapy. Diabetes Care, 2003, 26, 1589-1596, with the kind permission of the author)

Superoxide overproduction reduces eNOS activity, but through NF-B and protein kinase C (PKC) activates NAD(P)H and increases iNOS expression: the final effect is an increased NO generation. This condition favors the formation of the strong oxidant peroxynitrite, which in turn produces, in iNOS and eNOS, an uncoupled state, resulting in the production of superoxide rather than NO, and damages DNA. DNA damage is an obligatory stimulus for the activation of the nuclear enzyme poly(ADP-ribose) polymerase (PARP). Poly(ADP-ribose) polymerase activation in turn depletes the intracellular concentration of its substrate

NAD^+, slowing the rate of glycolysis, electron transport, and ATP formation, and produces an ADP-ribosylation of the GAPDH. This process results in acute endothelial dysfunction in diabetic blood vessels, which contributes to the development of diabetic complications. NF-B activation also induces a proinflammatory conditions and adhesion molecule overexpression. All these alterations produce the final picture of diabetic complications. SOD or catalase mimetics, L-propionyl-carnitine and lipoic acid, reducing mitochondrial overproduction of superoxide, and reducing DNA damage may be good candidates for causal intracellular antioxidants. This causal therapy would also be associated with LY 333531, PJ34, and FP15, which block protein kinase ß isoform, poly(ADP-ribose) polymerase, and peroxynitrite, respectively. Other current options may be thiazolinediones, statins, ACE inhibitors, and ATI inhibitors, which also have, at different levels, intracellular causal antioxidant activity. AGE, advanced glycosylation end product.

4.2 Crohn´s Disease

Crohn's disease (CD) belongs to idiopathic inflammatory bowel diseases (IBD) that also include idiopathic proctocolitis (IPC) and indeterminate colitis (IC), impossible to be ranked precisely into CD or IPC. These diseases cause the intestinal tissue to become inflamed, form sores and bleed easily. Symptoms include abdominal pain, cramping, fatigue, fever, diarrhoea sometimes bloody, malabsorption, loss of weight, failure to thrive in children. CD is characterized by an *autoimmune granulomatous chronic process affecting any part of the gastrointestinal tract, from the mouth to the anus* (Figure 19). *Patches of inflammation occur, with healthy tissue between the diseased areas* [143](Figure 20). The inflammation can extend through every layer of affected bowel tissue [143]. The generalized inflammation can also affect *extragastrointestinal organs* and their involvements are presented as skin affections (erythema nodosum, erythema multiforme), bone osteoporosis even osteonecrosis, joint inflammation under the picture of reactive arthritis or ankylosing spondylitis, liver affection as autoimmune hepatitis eventually primary sclerosing cholangitis, eye inflammation (episcleritis or anterior uveitis). Crohn's disease can not be cured by drugs or surgery, although either or both can help relieve symptoms [144].

Ulcerative colitis affects only the inner layer of the colon, or large bowel. It always starts in the rectum and may extend as a continuous inflammation from there into the rest of the colon. Usually ulcerative colitis can be controlled with medication. The disease can be completely eliminated by surgically removing the colon, but afterward, waste material may have to be stored and expelled through an external appliance [3, 144].

There is no known cause or cure for IBD. People are most frequently diagnosed between the ages of 15-25, or 45-55. IBD is particularly difficult for children and young adults since it often affects a person's self-concept, body image and lifestyle at a time when "being like everyone else" is so important. IBD is unpredictable. Most people experience periods of remission and flare-ups of the disease, often requiring long-term medication, hospitalisation or surgery [145]. Although IBD is found throughout the world, it seems to be more common in North America and northern Europe.

CD incidence keeps growing, and is high particularly in developed countries. In Europe, there is an incidence 9-10/100000 people per year, CD prevalence is about 20-80 persons per 100000 people. Both genders are affected equally.

Etiopathogenesis of CD is complex and includes genetic, immunological, infectious and other environmental factors. *The formation of generalized granulomatous inflammation is accompanied by ROS formation* [3, 146, 147, 148].

Initial inflammatory changes disrupt the protective intestinal barrier, then inflammatory cytokines are overproduced and inflammation progresses (cytokine phase). The next step includes tissue damage with increased inflammatory infiltration and simultaneous overproduction of ROS (Figure 21). The further phase of healing is characterized by connective tissue formation in the intestinal wall and results in consequent stenoses and/or fistulae creation.

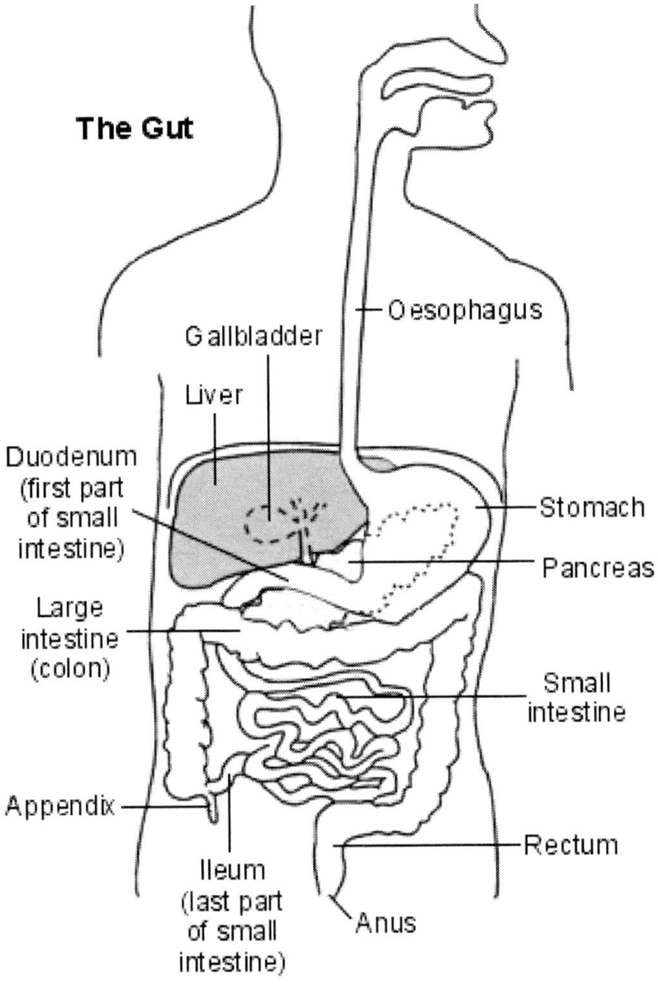

Figure 19. Distribution of inflammatory gastrointestinal affection in Crohn's disease

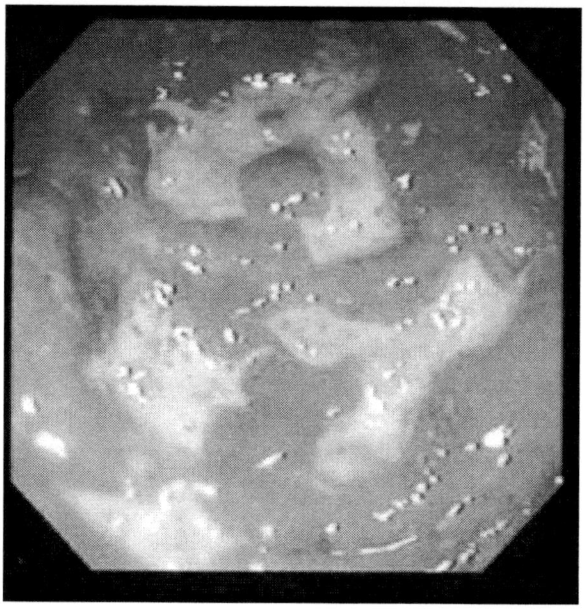

Figure 20. Inflammatory changes of gastrointestinal mucosa in Crohn's disease

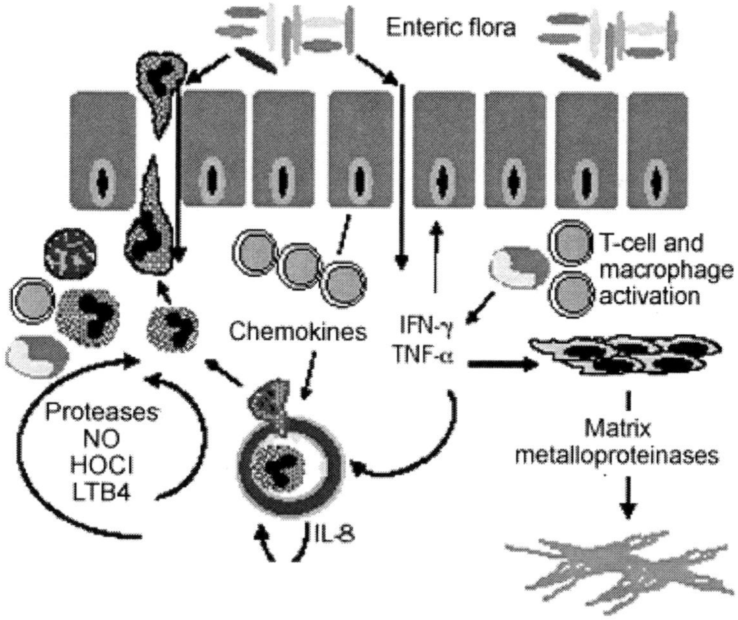

Figure 21. Immunological changes in the intestinal mucosa in CD (published by Shanahan, F. Crohn´s disease. The Lancet, 2002, 359, 62-69.

CD treatment is complex and encompasses anti-inflammatory (mesalazine), immunosuppressive (corticosteroids and azathioprine), and biological therapy with the aim to achieve the remission and to prevent disease complications. An appropriate nutritional support is indispensable, first total parenteral nutrition until the moment when the stabilisation of intestinal inflammation is achieved and the patient is able to stand the enteral nutrition without diarrhoea recurrence. The term of biological therapy is in CD reserved for the monoclonal anti-TNFα antibody that has success in refractory CD treatment. If conservative treatment in CD fails, the patient is indicated for surgical therapy with the management of Crohn's specific complications like stenosis, fistula, and abscess by bowel preservation. Limited resection and/or strictureplasty do not influence morbidity and rate and also time of recurrence [145].

ROS and IBD

As published long ago in 1991 by Yamada [149], the chronically inflamed intestine and/or colon is subjected to considerable oxidative stress whose source are the oxidants produced in phagocytic leukocytes (activated monocytes and polymorphonuclear leukocytes). These cells infiltrate in large numbers the intestinal mucosa and produce significant amounts of ROS in response to different inflammatory stimuli. Because the colonic mucosa contains relatively small amounts of antioxidant enzymes (SOD, catalase, GPx), the gut mucosa is overwhelmed during the time of active inflammation that results in intestinal injury [3, 149]. The complex review of oxidative stress as a pathogenic factor in inflammatory bowel disease brought Kruidenier in 2002 [146]. Here, the attention is paid to the origin of ROS and its impact on all cellular and extracellular components (Figure 22). Evidence of increased reactive oxygen metabolite levels is mentioned as it was found in biopsy specimens of IPC or CD correlated with clinical and endoscopic indices of disease activity. The consequences of oxidative stress on the gut are analysed, such as increased lipid peroxidation, presence of the protein carbonyl content as well as peroxynitrite-modified proteins in colonic biopsies, also the presence of DNA oxidation expressed as increased presence of 8hydroxy-deoxyguanosine in the inflammatory changed mucosa, increased apoptosis in the epithelium. In addition, the importance of different antioxidant defences is emphasized. Non-enzymatic antioxidants represented by glutathione and metallothionein are discussed in detail, similarly much attention is devoted to antioxidant enzymes (SOD, GPx, catalase), their activities in IBD mucosa and their expression regulation. It has been confirmed that mainly Mn-SOD is highly inducible under inflammatory conditions as IBD are. Much less information is available concerning the expression regulation of catalase and GPx.. The last part of this review describes some possibilities of antioxidant therapy in IBD and its limitations [150). The other works by Kruidenier et al. [151] contributed to the better knowledge of an imbalance between oxidant and antioxidant mechanisms at the tissue level in patients with IBD. These studies focused on thorough systemic examination of intestinal resection specimens of patients with CD or IPC and compared with normal control mucosa. They confirmed different gut mucosal SOD isoform expression, without major differences between CD and IPC. A marked stepwise increase in Mn-SOD (mitochondrial) levels was observed in non-inflamed and inflamed IBD mucosae, but a proportion of this enzyme was found to be enzymatically inactive. The Cu/Zn-SOD (cytosolic) content decreased in epithelium with inflammation. Extracellular EC-SOD was found in low amounts in normal control mucosa, moreover with tendency in IBD patients to be decreased with inflammation. In lamina propria, SOD expression was much lower and not effected by inflammation. Mn-SOD and Cu/Zn-SOD were found mainly in neutrophils and macrophages, and EC-SOD was localized in small vessels, stromal cells, and neutrophils. These findings were extended with further study for the assessment of catalase, GPx, GSH, myeloperoxidase, and metallothionein (OH· hydroxyl radical scavenger) in the intestinal resection specimens of patients with CD or IPC versus normal mucosa. Both in CD and IPC patients, intestinal inflammation was associated with increased activities of catalase, GPx, and MPO, whereas the mucosal GSH content was unaffected. Despite this overall increase in mucosal H_2O_2 metabolising enzyme capacity, there were found the important differences between epithelium and lamina propria. The risk of direct hydrogen peroxide damage in the lamina propria seemed to be attenuated by the increasing numbers of catalase and MPO positive monocytes/macrophages and neutrophils that infiltrated the inflamed areas. But MPO overexpression might increase the lamina propria levels of hypochlorous acid, a stable ROS with multiple pro-inflammatory effects. Epithelial cells expressing catalase and GPx were found unchanged during inflammation, and moreover hydroxyl radical scavenger metallothionein displayed decreased expression, thus epithelial antioxidant defence is low. Another study performed by Kruidenier et al. confirmed increased levels of peroxynitrite in the inflamed mucosa of IBD patients, and also elevated malondialdehyde concentration as a marker of lipoperoxidation [147]. All these results confirm an imbalanced and inefficient endogenous antioxidant response to ROS produced in the inflamed intestinal mucosa of IBD patients and pointed out the importance of oxidative stress in the pathogenesis of IBD [146, 147, 150, 151]. In another study [152], patients with CD had increased markers of lipid peroxidation as measured by plasma F_2 isoprostane, breath pentane and ethane output and significantly lower plasma antioxidant vitamins (ascorbic acid, α- and β-carotene, lycopene, and β-cryptoxanthin) when compared with control subjects. High level of GPx were found in a Turkish group of IBD patients indicating in this way stimulated response against oxidative stress. MDA levels in this study were normal in IBD individuals and this finding suggests the clearance of free radicals without leading to important lipid peroxidation [148]. A large group of IBD patients (94 with IPC, 97 with CD) was compared with 72 healthy controls with regard to blood total antioxidant capacity TAC and corrected TAC cTAC (TAC after subtraction of the interactions due to endogenous uric acid, bilirubin, and albumin). In both groups of IBD, TAC and cTAC were significantly reduced when compared with controls irrespective of disease activity [153]. The study on animal mice model with dextran sulphate sodium (DSS)-induced colitis used the preventive (before colitis induction) or treatment (after colitis induction) with GSH or CoQ. Colitis symptoms were reduced in both groups of animals, hence GSH or CoQ had a beneficial effect on acute signs of IBD. Controversy brought into the problem the histological evaluation that revealed increases in colonic dysplasia and ulceration after GSH or CoQ supplementation [154]. The more favourable result had another animal study with DSS induced colitis. Mice treated with three different antioxidants (S-adenosylmethionine, a GSH precursor; green tea polyphenols; a cysteine prodrug - 2(R,S)-n-propylthiazolidine-4(R)-carboxylic acid – PTCA). All the antioxidants significantly improved diarrhoea and colon lesions, in blood reduced GSH levels returned to normal when treated with antioxidants. Serum amyloid as acute phase protein and tumour necrosis factor-alpha were significantly increased in animals with florid colitis, but they improved with antioxidant treatment. These results may support a beneficial role of antioxidant therapy in IBD individuals [155]. Another recent study used the treatment with N-acetylcysteine (NAC) against toxic damage in the rat colitis induced with acetic acid. NAC was applied locally (into colon) and systemically (intraperitoneally). Treatment with higher levels of NAC (100mg/kg for 7 days) significantly decreased the degree of colonic injury and NAC is judged as having a role in the treatment of IBD [156]. Italian authors published an article on IBD patients and their plasma vitamin A, E, and carotenoid concentrations. They found significantly reduced antioxidant levels in IBD patients (both IPC and CD), particularly in those with active disease, when compared with healthy controls. 8-hydroxy-deoxy-guanosine (8-OHdG) were also assessed in the patients´leucocytes. A significantly increased levels of 8-OHdG were found without regarding the disease activity and antioxidant levels [157].

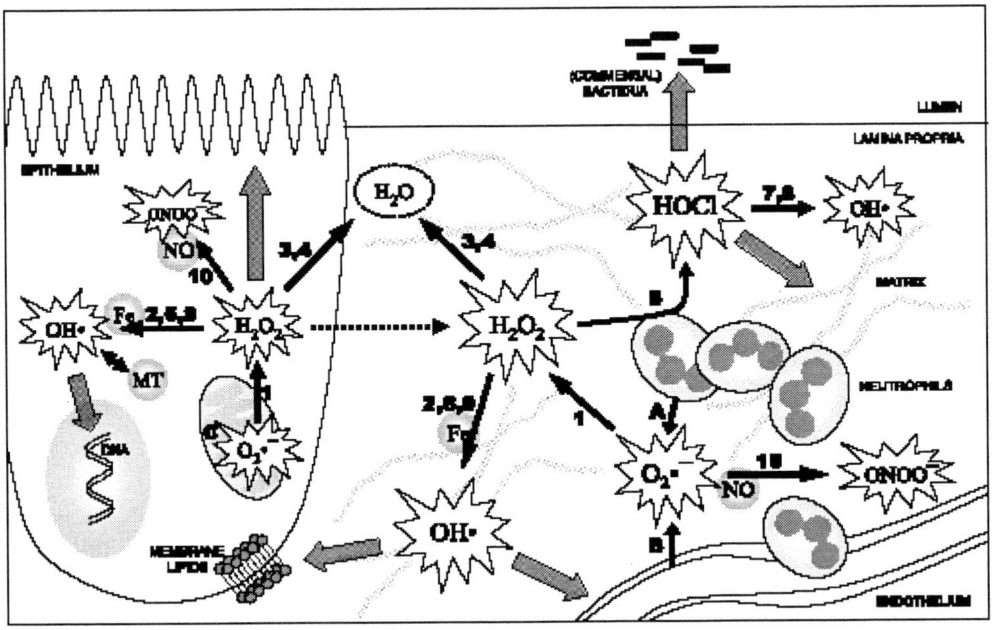

Figure 22. Schematic representation of ROS in intestinal inflammation (published by Kruidenier, L; Verspaget, HW. Oxidative stress as a pathogenic factor in inflammatory bowel disease — radicals or ridiculous? Alimentary Pharmacology and Therapeutics, 2002, 16, 1997-2015, with the kind permission of the author)

A- neutrophil NADPHoxidase, B-xanthine oxidase, C-mitochondrial NADPH cytochrome p450 reductase

1- formation of hydrogen peroxide from superoxide, 2-formation of OH· and OH- from hydrogen peroxide (Fenton reaction)
2- formation of oxygen and water from hydrogen peroxide catalysed by catalase or GPx
3- formation of water nad NADP+ from hydrogen peroxide, H+ and NADPH
4- formation of hypochlorous acid from hydrogen peroxide and chlorine (catalysing enzyme myeloperoxidase)
5- formation of O_2, OH· and OH- from hydrogen peroxide and superoxide (iron-catalysed Haber-Weiss reaction)
6- formation of oxygen, chlorine and hydroxyl radical from hypochlorous acid and superoxide
7- formation of OH· and OH- and oxidized iron from reduced iron ions and hypochlorous acid
8- formation of nitrogen dioxide, hydroxyl radical and H+
9- formation of peroxynitrite anion and H+ from nitric oxide and superoxide

No known enzyme exists to facilitate the detoxification of hydroxyl radical OH· , OH·-induced tissue damage may be prevented by the binding of transition metal ions by albumin,k ceruloplasmin, ferritin, transferrin and metallothionein.

ROS, DNA Damage, DNA Repair and IBD

An association between IPC and an elevated risk for colorectal cancer is well established and this carcinogenesis is probably driven by chronic inflammation. The available evidence suggests that DNA damage caused by oxidative stress in the characteristic damage-regeneration cycle is a major contributor to colorectal cancer development in IPC patients [158]. Oxidative DNA damage (8-OhdG) in mucosa of ulcerative colitis has been examined in the D´Inca study [159]. Patients with IPC and dysplasia had significantly higher mucosal 8-OhdG concentrations, in particular in older patients, in patients with long-standing disease, and active disease when compared with sporadic colon cancer and irritable bowel syndrome. Also the findings in patients with CD demonstrated increased levels of 8-OhdG, this time in peripheral leucocytes [D´Odorico]. An older study on a small number of patients with IPC [160] showed deficient repair of radiation-induced DNA damage compared with a group of healthy controls. The development of colorectal cancer is the most serious long-term complication faced by patients with longstanding extensive ulcerative colitis, with an incidence 20-fold higher than colorectal carcinoma (CRC) in the general population. Thus, more attention is paid to the intensity of DNA repair, expression of DNA repair genes (BER or MMR), and their association with IPC [161,162, 163]. The proper course of the cell cycle is controlled by protein p53 that is overexpressed in the G1 stage of the cell cycle when DNA damage is present. In order to allow DNA repair in stressed or injured cells, protein p53 blocks the continuation of the cell cycle and DNA damage can be repaired. When the expression of p53 was measured in inflamed and regenerated mucosa of patients with IBD, the increased number of cells expressing p53 was found in patients with IPC than with CD. This finding supports the idea of importantly changed DNA and the cell cycle arrest mediated through p53 [164]. Oxidative stress induces DNA strand breaks and their accumulation leads to the stimulation of poly(ADP-ribose)polymerase (PARP), that further initiates BER pathway, but also stimulates pro-inflammatory pathways as mentioned previously. The study on IL-10 deficient animal models showed, that the application of PARP inhibitor (3-aminobenzamide) led to the normalization of colonic permeability and downregulation of proinflammatory cytokines, such as tumour necrosis factor-α and interferon [73].

The information about the intensity of DNA repair in CD patients is lacking.

Oxidative stress undoubtedly contributes to the pathogenesis of both chronic lifelong diseases - diabetes mellitus and Crohn's disease though the origin of oxidative stress differs. In DM, oxidative stress is mostly of metabolic origin, in CD, oxidative stress is in particular of inflammatory origin. The extensive research of both diseases has brought recently an enormous knowledge of molecular genetics and participating genes, immunological processes and their consequences, metabolic changes with special attention to oxidative stress. What remains unpredictable is the future course of either diabetes or Crohn's disease in newly diagnosed patients.

5. Our Study Examining Oxidative Stress, DNA Damage and DNA Repair in Patients with Diabetes Mellitus and Crohn Disease

Many previously published reports established the fact of increased oxidative stress in patients with diabetes mellitus and inflammatory bowel diseases (IBD), in particular Crohn's disease (CD). Also our previously published article (JDC) reported increased parameters of oxidative stress in children with type 1 diabetes mellitus (T1DM), and similarly their non-diabetic siblings, when compared with age-matched healthy children. *Though the finding of increased oxidative DNA damage in diabetic individuals as well as in subjects suffering from IBD has been well documented in several studies, the information about the intensity of DNA repair in these patients is completely lacking.*

The acknowledged existence of interindividual differences in DNA repair [165] *and* our acquaintance with *a well established method comet assay* (single cell gel electrophoresis used for the assessment of DNA strand breaks and in a modified version for the measurement of DNA repair capacity) [65] *initiated our hypothesis* (Figure 23).

5.1 Hypothesis

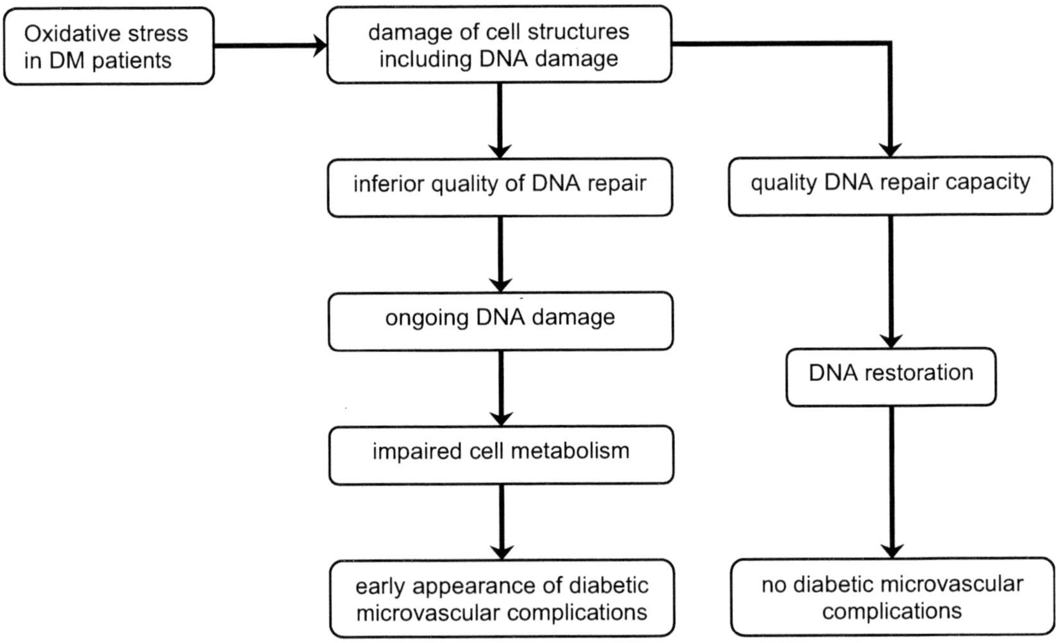

Figure 23. Hypothesis of influence of DNA repair on the course of DM or IBD (in DM diabetic microvascular complications and macrovascular complications, in IBD patients the presence of fistulae, stenosis, abscess)

Summarizing the hypothesis: these patients with free radical diseases, such as diabetes or IBD, that would have low DNA repair capacity could be expected as those having an early development of complicated course of disease and vice versa, those ones having good or excellent DNA repair capacity should not have an early development of disease complications.

In order to get the basic information about the intensity of DNA repair capacity in patients with diabetes mellitus and Crohn's disease, adult and paediatric patients with type 1 diabetes mellitus, adults with type 2 diabetes, adults and children with Crohn's disease were recruited and examined for the intensity of oxidative stress (parameters of OS) and for oxidative DNA damage (DNA strand breaks) and DNA repair capacity (DNArc).

5.2 Study Material

T1 diabetes mellitus patients: 53 adult patients, 28 women, 25 men, mean age 38.25±11.02 years, mean disease duration 16.49±3.22 years, mean HbA1c concentration 8.36±1.12 % (normal ranges 4.3-5.8% DCCT, performed 2002) were enrolled in the study. Among them 23 persons without any diabetic microvascular complication (DMC), 30 remaining persons having 1 or more diabetic complications - maximum 4 complications (15 subjects): diabetic retinopathy (18 subjects), diabetic nephropathy (22 subjects) diabetic neuropathy (11 subjects) and diabetic foot (3 patients). Diabetic retinopathy was diagnosed by a specialized ophthalmologist, diabetic nephropathy was defined as microalbuminuria higher than 20μg/min and/or proteinuria higher than 0.20g/24h, diabetic neuropathy was examined using a neurological disability score (NDS), electromyography (EMG), biothesiometer and monofilamenta and diabetic foot was evaluated according to International Consensus on the Diabetic Foot. 5 patients with DMC had simultaneous macrovascular complications (coronary heart disease, or peripheral vascular disease, or cerebral ischaemia).

These 2 groups of patients (without complications and with complications) did not substantially differ in age, sex, and diabetes control, but they differ in disease duration (14.70±3.11 years x 17.63±2.57 years, $p<0.01$). All patients were on diet, and treated with intensified insulin therapy or on insulin pump, other medicaments were applied according to the present diabetic complications.

Type 2 diabetes adults (T2DM): 14 patients with T2DM, 6 women, 8 men, mean age 58.0±5.6 years, mean disease duration 11±6.06 years, HbA1c 9.9±2.5% DCCT, treated with insulin, and/or PAD, + diet. 5 patients had macrovascular complications (cardiac artery disease or peripheral vascular disease), 5 patients had microvascular complications (retinopathy in 4 cases, once nephropathy, neuropathy in 3 patients), 3 patients had both types of complications.

Crohn's disease patients: 17 adult patients, 11 women, 6 men, mean age 37±11.36 years, mean disease duration 10.53±7.24 years, CDAI index 68.18±41.10 (normal ranges up to 150 as inactive disease, above 150 active disease) were examined. 11 patients underwent one or more operations for CD complications (stenoses, fistulae), all subjects were on intensive treatment including salicylates, corticosteroids and/or immunosuppressive drugs (Imuran). 1 patient was treated with biologicals (Remicade).

T1DM children: 20 children, all individuals were without diabetic microvascular complications, 8 girls and 12 boys, mean age 13.3±2.9 years, mean disease duration 2.94±2.72, mean HbA1c 9.50±2.52% (DCCT) (study performed in 2002-2003) were enrolled. All children were on diet and treated with intensified insulin therapy or on insulin pump.

17 children with Crohn's disease: 7 girls, 10 boys, mean age 14.29±SD 2.52 years, mean disease duration 3±1.43 years, PCDAI index (activity of disease) was 35.69±16.60 (normal up to 30), CDAI index (activity of disease compared with adults) was 112.94±82,7 (normal up to 150). All patients were treated with salicylates, and/or corticosteroids, at the time of blood collection, none, at the time of blood sample collection, was treated with biologicals. 3 patients underwent surgical treatment for stenosis, fistula, and abscess complications.

Control group of healthy adults: healthy control subjects were previously recruited by the corresponding laboratories and their results served as normals for appropriate methods (for markers of oxidative stress 46 women and 42 men, total mean age 34.80±10.32 years, for DNA strand breaks and DNA repair capacity 20 women and 22 men, mean age 45.20±8.31 years).

Control group consisted of 11 healthy children randomly chosen among children examined for accidental heart murmur (heart defect excluded using echocardiography) 5 girls, 6 boys, mean age 13.7±3.8 years.

T1DM and CD children were comparable with regard to their age and sex with the control group of children.

5.3 Methods

Methods used for the patients´ assessment: blood samples were examined for markers of oxidative stress, such as superoxide dismutase SOD in erythrocytes (U/g Hb), glutathione peroxidase GPx in blood (U/g Hb), antioxidant plasmatic capacity AOC (mmol/l), reduced glutathione GSH in erythrocytes (mmol/l ery), plasmatic malondialdehyde MDA (μmol/l).Kits from Randox (Crumlin, Great Britain), adapted to an automated Hitachi 717 analyser (Roche, Mannheim, Germany) were used for determination of superoxide dismutase in erythrocytes, glutathione peroxidase in whole blood, and finally for plasma antioxidant capacity. Reduced glutathione concentration in erythrocytes was estimated with kits from Oxis Int. (Bonnenie, Marue, France) while plasma malondialdehyde as a product of lipid peroxidation was determined photometrically as TBARS (thiobarbituric acid reactive substances) [125, 166].

DNA damage and DNA repair capacity in patient's peripheral lymphocytes were examined with comet assay (single cell gel electrophoresis) and its modified version (Figure 24, 25, 26).

DNA strand breaks (DNAsb) measured by X-ray-calibrated comet assay (alkaline single-cell gel electrophoresis) [65], in peripheral blood lymphocytes isolated from heparinized blood samples were used as a parameter of oxidative DNA damage. Results are expressed as strand breaks per 10^9 Daltons of the DNA. Briefly, cells embedded in a thin layer of agarose on a microscope slide are lysed with detergent and high salt, and the resulting nucleoids electrophoresed at high pH. DNA is pulled out of the nucleoid to form a "comet tail". Comets are visualized by fluorescence microscopy, after staining with ethidiumbroide. The relative amount of DNA in the tail compared with the head reflects the number of DNA breaks present.

The individual DNA repair capacity (DNArc) restoring oxidative DNA damage was measured by modified comet assay using cell extracts from patients′ lymphocytes. In this case, cultured cells (HeLa) treated with a photosensitiser Ro 19-8022 Hoffman-La Roche and visible light are used as a target cells with a defined amount of oxidative damage. These cells embedded in agarose are treated for 45 min. with cell extracts prepared from lymphocytes isolated from tested patients. The number of DNA breaks (expressed as strand breaks per 10^9 Daltons) formed in the 8-oxoguanine-containing DNA of target cells by cell extracts expresses the capacity of the examined lymphocytes to initiate the repair of oxidised bases (8-oxoguanines) [65, 167].

To express the relationship between the intensity of individual DNA repair capacity and the existing level of oxidative DNA damage, a *DNA repair index* (DNRI) where DNArc represents the number of strand breaks/10^9 Daltons induced by cell extract in DNA of target (HeLa) cells containing 8-oxoguanine and DNAsb is the number of strand breaks/10^9 Daltons measured in DNA of tested lymphocytes [136].

Statistical evaluation: data were expressed as means±standard deviation. Wilcoxon unpaired test, Spearman and Kruskal-Wallis test and rank correlation were used in statistical evaluation of the results. Statistical significance was implied by p-value <0.05.

The Local Ethics Committee approved the study, and patients′ informed consent was obtained from all participants before entering the study.

5.4 Results

All the graphs are expressed in % of values. One group, usually healthy adults or healthy children, were indicated as a baseline 100% value and statistical average and standard deviation of all other groups were expressed as the percentage of the baseline value.

Markers of oxidative stress includes superoxide dismutase SOD, glutathione peroxidase GPx, antioxidant plasmatic capacity AOC, reduced glutathione GSH, malondialdehyde MDA.

Evaluation of DNA damage is indicated as DNAsb. DNA repair capacity as DNArc. Statistical significance $^{*}p<0.05$ $^{**}p<0.01$ $^{***}p<0.001$

If standard deviation surpasses the size of the graph, its value is mentioned below the graph.

Axis X - examined parameters axis Y - % of values

This pilot study brings some new information about the intensity of DNA damage and DNA repair capacity in seven different groups of individuals, among them five groups of patients with chronic lifelong diseases and still among them, two groups of pediatric children. As we would like to get some knowledge about the development of the assessed parameters not only with regard to the patients′ diagnosis, but also with regard to the patients′age (having in mind the theory of aging), we dared to compare the results of diseased children with diseased adults, and also to relate all the results to a baseline value of healthy adults. Concerning children, we accomplished the comparison between both groups of pediatric patients with healthy controls.

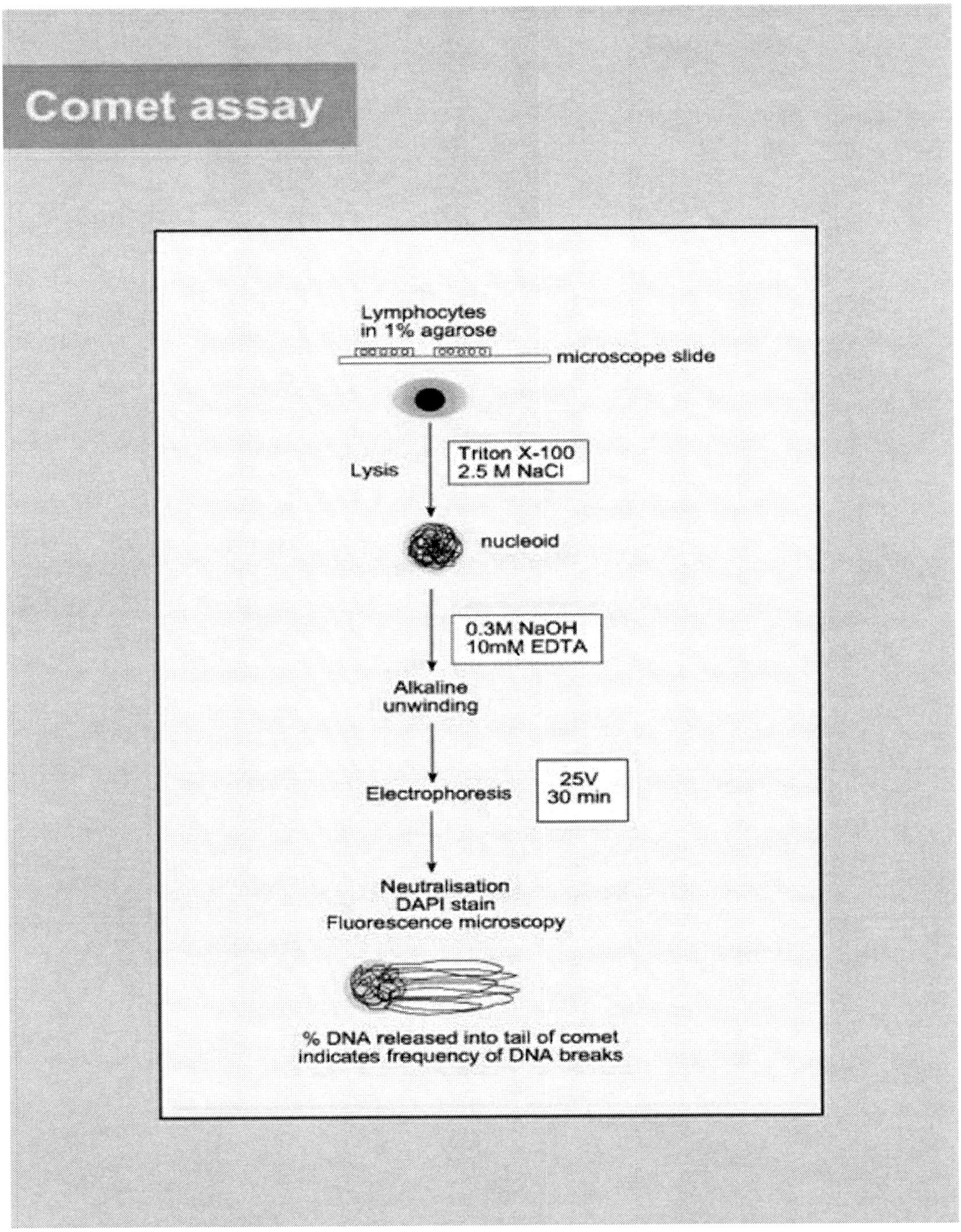

Figure 24. Comet assay for the evaluation of DNA strand breaks (by AR Collins)

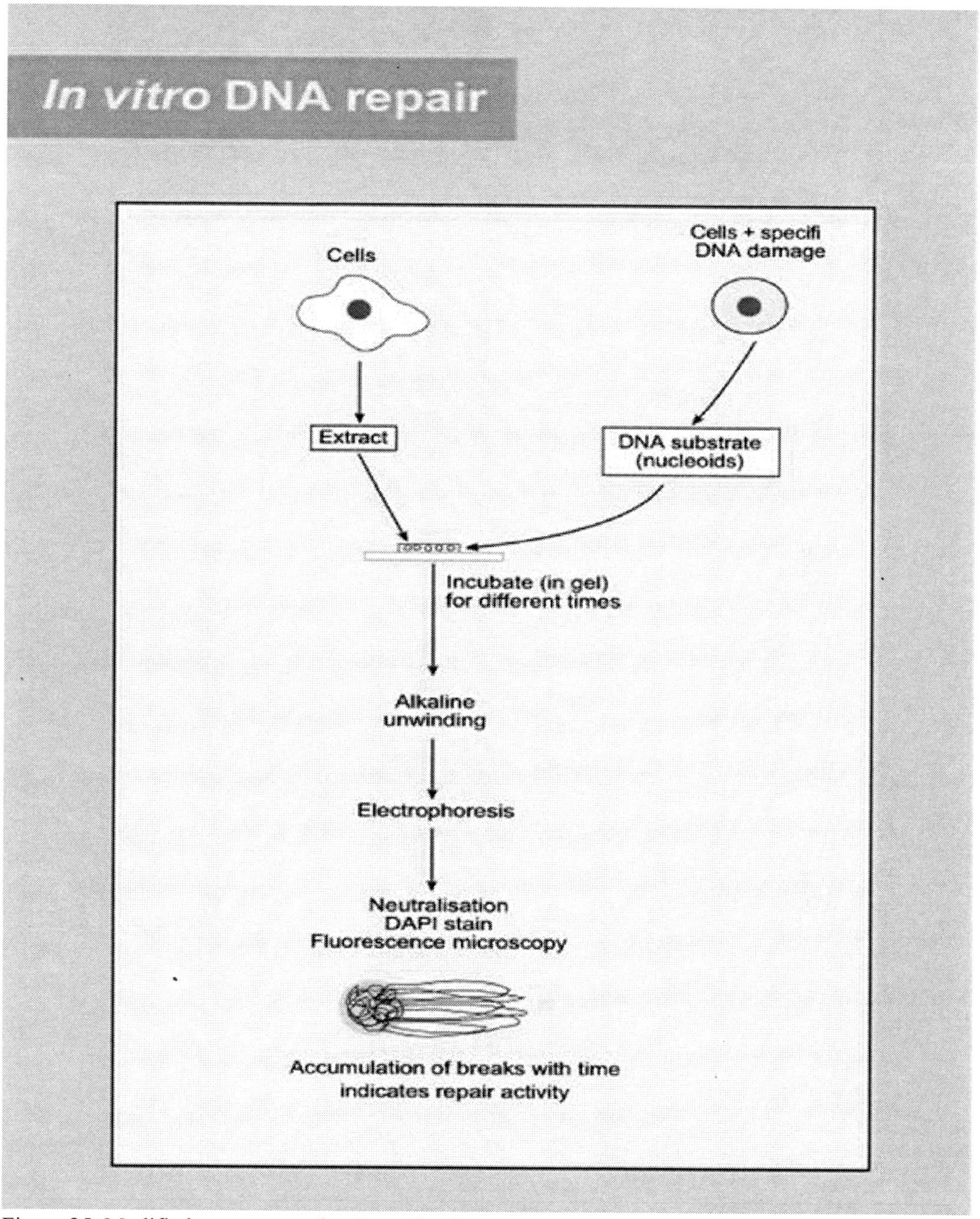

Figure 25. Modified comet assay for the evaluation of DNA repair (by AR Collins)

1 2 3

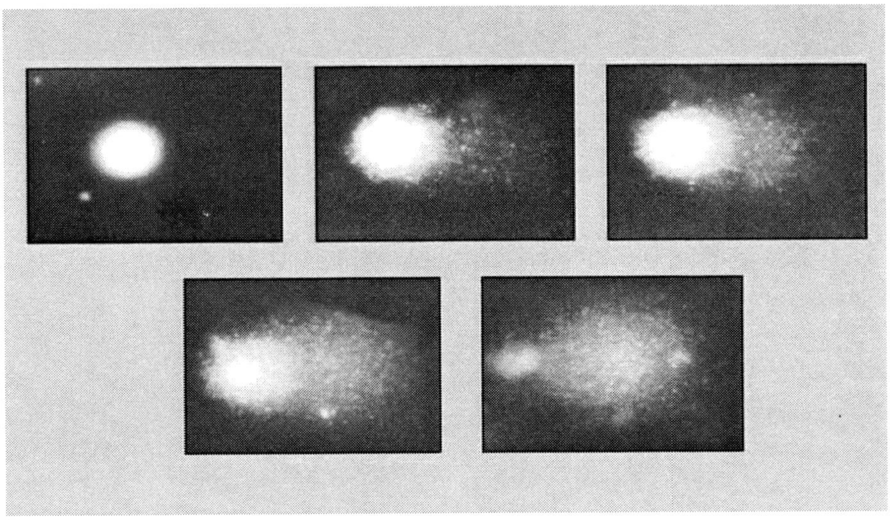

4 5

Figure 26. Comet assay - different degrees of DNA damage (1. nucleoid without damage, 3. nucleoid with comet and present DNA breaks 5. completely destroyed nucleoid (published by AR Collins. The comet assay for DNA damage and repair: principles, applications, and limitations. Mol Biotechnol, 2004, 26, 249-61, with the kind permission of the author)

5.4.1 Study of Oxidative Stress, DNA Damage and DNA Repair Capacity of Lymphocytes in Healthy Adults and Healthy Children

The level of SOD was significantly higher in healthy children than in adults ($p<0.001$), on the other hand GPx was lower ($p<0.001$), the remaining parameters of oxidative stress (AOC, GSH, MDA) did not differ substantially. DNA strand breaks were comparable in both groups (a large variance of results in children influences the statistical significance), but DNA repair capacity was significantly higher in children ($p<0.001$) together with DNRI ($p<0.001$).

The activities of antioxidant enzymes and levels of other antioxidant substances do not change substantially with age. Our group of healthy children had higher SOD and lower GPx when compared with healthy adults. This result corresponds with the finding of SOD and catalase activation in physically active children [168]. Similar activation of catalase and glutathione reductase and reversely decrease glutathione peroxidase in healthy men after an extreme cycling performance was found by Aguilo [169]. It could be expected that our healthy children had certainly more physical activity than healthy adults. Oxidative damage of healthy children was lower than in adults, but their DNA repair capacity and DNRI were significantly higher than in healthy adults. This finding certainly correlates with age difference between children and adults, and thus age-related decreased activity of DNA repair enzymes, as published by several authors and implied in the theory aging [83, 84, 170, 171, 172]. Raji [173] confirmed an increased DNA repair in children. Chen [174] found age-associated decrease of oxidative repair enzymes, namely human 8-oxoguanine DNA glycosylase.

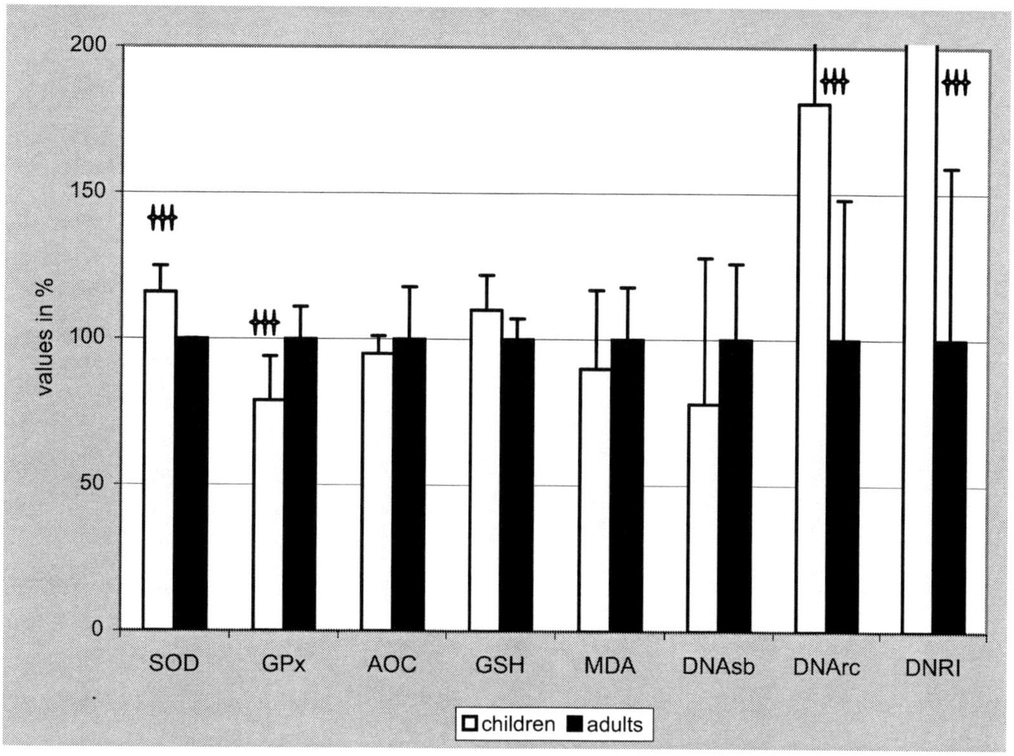

Figure 27. Markers of oxidative stress, DNA damage and repair. Mean values of healthy adults=100%, DNArc SD in healthy children SD±36%, mean DNRI in healthy children 1044% of the value of healthy adults, DNRI SD in healthy children SD 3026% of the value of healthy adults

5.4.2 Comparison of T1DM Patients versus Healthy Population

T1DM patients showed lower GPx (both groups $p<0.01$) and lower antioxidant plasmatic capacity (both groups $p<0.01$). Their MDA was very high (both T1DM groups $p<0.001$). SOD was significantly high in T2DM adults ($p<0.001$), on the other hand GSH as the important intracellular antioxidant was significantly decreased ($p<0.01$) in the same group of patients. Their MDA was substantially low ($p<0.01$). Metabolic compensation (evaluated as the value of HbA1c) of T1DM adults was significantly better (HbA1c 8.36±1.12 % DCCT) than this one of T2DM adults (HbA1c 9.9±2.5% DCCT, $p<0.05$) and T1DM children (HbA1c 9.50±2.52% DCCT) ($p<0.05$), (it is not shown in the figure).

The findings of lower GPx and AOC and high MDA both in adults and children with T1DM correspond with the results of other authors [130, 175, 176]. Results of patients with T2DM showed stimulation of antioxidant enzymes and low GSH. Low MDA could be explained by MDA incorporation into LDL that are usually elevated in T2DM [177].

The results of T1DM patients behaved differently. Significantly increased DNA repair capacity was found in both adult and pediatric groups of T1DM individuals when compared with adult healthy controls ($p<0.001$ both), and along with it, DNRI was also extremely elevated (both groups $p<0.001$).

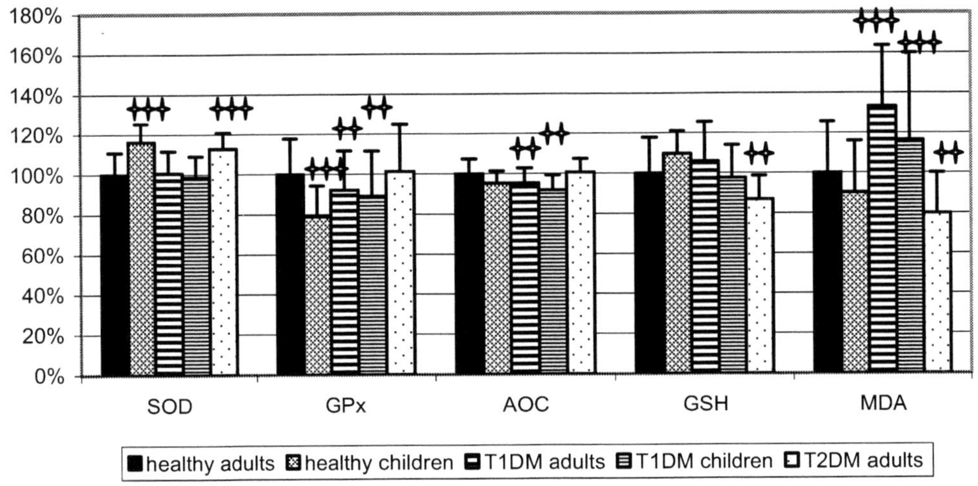

Figure 28. Markers of oxidative stress. Mean values of healthy adults=100%

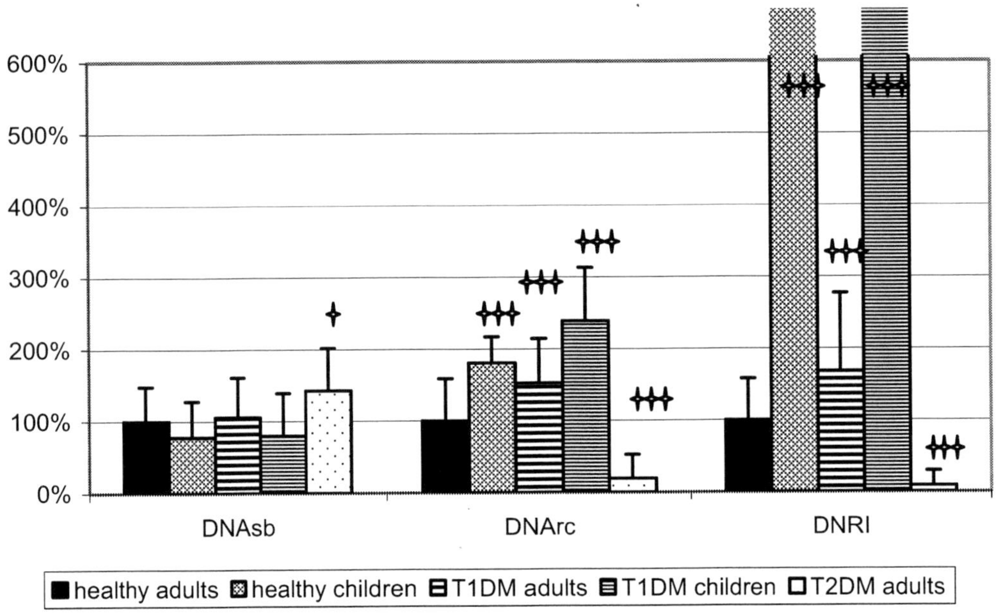

Figure 29. DNA damage and repair. Mean values of healthy adults=100%, DNRI in healthy children mean 1144% SD 3026% , T1DM children DNRI mean 919% SD 1307%

There is an apparent finding of significantly elevated DNA strand breaks in patients with T2 diabetes ($p<0.05$). On the other hand, their DNA repair capacity showed an extremely low level of repairing strand breaks ($p<0.001$) and similarly DNRI is extremely low ($p<0.001$).

Several studies confirmed oxidative DNA damage in diabetic patients using different methods, mainly with increased loss of oxidized bases into urine or an increased number of DNA strand breaks [3, 126, 127, 129]. In our study, the differences in DNA damage between healthy controls and T1DM (adults, children) were not statistically significant. T2DM patients had significantly elevated DNA strand breaks. Similar results were described by Sardas [131] who found worse DNA damage in T2DM than in T1DM. Krapfenbauer [126] also confirmed increased DNA oxidation in both types of diabetes. On the other hand, our T2DM patients had a very low DNA repair. It could be explained either by the older age of this group, or the problem could be hypothetically also in the genetically or environmentally influenced bad DNA repair. Similar results were presented by Blasiak et al.[99] in a case-control study and he found also low DNA repair in T2DM subjects. This fact could represent a link to susceptibility of T2DM patients to carcinogenesis. Generally, low DNA repair can lead to extreme DNA damage, and thus initiate apoptosis, or inaccurate repair of damaged DNA leads to mutations and genomic instability and finally to carcinogenesis [2, 3, 53, 55, 56, 57].

5.4.3. Comparison of T1DM Adult Group versus T1DM Children

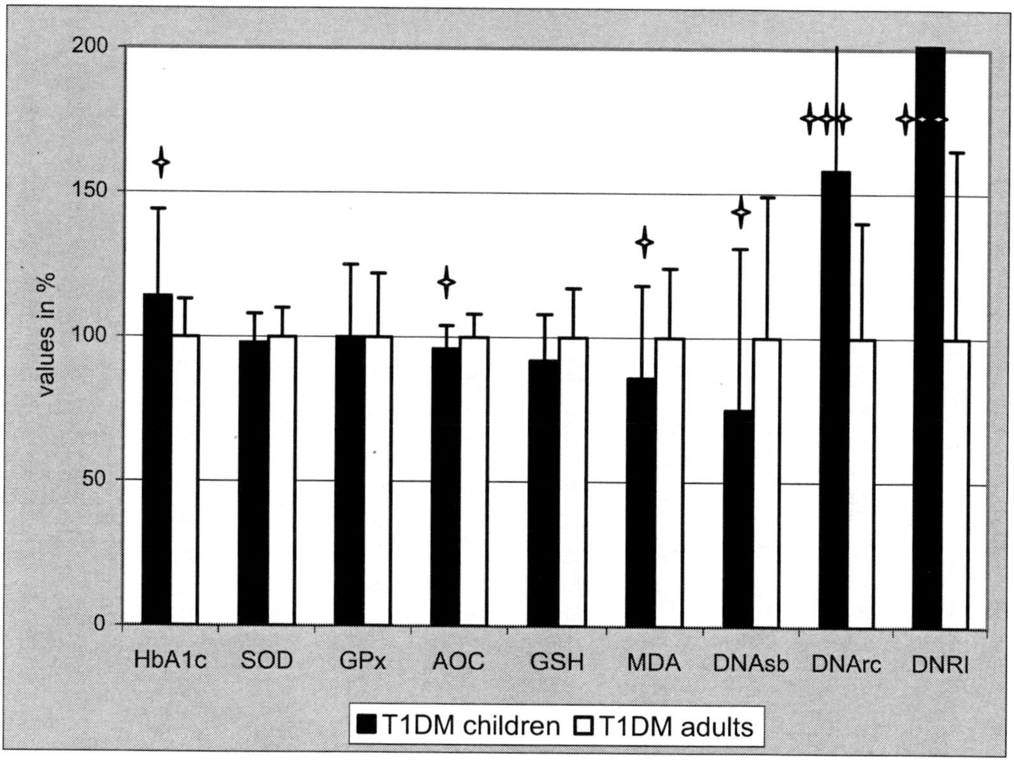

Figure 30. Markers of oxidative stress, DNA damage and repair. Mean values of T1DM adults=100%, DNArc diabetic children SD±49%, DNRI children mean 538%, SD 755%. This graph matches results of diabetic children and adults with T1DM. Though a worse diabetes compensation in children measured as glycated hemoglobin HbA_{1c} (significantly higher, $p<0.05$) and lower levels of AOC ($p<0.05$), diabetic children had favourable low levels of MDA ($p<0.05$), i.e. low lipid peroxidation. They showed also significantly lower DNA damage ($p<0.05$) and stimulated DNA repair ($p<0.001$), as well as DNRI (also $p<0.001$).

The presented results cannot be compared with a similar study in T1DM children and adults. Nevertheless, it is obvious that young organisms coped better with the requirements of hyperglycemic state and oxidative load. The influence of a shorter disease duration

(2.94±2.72 years in children versus 16.49±3.22 years in adults, $p<0.001$) could also influence the presented results. Genetically conditioned individual DNA repair of oxidative damage (via BER) might also affect the results. Unfortunately, the matched results of DNAsb, DNArc and DNRI measured in each patient after a 2-year interval are not yet available, hence it is impossible to declare an attitude towards this question.

5.4.4 Comparison of T1DM Adults Divided into 2 Subgroups Based on the Abscence or Presence of Diabetic Microvascular Complications with T1DM Children (Published by Varvarovska, Biomedicine and Pharmacotherapy 2004, Citation 136)

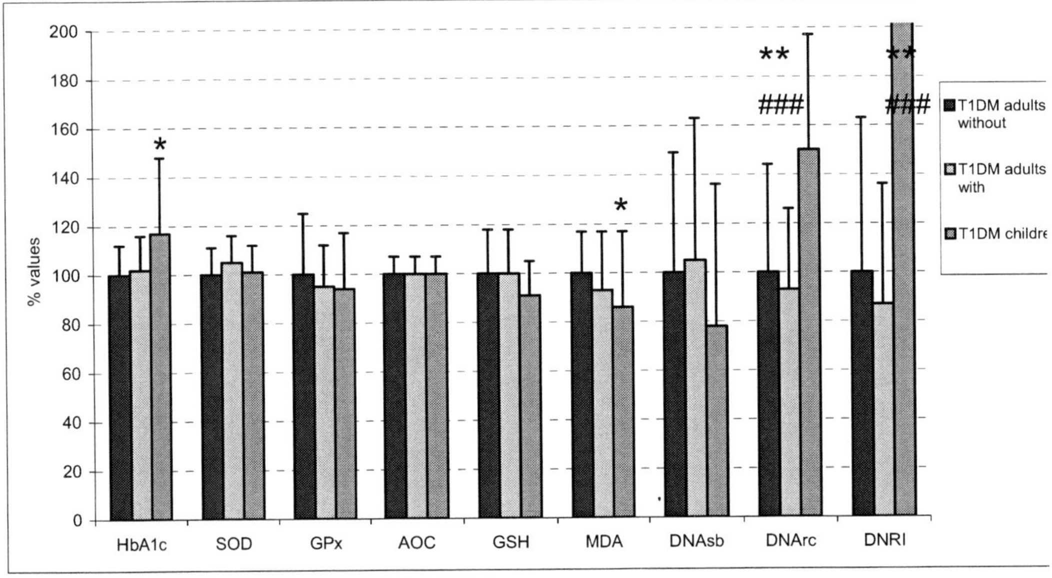

Figure 31. Markers of oxidative stress, DNA damage and repair. (mean values of adult diabetic patients without microvascular complications=100%) , published by Varvarovska (...) T1DM adults without= T1DM patients without diabetic microvascular complications (DMC), T1DM with=adults with DMC, mean values of T1DM adults without complications=100% $^{*}p<0.05$ $^{**}p<0.01$ T1DM children versus adult T1DM patients without diabetic microvascular complications; ### $p<0.001$ T1DM children versus adult T1DM with diabetic microvascular complications; DNRI children mean 489%, SD693%

In order to support our hypothesis, the group of adults T1DM patients was divided into 2 subgroups. The first one was composed of 23 patients without diabetic microvascular complications, the second group consisted of 30 adults having 1-4 complications (nephropathy, retinopathy, neuropathy, diabetic foot). We compared those 2 subgroups with T1DM children. Though the worse diabetes control (HbA_{1c}) and MDA in children (both values higher on $p<0.05$ versus T1DM adults without DMC), T1DM children displayed similar DNAsb like both adult subgroups. On the contrary, children's DNArc was significantly higher when compared with T1DM adults without DMC ($p<0.01$) and the comparison with T1DM adults with diabetic complications showed the statistical significance on $p<0.001$. DNRI behaved similarly like DNArc, i.e. statistical significance children versus T1DM without DMC $p<0.01$, and versus T1DM with DMC $p<0.001$. Hence, it could be concluded that T1DM children had better antioxidant defence against oxidative stress including superior DNA repair process. *Adult diabetic patients with microvascular complications showed the worst values of DNA assays and this might agree with our hypothesis, i.e. an individually bad DNA repair could contribute to the earlier development of diabetic microvascular complications.* However, it is also necessary to acknowledge a fact, that diabetic patients with DMC had longer disease duration (both subgroups $p<0.001$ versus diabetic children, not shown in the figure), so DNA repair could be exhausted after a long exposition to oxidative stress originated from the long-lasting hyperglycemia.

5.4.5 Study of CD Patients (Adults and Children) versus Healthy Adult Population

The values of SOD, GPx and GSH in CD patients cannot be compared with the findings in GIT mucosa, as markers of oxidative stress were measured in blood or erythrocytes. Nevertheless, it is obvious that CD patients had lower GPx activity, particularly CD children ($p<0.01$) when compared with healthy adults. Also total plasmatic antioxidant capacity was significantly low both in CD adults and children (both $p<0.01$). In CD adults, GSH is significantly higher ($p<0.01$), also their MDA low levels corresponds with the more localized and inflammatory pattern of the disease ($p<0.05$). In children, these two markers are presented in a similar way, but there are not significantly changed.

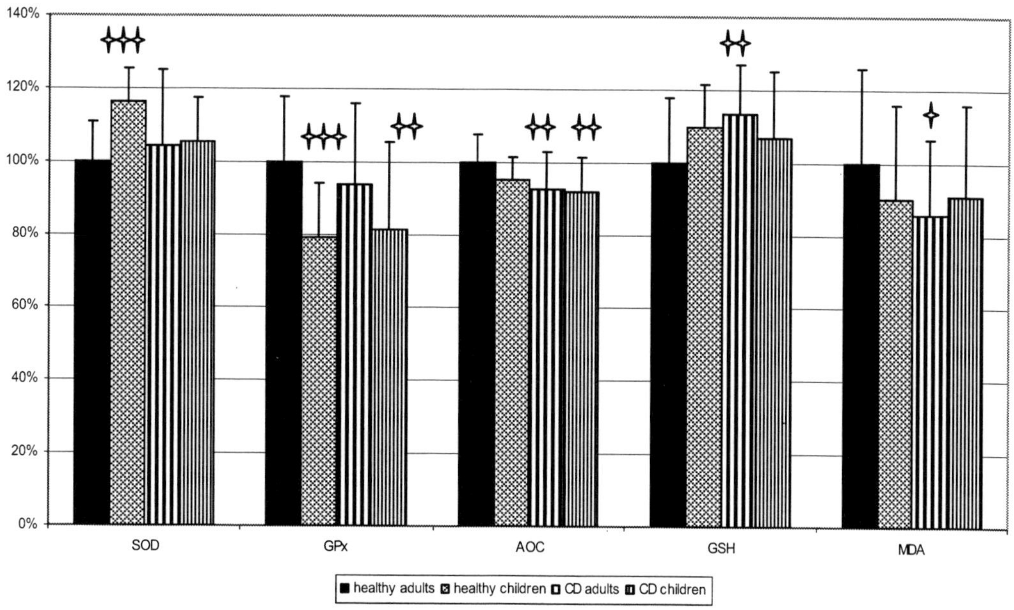

Figure 32. Markers of oxidative stress. Mean values of healthy adults=100%

In correlation with the scarce literary data, our patients had significantly decreased antioxidant plasmatic activity and lower GPx (mainly children) [153]. Lower GPx gives evidence of the worse antioxidant defence of CD patients. The levels of GSH was higher in CD adults (versus healthy adults) what might be in relationship with a special diet applied in those group of patients.

CD adults and children showed decreased levels of DNA damage (CD adults DNA sb $p<0.05$ versus healthy adults). On the contrary, the significantly increased DNA repair capacity was found in both groups of CD patients (adults $p<0.05$, children $p<0.001$). Similar finding was confirmed in DNRI (both groups $p<0.001$).

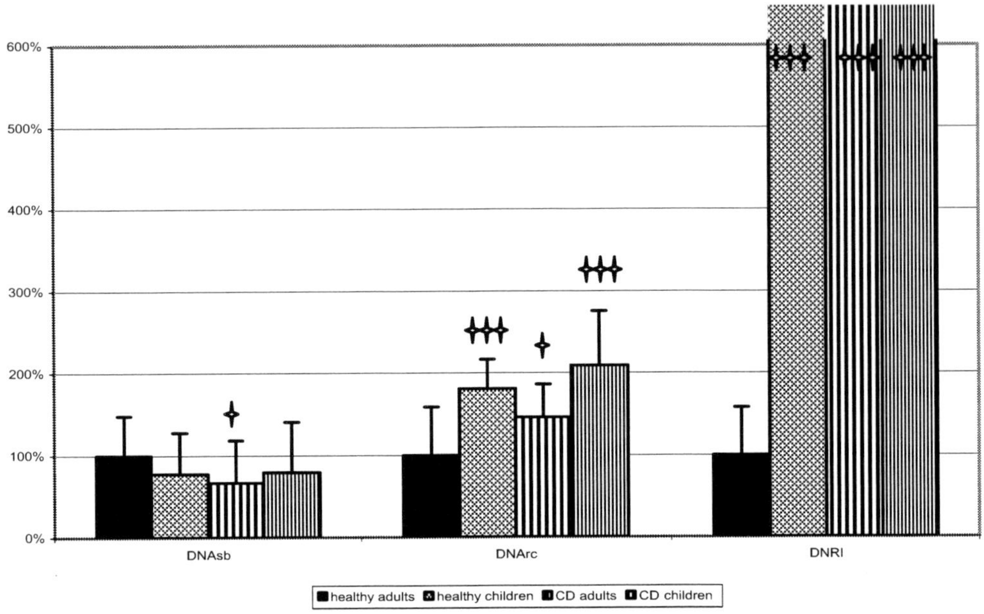

Figure 33. DNA damage and repair. Mean values of healthy adults=100%, healthy children DNRI mean 1144%, SD 3026%, CD adults DNRI mean 668%, SD 1256%, CD children DNRI mean 862%, SD 1240%

The studied group of CD adults and children did not display increased DNA damage as cited in the literature (157). Their levels of DNA repair capacity was significantly high mainly in children, it corresponds with the quality of young organism and is stimulated in inflammatory disease. These results are contradictory to the findings in idiopathic proctocolitis where DNA repair is usually low (but there is a susceptibility to carcinogenesis)[160, 161, 162, 163]. Our results of DNA repair cannot be compared with similar study in the literature.

CDAI index was higher in children, but not significantly (large variance). So their disease was more active (we dared to use CDAI index because pediatric patients were at the older school age or adolescents). CD children had shorter disease duration ($p<0.001$, not shown here). Markers of oxidative stress did not differ significantly from those of CD adults. DNAsb and DNRI in children were elevated, but not significantly. The intensity of DNA repair was significantly higher in children than in CD adults ($p<0.05$), certainly reflecting their younger age.

5.4.6 Comparison of Adult CD Patients with CD Children

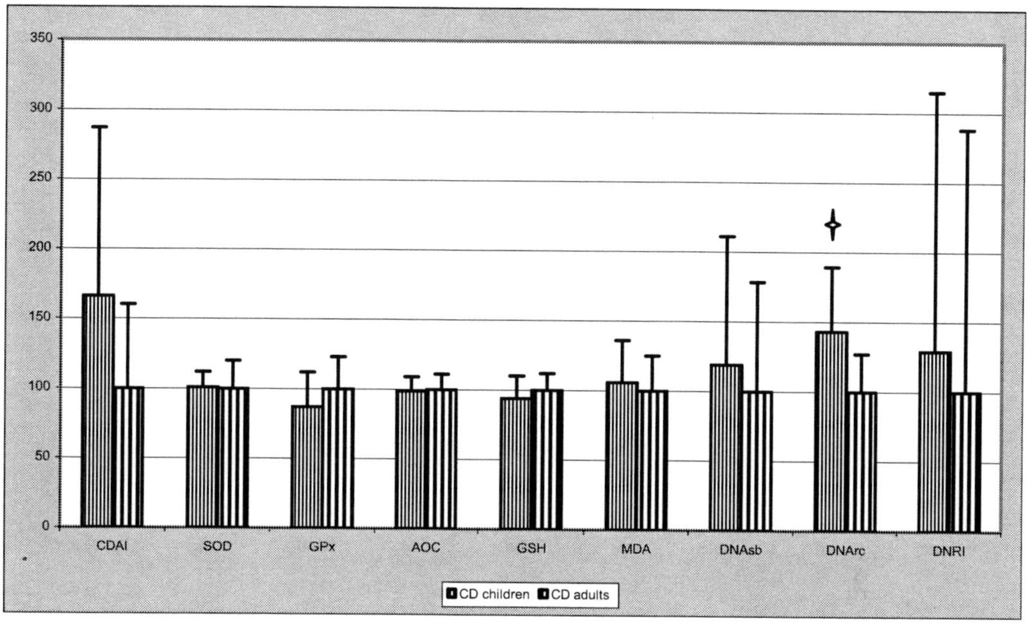

Figure 34. Markers of oxidative stress, DNA damage and repair. Mean values of CD adults=100%

5.4.7 Comparison of Adult Diabetic Patients and Patients with Crohn's Disease

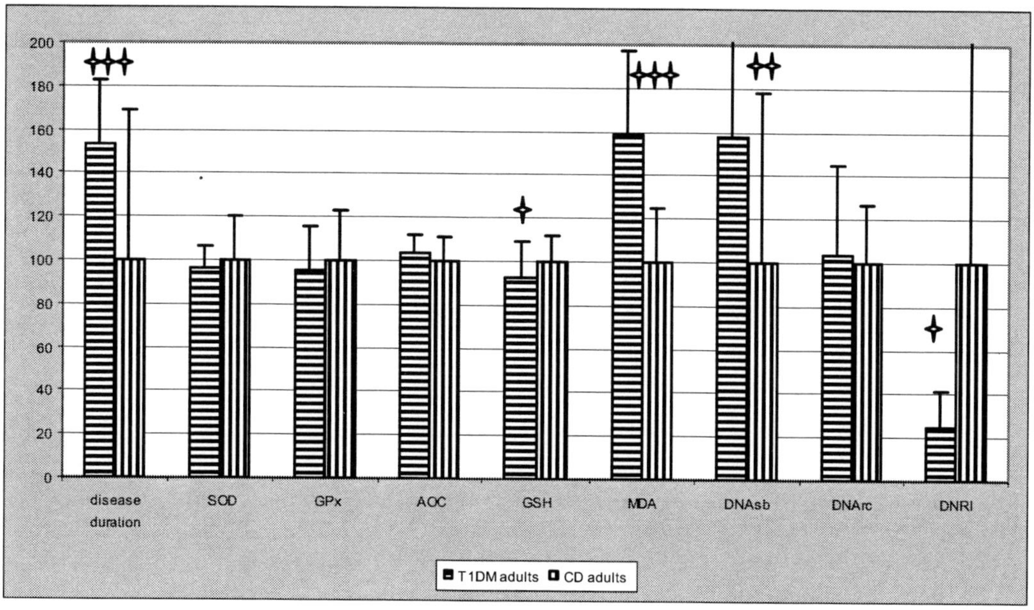

Figure 35. Markers of oxidative stress, DNA damage and repair. Mean values of CD adults=100%, T1DM adults DNAsb SD 78%, CD adults DNRI SD 188%

Patients with T1DM were comparable with CD patients with regard to their age, but they had longer disease duration ($p<0.001$). Markers of oxidative stress in T1DM adults displayed lower GSH ($p<0.05$) than CD adults, and also of course very high MDA ($p<0.001$). DNAsb were significantly higher in T1DM adults ($p<0.01$), but their DNArc did not differ substantially. So DNRI in diabetic adults was significantly lower than in CD patients ($p<0.05$).

The presented results displayed the more expressed consequencies of oxidative stress in T1DM patients than in CD adults. It is not excluded that besides the generalized influence of hyperglycemic state, the disease duration (longer in T1DM group) might influence the studied parameters.

5.4.8 Children with T1DM and CD Compared with Healthy Children

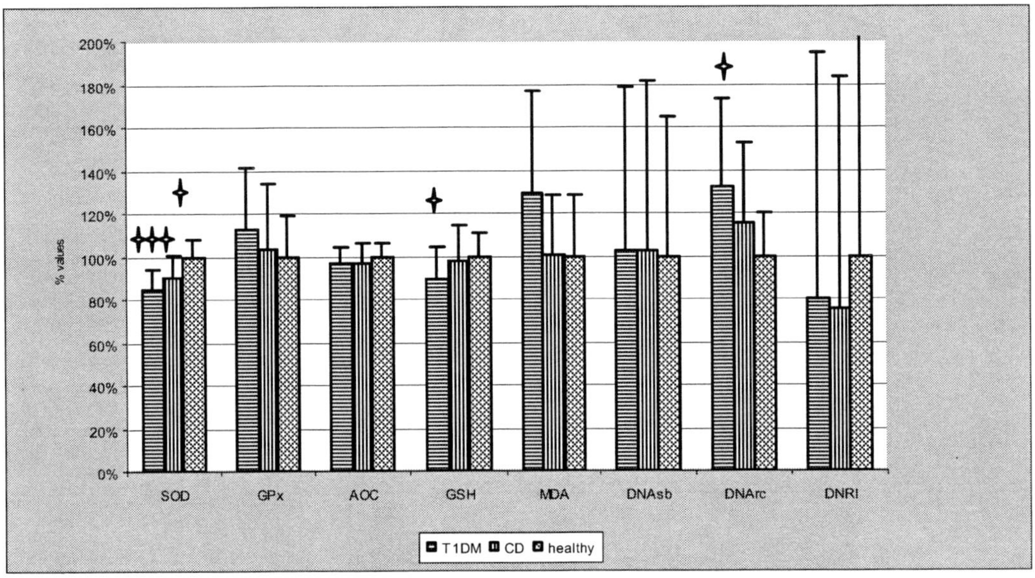

Figure 36. Markers of oxidative stress, DNA damage and repair. Mean values of healthy children=100%, DNRI healthy children SD 264%

The children with T1DM had the lowest levels of SOD, stimulated GPx (even if not statistically significant), importantly decreased GSH when compared with healthy children. DNA damage in diabetic children did not differ from the other groups, but DNA repair capacity was statistically increased ($p<0.05$). CD children did not differ from healthy children though similar tendencies in the examined parameters like in diabetic children were observed (SOD, GPX, AOC, GSH, DNArc and DNRI, but not MDA).

The results of children with T1DM demostrated the more intensive oxidative stress than in CD and healthy children. It is also obvious that DNA repair was apparently stimulated, and thus correcting the present DNA oxidative damage. Oxidative stress due generalized long-lasting hyperglycemic state overwhelms T1DM children and obviously leads to the more intensive oxidative stress than a patchy granulomatous inflammation in CD children. The results cannot be compared with similar findings in the literature.

Table 1. Comparison of T1DM and CD children versushealthy children

Children		T1DM	CD	Healthy
age	years	13.26±2.98	14.29±2.52	13.73±3.8
disease duration	years	2.94±2.72	2.99±1.43	
HbA1c	% (DCCT - <5%)	9.5±2.52		
PCDAI	Index (<30)		35.69±16.6	
SOD	U/g Hb	1227±131 ***	1312±148 *	1447±115
GPx	U/g Hb	53.68±13.44	49.05±14.40	47.52±9.21
AOC	mmol/l plasma	1.36±0.11	1.36±0.14	1.41±0.09
GSH	mmol/l ery	2.02±0.34 *	2.21±0.38	2.27±0.24
MDA	μmol/l plasma	2.49±0.93	1.94±0.54	1.93±0.55
DNAsb	breaks per 10^9daltons	0.43±0.32	0.43±0.33	0.42±0.27
DNArc	breaks per 10^9daltons	1.86±0.58 *	1.63±0.52	1.41±0.28
DNRI	index	13.88±19.74	13.02±18.72	17.28±45.69

5.4.9 Comparison between T1DM and CD Children

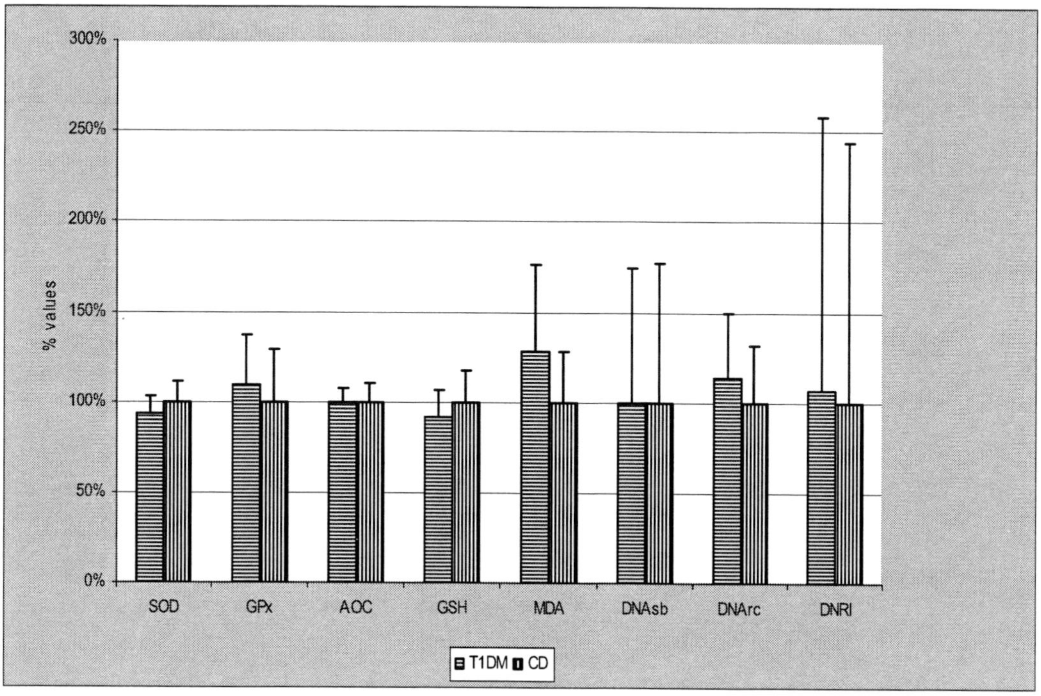

Figure 37. Markers of oxidative stress, DNA damage and repair. Values of CD children=100%; Mean values of CD children=100%. Comparison between T1DM children and CD children did not show any important differences. Both groups were comparable in their age, sex, and disease duration.

5.4.10 Comparison of all Groups of Patients versus Healthy Adults

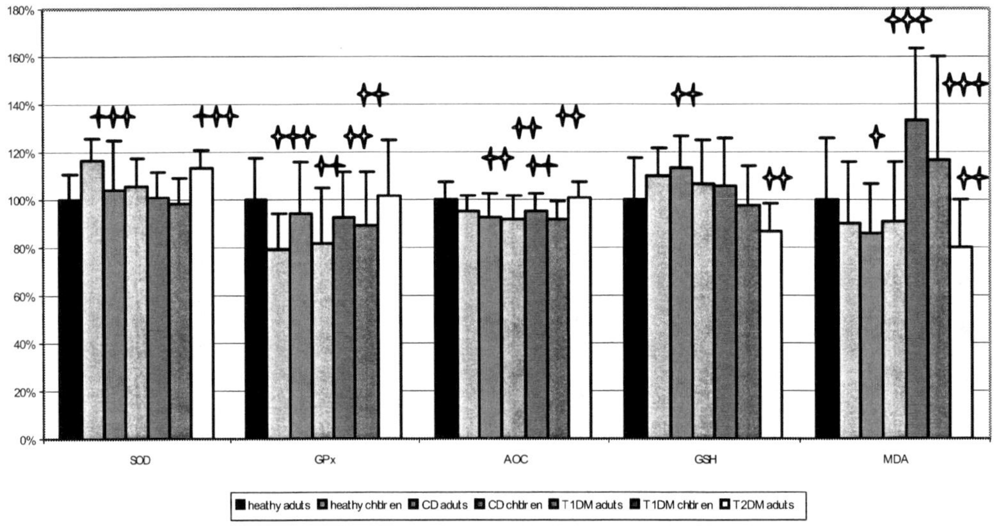

Figure 38. Markers of oxidative stress. Mean values of healthy adults=100%

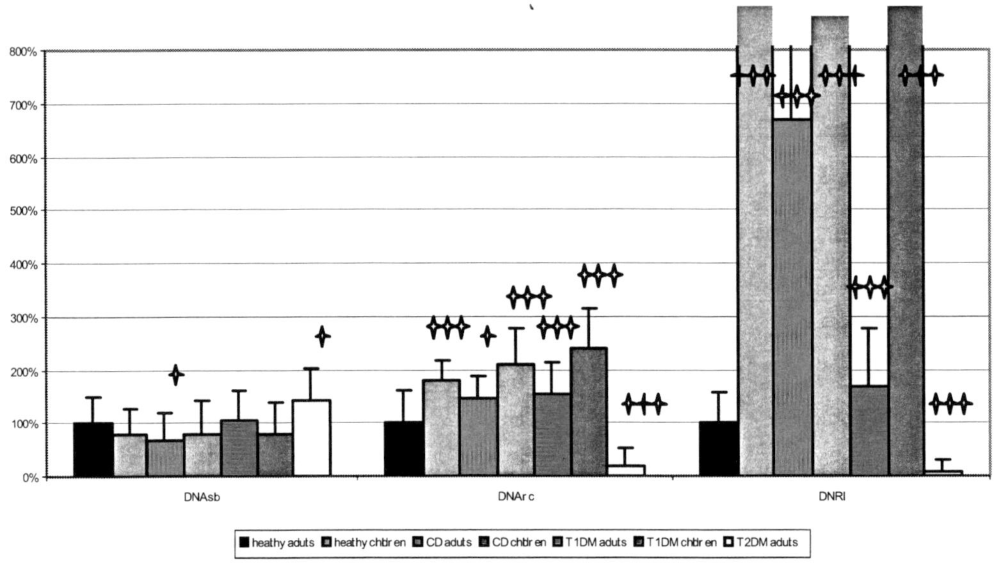

Figure 39. DNA damage and repair. Mean values of healthy adults=100%, DNRI healthy children mean 1144%, SD 3026%, DNRI CD adults mean 668%, SD 1256%, DNRI CD mean children 862%, SD 1240%, DNRI T1DM children mean 919%, SD 1307%

The summarizing graph brings a complex view on differences among healthy adults and children, CD adults and children, as well as T1DM adults and children, and finally T2DM adults. Both CD patients had significantly low total antioxidant plasma capacity ($p<0.01$), but on the other hand elevated GSH in CD adults ($p<0.01$). This finding can be influenced by a special diet in the majority of adult CD patients. CD children had SOD elevated only moderately, but significantly lower GPx ($p<0.01$). Similar finding was displayed in diabetic adults and children. In addition, they had also significantly low AOC. MDA was elevated in all T1DM patients in agreement with the disease character. In adult T2DM patients, extremely high SOD was found, and reversely low GSH ($p<0.01$) and MDA ($p<0.01$) as mentioned above.

It is evident that all groups of children differed from healthy adults in DNAsb, DNArc and DNRI. They had lower levels of DNAsb, i.e. less DNA damage. On the contrary, DNArc was significantly higher in healthy children ($p<0.001$), CD children ($p<0.001$), and mainly in T1DM children ($p<0.001$). Analogous assay tendency was found both in CD and T1DM adults versus healthy adult controls, i.e. lower DNAsb (CD adults $p<0.05$, similar but not significant finding in T1DM adults), DNArc increased in CD adults ($p<0.05$) and also in T1DM adults ($p<0.001$). DNRI reflected those presented results, i.e. they were elevated both in CD and T1DM adults ($p<0.001$). The completely different trend was observed in T2DM adults that showed high DNAsb ($p<0.05$), extremely low DNA repair capacity ($p<0.001$) and also DNRI ($p<0.001$).

It could be concluded that both *children and adults with Crohn´s disease or type 1 diabetes mellitus displayed stimulated DNA repair of oxidative DNA damage. On the other hand, adult patients with T2DM had very low DNA repair capacity and this might be linked with their susceptibility to carcinogenesis.*

CONCLUSION

Oxidative stress as predominance of reactive oxygen species in organism contributes substantially to many pathological processes in human body. An intensive research has brought a developing knowledge of oxidative stress and its impact on human metabolism. The short survey in the first theoretic part of this chapter summarizes current knowledge of oxidative stress, antioxidant defence, new antioxidant therapeutic possibilities. As oxidative stress injures DNA structure, oxidative DNA damage and DNA repair process has been reviewed with regard to different human diseases.

In the second part of this chapter, the authors present their study of oxidative stress, oxidative DNA damage and DNA repair in patients with diabetes mellitus type 1, type 2 and with Crohn´s disease. Summarizing the results, adult patients with type 1 diabetes mellitus had the signs of important oxidative stress, but compensated with a stimulated DNA repair. The subgroup of T1DM with diabetic microvascular complications had lower DNA repair, maybe due to exhaustion of repair machinery in a long disease duration or due to a decreased individual quality of DNA repair. When T1DM adults were compared with T1DM children, the young patients showed better results of parameters of oxidative stress and very high DNA repair, certainly in association with short disease duration and young age, though their diabetes control was not good. The adult patients with type 2 diabetes had very high oxidative DNA damage and extremely low DNA repair, these signs are assumed to be linked to the possible future carcinogenesis. Patients with Crohn´s disease (both children and adults) did not display such an intensive oxidative stress as diabetic patients did. It could be related to the fact that Crohn´s disease need not affect the whole organism like hyperglycemia in diabetes does. The results acquired in T1DM adult patients seems to support our hypothesis i.e. patients with bad DNA repair may have the development of diabetic microvascular complications. Nevertheless, large population studies in DM or IBD studying intensity of OS and expression of DNA repair enzymes are needed in order to get the correlation between individual repair enzymes expression and the long-term course and occurence of complications in DM or IBD.

ACKNOWLEDGEMENTS

The study was supported by the grant IGA MZ CR NR7919-3/2004 Individual DNA repair capacity induced by oxidative stress and its influence on the development and prognosis of some chronic non-infectious diseases, and the Research Aim MZ CR MSM 0021620814 Prevention, diagnostics, and the therapy of diabetes mellitus, metabolic and endocrine disorders of human organism.

We thank prof. F. Stožicky, MD, DrSc, Head of the Dpt. of Paediatrics, Faculty of Medicine Plzen, Charles University Prague, for his advice and encouragement.

REFERENCES

[1] Dröge, W. Free Radicals in the Physiological Control of Cell Function. *Physiol Rev,* 2002, 82, 47-95.

[2] Cooke, MS; Evans, MD; Dizdaroglu, M; Lunec, J. Oxidative DNA damage: mechanisms, mutation, and disease. *The FASEB Journal*, 2003, 17, 1195-1214.

[3] Stipek, S. *Antioxidants and free radicals in health and disease.* 1st Edition. Praha, Grada Publishing, 2000.

[4] Racek, J. *Oxidative stress and how to influence it.* 1st Edition. Praha, Galen, 2003.

[5] Forsberg, L; de Faire, U; Morgenstern, R. Oxidative Stress, Human Genetic Variation, and Disease. *Archives of Biochemistry and Biophysics,* 2001, 389, 84-93.

[6] McCord, JM; Edeas, MA. SOD, oxidative stress and human pathologies: a brief history and a future vision. *Biomed Pharmacother,* 2005, 59, 139-42.

[7] Muscoli, C; Cuzzocrea, S; Riley, DP; Zweier, JL; Thiemermann, C; Wang, ZQ; Salvemini, D. On the selectivity of superoxide dismutase mimetics and its importance in pharmacological studies. *British Journal of Pharmacology,* 2003, 140, 445-460.

[8] Day, BJ. Catalytic antioxidants: a radical approach to new therapeutics. *Drug Discovery Today,* 2004, 9, 557-566.

[9] Vouldoukis, I; Conti, M; Krauss, P; Kamaté, C; Blazquez, S; Tefit, M; Mazier, D; Calenda, A; Dugas, B. Supplementation with Gliadin-combined Plant Superoxide Dismutase Extract Promotes Antioxidant Defences and Protects Against Oxidative Stress. *Phytotherapy Research,* 2004, 18, 957-962.

[10] Hayes, JD. Glutathione transferases. *Annu Rev Pharmacol Toxicol,* 2005, 45, 51-88.

[11] Townsend, D; Tew, KD; Tapiero, H. The importance of glutathione in human disease. *Biomed Pharmacother,* 2003, 57, 145-155.

[12] Sgambato, A; Campisi, B; Zupa, A; Bochicchio, A; Romano, G; Tartarone, A; Galasso, R; Traficante, A; Cittadini, A. Glutathione S-transferase (GST)

polymorphisms as risk factors for cancer in a highly homogenous population from sosuthern Italy. *Anticancer Research,* 2002, 22, 3647-52.

[13] Dusinska, M; Ficek, A; Horska, A; Raslova, K; Petrovska, H; Vallova, B; Drlickova, M; Wood, SG; Stupakova, A; Gasparovic, J; Bobek, P; Nagyova, A; Kovacikova, Z; Blazicek, P; Liegebel, U; Collins, AR. Glutathione S-transferase polymorphisms influence the level of oxidative DNA damage and antioxidant protection in humans. *Mutat Research,* 2001, 482, 47-55.

[14] Tamer, L; Calkoglu, M; Ates NA; Zildirim, H; Ercan, B; Saritas, E; Ünlü, A; Atik, U. Glutathione-S-transferase gene polymorphisms (GSTT1, GSTM1, GSTP1) as as increased risk factors for asthma. *Respirology*, 2004, 9, 493-498.

[15] Rahman, SH; Nanny, Ch; Ibrahim, K; O'Reilly, D; Larvin, M; Kingsnorth, AJ; McMahon, MJ. Genetic Polymorphisms of GSTT1, GSTM1, GSTP1, MnSOD, and Catalase in Nonhereditary Chronic Pancreatitis: Evidence of Xenobiotic Stress and Impaired Antioxidant capacity. *Digestive Diseases and Sciences,* 2005, 50, 1376-1383.

[16] Rahman, SH; Ibrahim, K; Larvin, M; Kingsnorth, A; McMahon, MJ. Association of antioxidant enzyme gene polymorphisms and glutathione status with severe acute pancreatitis. *Gastroenterology,* 2004, 126, 1312-1322.

[17] Fukagawa, NK; Liang, P; Li, M; Ashikaga, T; Reddz, KR; Krawitt, EL. Glutathione-S-Transferase M1 null genotype in autoimmune hepatitis. Dig Dis Sci, 2001, 46, 2080-3.

[18] Yun, BR; El-Sohemy, A; Cornelis, MC; Bae, SC. Glutathione S-transferase M1, T1, and P1 genotypes and rheumatoid arthritis. *J Rheumatol,* 2005, 32, 992-7.

[19] Janssen, YM; Van Houten, B; Borm, PJ; Mossman, BT. Cell and tissue responses to oxidative damage. *Lab Invest,* 1993, 69, 261-274.

[20] Kidd, PM. Glutathione: Systemic Protectant Against Oxidative and Free Radical Damage. *Alternative Medicine Review,* 1997, 2, 155-176.

[21] Nobili, V; Pastore, A; Gaeta, LM; Tozzi, G; Comparcola, D; Sartorelli, MR; Marcellini, M; Bertini, E; Piemonte, F. Glutathione metabolism and antioxidant enzymes in patients affected by nonalcoholic steatohepatitis. *Clinica Chimica Acta,* 2005, 355, 105-111.

[22] Wu, G; Fang, YZ; Yang, S; Lupton, JR; Turner ND. Glutathione Metabolism and Its Implications for Health. J Nutr, 2004,134, 489-92.

[23] Valverde, M; Rojas, E; Kala, SV; Kala, G; Lieberman, MW. Survival and cell death in cells constitutively unable to synthesize glutathione. *Mutation Research,* 2005, Epub ahead of print.

[24] Rahman, I; MacNee, W. Oxidative stress and regulation of glutathione in lung inflammation. *Eur Respir J,* 2000, 16, 534-554.

[25] Tiitto, LH; Peltoniemi, MJ; Kaarteenaho-Wiik, RL; Soini, YM; Paakko, PK; Sormunen, RT; Kinnula, VL. Cell-specific regulation of gamma-glutamylcysteine synthetase in human interstitial lung diseases. *Hum Pathol,* 2004, 35, 832-9.

[26] Hudson, VM. New insights into the pathogenesis of cystic fibrosis: pivotal role of glutathione system dysfunction and implications for therapy. *Treat Respir Med,* 2004, 3, 353-63.

[27] Day, BJ; van Heeckeren, AM; Min, E; Velsor, LW. Role for Cystic Fibrosis Transmembrane Conductance Regulator Protein in a Glutathione Response to Bronchopulmonary Pseudomonas Infection. *Infection and Immunity,* 2004, 72, 2045-2051.

[28] Witschi, A; Reddy, S; Stofer, B; Lauterburg, BH. The systemic availability of oral glutathione. *Eur J Clin Pharmacol,* 1992, 43, 667-9.

[29] Shah, P. Food Sources that Boost Glutathione Naturally. 2004 . Available from: http://www.1whey2health.com/food-sources-glutathione.htm.

[30] Brok, J; Buckley, N; Gluud, C. Interventions for paracetamol (acetaminophen) overdoses. *Cochrane Database Syst Rev,* 2002, 3, CD003328.

[31] Bagshaw, SM; Ghali, WA. Acetylcysteine for prevention of contrast-induced nephropathy after intravascular angiography: A systematic review and meta-analysis. 2004 october. Available from: http://www.biomedcentral.com/1741-7015/2/38

[32] Dekhuijzen, PNR. Antioxidant properties of N-acetylcysteine: their relevance in relation to chronic obstructive pulmonary disease. *Eur Respir J,* 2004, 23, 629-636.

[33] Spapen, HD; Diltoer, MW; Nguyen, DN; Hendrickx, I; Huyghens, LP. Effects of N-acetylcysteine on microalbuminuria and organ failure in acute severe sepsis: results of a pilot study. *Chest,* 2005, 127, 1413-9.

[34] Hein, OV; Őhring, R; Schilling, A; Oellerich, M; Armstrong, VW; Kox, WJ; Spies, C. N-acetylcysteine decreases lactate signal intensities in liver tissue and improves liver function in septic shock patients, as shown by magnetic resonance spectroscopy: extended case report. *Critical Care,* 2004, 8, R66-71.

[35] Del Sorbo, L; Zhang, H. Is there a place for N-acetylcysteine in the treatment of septic shock? *Critical Care,* 2004, 8, 93-5

[36] Grinberg, L; Fibach, E; Amer, J; Atlas, D. N-acetylcysteine amide, a novel cell-permeating thiol, restores cellular glutathione and protects human red blood cells from oxidative stress. *Free Radical Biology and Medicine,* 2005, 38, 136-145.

[37] Das, DK. Thioredoxin regulation of ischemic preconditioning. *Antioxid Redox Signal,* 2004, 6, 405-12.

[38] Nakamura, T; Nakamura, H; Hoshino, T; Ueda, S; Wada, H; Yodoi, J. Redox regulation of lung inflammation by thioredoxin. *Antioxid Redox Signal,* 2005, 7, 60-71.

[39] Alberts, B; Johnson, A; Lewis, J; Raff, M; Roberts, K; Walter, P. Molecular biology of the cell. Fourth Edition. New York, Garland Science, Taylor and Francis Group, 2002.

[40] Okuyama, H; Shimahara, Y; Nakamura, H; Araya, S; Kawada, N; Yamaoka, Y; Yodoi, J. Thioredoxin prevents thioacetamide-induced acute hepatitis. *Comparative Hepatology,* 2004, 3 (Suppl 1), S 6.

[41] Bonakdar, RA; Guarneri, E. Coenzyme Q10. *American Family Physician,* 2005, 72, 1065-70.

[42] Langsjoen, PH. Introduction to coenzyme Q10. 1994. Available from: http://faculty.washington.edu/~ely/coenzq10.html

[43] Haargraves, IP; Duncan, AJ; Heales, SJ; Land, JM. The effect of HMG-CoA reductase inhibitors on coenzyme Q10: possible biochemical/clinical implications. *Drug Saf,* 2005, 28, 659-76.

[44] Wang, XL; Rainwater, DL; Mahaney, MC; Stocker, R. Cosupplementation with vitamin E and coenzyme Q10 reduces circulating markers of inflammation in baboons. *Am J Clin Nutr,* 2004, 80, 649-55.

[45] Carcamo, JM; Pedraza, A; Borquez-Ojeda, O; Zhang, B; Sanchez, R; Golde, DW. Vitamin C Is a Kinase Inhibitor: Dehydroascorbic Acid Inhibits IκBα Kinase β. *Molecular and Cellular Biology,* 2004, 24, 6645-6652.

[46] Hart, JA; Kracoff, G; Ottariono, S; Ullmann-Weil, M. Vitamin E. 2002 april. Available from: http://www.umm.edu/altmed/ConsSupplements/Print/VitaminEcs.html .

[47] Niki, E; Noguchi, N. Dynamics of Antioxidant Action of Vitamin E. *Acc Chem Res,* 2004, 37, 45-51.

[48] Li, HL; Wang, AB; Huang, Y; Liu, DP; Wei, C; Williams, GM; Zhang, CN; Liu, G; Liu, YQ; Hao, DL; Hui, RT; Lin, M; Liang, CC. Isorhapontigenin, a new resveratrol analog, attenuates cardiac hypertrophy via blocking signaling transduction pathways. *Free Radic Biol Med,* 2005, 38, 243-57.

[49] Borek, C. Dietary Antioxidants and Human Cancer. *Integrative cancer therapies,* 2004, 3, 333-341.

[50] Valko, M; Izakovic, M; Mazur, M; Rhodes, CJ; Telser, J. Role of oxygen radicals in DNA damage and cancer incidence. *Molecular and Cellular Biochemistry,* 2004, 266, 37-56.

[51] Delmas, D; Jannin, B; Latruffe, N. Resveratrol: Preventing properties against vascular alterations and ageing. *Mol Nutr Food Res,* 2005, 49, 377-395.

[52] Wang, QL; Lin, M; Liu, GT. Antioxidative activity of natural isorhapontigenin. *Jpn J Pharmacol,* 2001, 87, 61-66.

[53] Bernstein, C; Bernstein, H; Payne, CM; Garewal, H. DNA repair/pro-apoptotic dual-role proteins in five major DNA repair pathways: fail-safe protection against carcinogenesis. *Mutation Research,* 2002, 511, 145-178.

[54] Hansen, WK; Kellez, MR. Review of Mammalian DNA Repair and Translational Implications. *The Journal of Pharmacology and Experimental Therapeutics,* 2000, 295, 1-9.

[55] Smith, PJ; Jones, CJ. *DNA Recombination and Repair.* 1st Edition, New York, Oxford University Press, 1999.

[56] Wood, RD; Mitchell, M; Sgouros, J; Lindahl, T. *Human DNA Repair Genes*. Science, 2001, 291, 1284-1289.

[57] Wood, RD; Mitchell, M; Lindahl, T. Human DNA repair genes. *Mutat Res,* 2005, 577, 275-83.

[58] Huberman JA. DNA repair pathways. Lectures. 2005, October-November. Available from: http://saturn.roswellpark.org/cmb/huberman/DNA-Repair/lecture-intro.html.

[59] Herbert, KE; Mistry P. DNA Oxidation: Basics of Repair. Virtual Free Radical School. 2003, May. Available from: www.medicine.uiowa.edu/frrb/V irtualSchool/Herbert-DNA-Repair.ppt.

[60] Passarge E. Color Atlas of Genetics. 2nd Edition. New York., Thieme New York, 2001.

[61] Thompson, LH; Schild, D. Recombinational DNA repair and human disease. *Mutation Research,* 2002, 509, 49-78.

[62] Duker, NJ. Chromosome breakage syndromes and cancer. *Am J Med Genet,* 2002, 115, 125-9.

[63] Welcsh, PL; King, MC. BRCA1 and BRCA2 and the genetics of breast and ovarian cancer. *Human Molecular Genetics,* 2001, 10, 705-713.

[64] Evans, MD; Dizdaroglu, M; Cooke, MS. Oxidative DNA damage and disease: induction, repair and significance. *Mutation Research,* 2004, 567, 1-61.

[65] Collins, A; Dusinska, M; Franklin, M; Somorovska, M; Petrovska, H; Duthie, S; Fillion, L; Panayiotidis, M; Raslova, K; Vaughan, N. Comet assay in human

biomonitoring studies: reliability, validation, and applications. *Environ Mol Mutagen,* 1997, 30, 139-46.

[66] Powell, CL; Swenberg, JA; Rusyn, I. Expression of base excision DNA repair genes as a biomarker of oxidative DNA damage. *Cancer Letters,* 2005, 229, 1-11.

[67] Cheadle, JP; Sampson, JR. Exposing the MYtH about base excision repair and human inherited disease. *Human Molecular Genetics,* 2003, 12, R159-R165.

[68] Fukae, J; Takanashi, M; Kubo, S; Nishioka, K; Nakabeppu, Y; Mori, H; Mizuno, Y; Hattori, N. Expression of 8-oxoguanine DNA glycosylase (OGG1) in Parkinson´s disease and related neurodegenerative disorders. *Acta Neuropathologica,* 2005, 109, 256-62.

[69] Mathonnet, G; Labuda, D; Meloche, C; Wambach, T; Krajinovic, M; Sinnet, D. Variable continental distribution of polzmorphisms in the coding regions of DNA-repair genes. *J Hum Genet,* 2003, 48, 659-664.

[70] Collins, AR; Dusinska, M; Horvathova, E; Munro, EW; Savio, M; Stetina, R. Inter-individual differences in repair of DNA base oxidation, measured in vitro with the comet assay. *Mutagenesis*, 2001, 16, 297-301.

[71] Stevnsner, T; Thorslund, T; de Souza/Pinto, NC; Bohr, VA. Mitochondrial repair of 8-oxoguanine and changes with aging. *Experimental Gerontology,* 2002, 37, 1189-1196.

[72] Larsen, NB; Rasmussen, M; Rasmussen, LJ. Nuclear and mitochondrial DNA repair: similar pathways? *Mitochondrion*, 2005, 5, 89-108.

[73] Bürkle, A. Physiology and pathophysiology of poly(ADP-ribosyl)ation. *BioEssays,* 2001, 23, 795-806.

[74] Virag, L. Structure and Function of Poly(ADP-ribose) Polymerase-1: Role in Oxidative Stress-Related Pathologies. *Current Vascular Pharmacology,* 2005, 3, 209-214.

[75] Erdelyi, K; Bakondi, E; Gergely, P; Szabo, C; Virag, L. Pathophysiologic role of oxidative stress-induced poly(ADP-ribose) polymerase-1 activation: focus on cell death and transcriptional regulation. *Cell Mol Life Sci,* 2005, 62, 751-759.

[76] Wiesmüller, L. Genetic stabilization by p53 involves growth regulatory and repair pathways. *Journal of Biomedicine and Biotechnology,* 2001, 1, 7-10.

[77] Beneke, S; Diefenbach, J; Bürkle, A. Poly(ADP-ribosyl)ation inhibitors: promising drug candidates for a wide variety of pathophysiologic conditions. *Int J Cancer,* 2004, 111, 813-818.

[78] Woon, EC; Threadgill, MD. Poly(ADP-ribose)polymerase inhibition – where now? *Curr Med Chem,* 2005, 12, 2373-92.

[79] Szabo, C. Pharmacological inhibiton of poly(ADP-ribose)polymerase in cardiovascular disorders: future directions. *Curr Vasc Pharmacol,* 2005, 3, 301-303.

[80] Inotek News. 2003, April. Available from: www.inotekcorp.com/news/apr-26-2003.htm

[81] De Magalhaes, JP. From cells to ageing: a review of models and mechanisms of cellular senescence and their impact on human ageing. *Experimental Cell Research,* 2004, 300, 1-10.

[82] Chen, SK; Hsieh, WA; Tsai, MH; Chen, CH; Hong, AI; Wei, YH; Chang, WP. Age-associated Decrease of Oxidative Repair Enzymes, Human 8-Oxoguanine DNA Glycosylases (hOgg1), in Human Aging. *J Radit Res,* 2003, 44, 31-35.

[83] Szczesny, B; Bhakat, KK; Mitra, S; Boldogh, I. Age-dependent modulation of DNA repair enzymes by covalent modification and subcellular distribution. *Mechanisms of Ageing and Development,* 2004, 125, 755-765.

[84] Szczesny, B; Hazra, TK; Papaconstantinou, J; Mitra, S; Boldogh, I. Age-dependent deficiency in import of mitochondrial DNA glycosylases required for repair of oxidatively damaged bases. *PNAS,* 2003, 100, 10670-10675.

[85] Lee, JW; Harrigan, J; Opresko, PL; Bohr, VA. Pathways and functions of the Werner syndrome protein. *Mechanisms of Ageing and Development,* 2005, 126, 79-86.

[86] Mohaghegh, P; Hickson, ID. Premature aging in RecQ helicase-deficient human syndromes. *The International Journal of Biochemistry and Cell Biology,* 2002, 34, 1496-1501.

[87] Opresko, PL; Cheng, WH; von Kobbe, C; Harrigan, JA; Bohr, VA. Werner syndrome and the function of the Werner protein; what they can teach us about the molecular aging process. *Carcinogenesis,* 2003, 24, 791-802.

[88] Browner, WS; Kahn, AJ; Ziv, E; Reiner, AP; Oshima J; Cawthon, RM; Hsueh, WC; Cummings, SR. The genetics of Human Longevity. *Am J Med,* 2004, 117, 851-860.

[89] Szibor, M; Holtz, J. Mitochondrial ageing. Basic Res Cardiol, 2003, 98, 210-218.

[90] Wei, YH; Lee, HC. Oxidative stress, Mitochondrial DNA Mutation, and Impairment of Antioxidant Enzymes in Aging. *Exp Biol Med,* 2002, 227, 671-682.

[91] Sastre, J; Pallardo, FV; Vina, J. The Role of Mitochondrial Oxidative Stress in Aging. *Free Radical Biology and Medicine,* 2003, 35, 1-8.

[92] Caporaso N. The Molecular Epidemiology of Oxidative Damage to DNA and Cancer. *J Natl Cancer Inst,* 2003, 95, 1263-5.

[93] Dixon, K; Kopras, E. Genetic alterations and DNA repair in human carcinogenesis. *Seminars in Cancer Biology,* 2004, 14, 441-448.

[94] Collins, A; Harringtion, V. Repair of oxidative DNA damage: assessing its contribution to cancer prevention. *Mutagenesis,* 2002, 17, 489-493.

[95] Shackelford, ER; Manuszak, RP; Heard, SC; Link, CJ; Wang, S. Pharmacological manipulation of ataxia-teleangiectasia kinase activity as a treatment for Parkinson´s disease. *Med Hypotheses,* 2005, 64, 736-41.

[96] Martinet, W; Knaapen, MWM; De Meyer, GRY; Herman, AG; Kockx, MM. Elevated Levels of Oxidative DNA Damage and DNA Repair Enzymes in Human Atherosclerotic Plaques. *Ciruclation,* 2002, 106, 927-932.

[97] Martinet, W; Knaapen, MWM; De Meyer, GRY; Herman, AG; Kockx, MM. Oxidative DNA Damage and Repair in Experimental Atherosclerosis Are Reversed by Dietary Lipid Lowering. *Circ Res,* 2001, 88, 733-739.

[98] Hofseth, LJ; Khan, MA; Ambrose, M; Nikolayeva, O; Xu-Welliver, M; Kartalou, M; Hussain, SP; Roth, RB; Zhou, X; Mechanic, LE; Zurer, I; Rotter, V; Samson, LD; Harris, CC. The adaptive imbalance in base excision-repair enzymes generates microsatellite instability in chronic inflammation. J Clin Invest, 2003, 112, 1887-94. Erratum in: *J Clin Invest,* 2004, 113, 490.

[99] Blasiak, J; Arabski, M; Krupa, R; Wozniak, K; Zadrozny, M; Kasznicki, J; Zurawska, M; Drzewoski, J. DNA damage and repair in type 2 diabetes mellitus. *Mutat Res,* 2004, 554, 297-304.

[100] Miyako, K; Kohno, H; Ihara, K; Kuromaru, R; Matsuura, N; Hara, T. Association study of human MTH1 gene polymorphisms with type 1 diabetes mellitus. *Endocr J,* 2004, 51, 493-8.
[101] Vodicka, P; Koskinen, M; Stetina, R; Soucek, P; Vodickova, L; Matousu, Z; Kuricova, M; Hemminki, K. The role of various biomarkers in the evaluation of styrene genotoxicity. *Cancer Detect Prev,* 2003, 27, 275-84.
[102] The Expert Committee on the Diagnosis and Classification of Diabetes Mellitus. Report of the Expert Committee on the Diagnosis and Classification of Diabetes Mellitus. *Diabetes Care,* 2003, 26, S 5-20.
[103] Brownlee, M. Glycation products and the pathogenesis of diabetic complications. *Diabetes Care,* 1992, 15, 1835-1843.
[104] Brownlee, M. Biochemistry and molecular cell biology of diabetic complications. Nature, 2001, 414, 813-820.
[105] Brownlee, M. The Pathobiology of Diabetic Complications. *Diabetes,* 2005, 54, 1615-1625.
[106] Ceriello, A. New insights on oxidative stress and diabetic complications may lead to a "causal" antioxidant therapy. *Diabetes Care,* 2003, 26, 1589-96.
[107] Skyler, JS. *Atlas of Diabetes.* 2nd Edition. Philadelphia, Lippincott, Williams and Wilkins, 2002.
[108] VanderJagt, DJ; Harrison, JM; Ratliff, DM; Hunsaker, LA; Vander Jagt, DL. Oxidative stress indices in IDDM subjects with and without long-term diabetic complications. *Clinical Biochemistry,* 2001, 34, 265-270.
[109] Holeček, V; Racek, J. The importance of free radicals and advanced glycosylation end-products (AGE) in diabetes mellitus. *Klin Biochem Metab,* 1995, 3, 18-22.
[110] Jakus, V. The role of free radicals, oxidative stress and antioxidant systems in diabetic vascular disease. *Bratisl Lek Listy* 2000, 101, 541-551.
[111] Jakus, V; Carsky, J; Hrnciarova, M. Importance of advanced glycosylation end-products AGE. *Bratisl Lek Listy,* 1998, 99, 368-375.
[112] Jakus, V; Rietbrock, N. Advanced Glycation End-Products and the Progress of Diabetic Vascular Complications. *Physiol. Res,* 2004, 53, 131-142.
[113] Vlassaara, H. Recent progression in the biologic and clinical significance of advanced glycosylation end products. *J Lab Clin Med* 1994, 124, 19-30.
[114] Rahbar, S; Figarola, JL. Inhibitors and Breakers of Advanced Glycation Endproducts (AGEs): A Review. Curr Med Chem-Immun, *Endoc and Agents,* 2002, 2, 135-161.
[115] Kalousova, M; Zima, T; Tesar, V; Dusilova/Sulkova, S; Skrha, J. Advanced glycoxidation end products in chronic disease – clinical chemistry and genetic background. *Mutation Research,* 2005, 579, 37-46.
[116] Jenkins, AJ; Best, JD; Klein, RL; Lyons, TJ. Lipoproteins, glycoxidation and diabetic angiopathy. *Diabetes Metab Res Rev,* 2004, 20, 349-368.
[117] Aljada, A; Ghanim, H; Mohanty, P; Syed, T; Bandyopadhyay, A; Dandona, P. Glucose intake induces an increse in activator protein 1 and early growth response 1 binding activities, in teh expression of tissue factor and matrix metalloproteinase in mononuclear cells, and in plasma tissue factor and matrix metalloproteinase concentrations. *Am J Clin Nutr,* 2004, 80, 51-7.
[118] Tsukuhara, H; Sekine, K; Uchiyama, M; Kawakami, H; Hata, I; Todoroki, Y; Hiraoka, M; Kaji, M; Yorifuji, T; Momoi, T; Yoshihara, K; Beppu, M; Mayumi, M. Formation

of Advanced Glycosylation End Products and Oxidative Stress in Young Patients with Type 1 Diabetes. *Pediatric Research,* 2003, 54, 419-424.

[119] Hempe, JM; Gomez, R; McCarter, RJ Jr; Chalew, SA. High and low hemoglobin glycation phenotypes in type 1 diabetes. a challenge for interpretation of glycemic control. *J Diabetes Complications,* 2002, 16, 313-320.

[120] Bartos, V; Pelikanova, T. et al. *Diabetology in practice.* 3rd Edition, Prague, Maxdorf-Jessenius, 2003.

[121] Svacina, S. Vascular complications of diabetes. Trends in current diabetology. 1st Edition, Prague, Galen, 2005.

[122] Williams, ME. New therapies for advanced glycation end product nephrotoxicity: Current challenges. *American Journal of Kidney Diseases,* 2003, 41 (S1), S42-47.

[123] Chistyakov, DA; Savostanov, KV; Zotova, EV; Nosikov, VV. Polymorphisms in the Mn-SOD and EC-SOD genes and their relationship to diabetic neuropathy in type I diabetes mellitus. *BMC Medical Genetics*, 2001, 2, 4.

[124] Ceriello, A. M; Morocutti, A; Mercuri, F; Quagliaro, L; Moro, M; Damante, G; Viberti GC. Defective Intracellular Antioxidant Enzyme Production in Type 1 Diabetic Patients With Nephropathy. *Diabetes*, 2000, 49, 2170-2177.

[125] Varvarovska, J; Racek, J; Stozicky, F; Soucek, J; Trefil, L; Pomahacova, R. Parameters of oxidative stress in children with Type 1 diabetes mellitus and their relatives. *J Diabetes Complications*, 2003, 17, 7-10.

[126] Krapfenbauer, K; Bimbacher, R; Vierhapper, H; Herkner, K; Kampel, D; Lubec, G. Glycoxidation, and protein and DNA oxidation in patients with diabetes mellitus. *Clinical Science,* 1998, 95, 331-7.

[127] Collins, AR; Raslova, K; Somorovska, M; Petrovska, H; Ondrusova, A; Vohnout, B; Fabry, R; Dusinska, M. DNA damage in diabetes: correlation with a clinical marker. *Free Radic Biol Med,* 1998, 25, 373-7.

[128] Wu, LL; Chiou, CC; Chang, PY; Wu, JT. Urinary 8-OHdG: a marker of oxidative stress to DNA and a risk factor for cancer, atherosclerosis and diabetics. *Clin Chim Acta,* 2004, 339, 1-9.

[129] Samcova, E; Kvasnicova, V. Oxidative stress and 8-hydroxy-2′-deoxyguanosine as a biomarker of oxidative DNA damage. *DMEV*, 2000, 3, 194-198.

[130] Dincer, Y; Akcay, T; Ilkova, H; Alademir, Z; Ozbay, G. DNA damage and antioxidant defense in peripheral leukocytes of patients with Type I diabetes mellitus. *Mutat Res,* 2003, 527, 49-55.

[131] Sardas, S; Yilmaz, M; Oztok, U; Cakir, N; Karakaya, AE. Assessment of DNA strand breakage by comet assay in diabetic patients and the role of antioxidant supplementation. *Mutat Res,* 2001, 490, 123-129.

[132] Du, X; Matsumura, T; Edelstein, D; Rossetti, L; Zsengeller, Y; Szabo, C; Brownlee, M. Inhibition of GAPDH activity by poly(ADP-ribose)polymerase activates three major pathways of hyperglycemic damage in endothelial cells. *J Clin Invest,* 2003, 112, 1049-1057.

[133] Zheng, L; Szabo, C; Kern, TS. Poly(ADP-Ribose) Polymerase Is Involved in the Development of Diabetic Retinopathy via Regulation of Nuclear Factor-κB. *Diabetes,* 2004, 53, 2960-2967.

[134] Miyako, K; Kohno, H; Ihara, K; Kuromaru, R; Matsuura, N; Hara, T. Association Study of Human *MTH1* Gene Polymorphisms with Type 1 Diabetes mellitus. *Endocrine Journal,* 2004, 51, 493-498.

[135] Tyrberg, B; Anachkov, KA; Dib, SA; Wang-Rodriguez, J; Yoon, KH; Levine, F. Islet expression of the DNA repair enzyme 8-oxoguanosine DNA glycosylase (OggI) in human type 2 diabetes. *BMC Endocrine Disorders,* 2002, 2, 2.

[136] Varvarovska, J; Racek, J; Stetina, R; Sykora, J; Pomahacova, R; Rusavy, Z; Lacigova, S; Trefil, L; Siala, K; Stozicky, F. Aspects of oxidative stress in children with type 1 diabetes mellitus. *Biomed and Pharmacother,* 2004, 58, 539-45.

[137] Schultz Johansen, J; Harris, AK; Rychly, DJ; Ergul, A. Oxidative stress and the use of antioxidants in diabetes: Linking basic science to clinical practice. *Cardiovascular Diabetology,* 2005, 4, 5.

[138] Da Ros, R; Asaloni, R; Ceriello, A. Antioxidant therapy in diabetic complications: what is new? *Curr Vasc Pharmacol,* 2004, 2, 335-41.

[139] Da Ros, R; Asaloni, R; Ceriello, A. Molecular targets of diabetic vascular complications and potential new drugs. *Curr Drug Targets,* 2005, 6, 503-9.

[140] Reusch, JEB. Diabetes, microvascular complications, and cardiovascular complications: what is it about glucose? *J Clin Invest,* 2003, 112, 986-988.

[141] Li, F; Drel, VR; Szabo, C; Stevens, MJ; Obrosova, IG. Low-Dose Poly(ADP-Ribose) Polymerase Inhibitor-Containing Combination Therapies Reverse Early Peripheral Diabetic Neuropathy. *Diabetes*, 2005, 54, 1514-1522.

[142] Obrosova, IG; Pacher, P; Szabo, C; Zsengeller, Z; Hirooka, H; Stevens, MJ; Yorek, MA. Aldose Reductase Inhibition Counteracts Oxidative-Nitrosative Stress and Poly(ADP-Ribose) Polymerase Activation in Tissue Sites for Diabetes Complications. *Diabetes,* 2005, 54, 234-242.

[143] Shanahan, F. Crohn´s disease. *The Lancet*, 2002, 359, 62-69.

[144] Matulka, M. Immunology of inflammatory bowel diseases. *Alergie*, 2001, 3, 65-70.

[145] Ruf, G. Surgical therapy of complicated inflammatory bowel disease. *Schweiz Rundsch Med Prax,* 2005, 94, 1681-5.

[146] Kruidenier, L; Verspaget HW . Oxidative stress as a pathogenic factor in inflammatory bowel disease—Radicals or ridiculous? *Aliment Pharmacol Ther,* 2002, 16, 1997–2015.

[147] Kruidenier, L; Kuiper, I; Lamers, CB; Verspaget, HW. Intestinal oxidative damage in inflammatory bowel disease: semi-quantification, localization, and association with mucosal antioxidants. *J Pathol,* 2003, 201, 28-36.

[148] Tuzun, A; Erdil, A; Inal, V; Aydin, A; Bagci, S; Yesilova, Y; Sayal, A; Karaeren, N; Dagalp, K. Oxidative stress and antioxidant capacity in patients with inflammatory bowel disease. *Clin Biochem,* 2002, 35, 569-72.

[149] Yamada, T; Grisham, MB. Role of neutrophil-derived oxidants in the pathogenesis of intestinal inflammation. *Klin Wochenschr,* 1991, 69, 988-94.

[150] Kruidenier, L; Kuper, I; van Duijn, W; Marklund, SL; van Hogezand, RA; Lamers, CB; Verspaget, HW. Differential mucosal expression of three superoxide dismutase isoforms in inflammatory bowel disease. *J Pathol,* 2003, 201, 7-16.

[151] Kruidenier, L; Kuiper, I; Van Duijn, W; Mieremet-Ooms, MA; van Hogezand, RA; Lamers, CB; Verspaget, HW. Imbalanced secondary mucosal antioxidant response in inflammatory bowel disease. *J Pathol*, 2003, 201, 17-27

[152] Wendland, BE; Aghdassi, E; Tam, C; Carrrier, J; Steinhart, AH; Wolman, SL; Baron, D; Allard, JP. Lipid peroxidation and plasma antioxidant micronutrients in Crohn disease. *Am J Clin Nutr,* 2001, 74, 259-64.

[153] Koutroubakis, IE; Malliaraki, N; Dimoulios, PD; Karmiris, K; Castanas, E; Kouroumalis, EA. Decreased total and corrected antioxidant capacity in patients with inflammatory bowel disease. *Dig Dis Sci,* 2004, 49, 1433-7.

[154] Liu, C; Russell, RM; Smith, DE; Bronson, RT; Milburz, PE; Furukawa, S; Wang, XD; Blumberg, JB. The effect of dietary glutathione and coenzyme Q10 on the prevention and treatment of inflammatory bowel disease in mice. *Int J Vitam Nutr Res,* 2004, 74, 74-85.

[155] Oz, HS; Chen, TS; McCLain, CJ; de Villiers, WJ. Antioxidants as novel therapy in a murine model of colitis. *J Nutr Biochem,* 2005, 16, 297-304.

[156] Akgun, E; Caliskan, C; Celik, HA; Ozutemiz, AO; Tuncyurek, M; Aydin, HH. Effects of N-acetylcysteine Treatment on Oxidative Stress in Acetic Acid-induced Experimental Colitis in Rats. *The Journal of International Medical Research,* 2005, 33, 196-206.

[157] D′Odorico, A; Bortolan, S; Cardin, R; D′Inca′, R; Martines, D; Ferronato, A; Sturniolo, GC. Reduced plasma antioxidant concentrations and increased oxidative DNA damage in inflammatory bowel disease. *Scan J Gastroenterol,* 2001, 36, 1289-94.

[158] Seril, DN; Liao, J; Yang, GY; Yang, CS. Oxidative stress and`ulcerative colitis-associated carcinogenesis: studies in humans and animal models. *Carcinogenesis,* 2003, 24, 353-362.

[159] D′Inca, R; Cardin, R; Benazzato, L; Angriman, I; Martines, D; Sturniolo, GC. Oxidative DNA damage in the mucosa of ulcerative colitis increases with disease duration and dysplasia. *Inflamm Bowel Dis,* 2004, 10, 23-7.

[160] Sanford, KK; Price, FM; Brodeur, C; Makrauer, FL; Parshad, R. Deficient DNA repair in chronic ulcerative colitis. *Cancer Detect Prev,* 1997, 21, 540-5.

[161] Pokorny, RM; Hofmeister, A; Galandiuk, S; Diety, AB; Cohen, ND; Neibergs, HL. Crohn′ s disease and ulcerative colitis are associated with the DNA repair gene MLH1. *Ann Surg,* 1997, 225, 718-23.

[162] Hofseth, LJ; Khan, MA; Ambrose, M; Nikolayeva, O; Xu-Welliver, M; Kartalou, M; Hussain, SP; Roth, RB; Zhou, X; Mechanic, LE; Zurer, I; Rotter, V; Samson, LD; Harris CC. The adaptive imbalance in base excision-repair enzymes generates microsatellite instability in chronic inflammation. *J Clin Invest,* 2003, 112, 1887-94. Erratum in: J Clin Invest, 2004, 113, 490.

[163] Guo, HH; Loeb, LA. Tumbling down a different pathway to genetic instability. *J Clin Invest,* 2003, 112, 1793-5.

[164] Krishna, M; Woda, B; Savas, L; Baker, S; Banner, B . Expression of p53 antigen in inflamed and regenerated mucosa in ulcerative colitis and Crohn′ s disease. *Mod Pathol,* 1995, 8, 654-7.

[165] Collins AR, Dusinska M, Horvathova E, Munro EW, Savio M, Stětina R. Inter-individual differences in repair of DNA base oxidation, measured in vitro with the comet assay. *Mutagenesis,* 2001, 16, 297-301.

[166] Racek, J; Eiselt, J; Opatrny, K Jr. Transitional elements and free radicals. *Cas Lek Cesk,* 2002 141, 479-82.

[167] Comet Assay Interest Group. Comet assay (single cell gel electrophoresis SCGE). 2005. Available from: http://www.comet.itrcindia.org
[168] Rovnakova, D. Oxidative stress in children after physical activity – thesis. Faculty of Medicine, UPJS, Kosice, Slovakia, 2002.
[169] Aguilo, A; Tauler, P; Fuentespina, E; Tur, JA; Cordova, A; Pons, A. Antioxidant response to oxidative stress induced by exhaustive exercise. *Physiology and Behavior,* 2005, 84, 1-7.
[170] Barja, G. Free radicals and aging. *Trends in Neurosciences,* 2004, 27, 595-600.
[171] Dufour, E; Larsson, NG. Understanding aging: revealing order out of chaos. *Biochim Biophys Acta*, 2004, 1658, 122-32.
[172] Weirich-Schwaiger, H; Weirich, HG; Gruber, B; Schweiger, M; Hirsch-Kauffmann, M. Correlation between senescence and DNA repair in cells from young and old individuals and in premature aging syndromes. *Mutat Res,* 1994, 316, 37-48.
[173] Raji, NS: Surekha, A; Rao, KS. Improved DNA-repair parameters in PHA –stimulated peripheral blood lymphocytes of human subjects with low body mass index. *Mech Ageing Dev,* 1998, 104, 133-48.
[174] Chen, SK; Hsieh, WA; Tsai, MH; Chen, ChCh; Hong, AI; Wei, YH; Chang, WP. Age-associated Decrease of Oxidative Repair Enzymes, Human 8-Oxoguanine DNA Glycosylases (hOgg1) in Human Aging. *J Radiat Res,* 2003, 44, 31-35.
[175] Dincer Y, Akcay T, Alademir Z, Ilkova H.: Effect of oxidative stress on glutathione pathway in red blood cells from patients with insulin-dependent diabetes mellitus. M*etabolism,* 2002, 51, 1360-1362.
[176] Ruiz C, Alegria A, Barbera R, Farre R, Lagard MJ: Lipid peroxidation and antioxidant enzyme activities in patients with type 1 diabetes mellitus. *Scand J Clin Lab Invest,* 1999, 59, 99-105.
[177] Haberland, ME; Fogelman, AM; Edwards, PA. Specifity of receptor-mediated recognition of malondialdehyde-modified low density lipoproteins. *Proc Natl Acad Sci,* 1982, 79, 1712-1716.

INDEX

A

B

C

D

E

F

G

H

I

J

K

L

M

N

Q

R

S

T

U

V